Damage Control in Trauma Care

Juan Duchesne • Kenji Inaba
Mansoor Ali Khan
Editors

Damage Control in Trauma Care

An Evolving Comprehensive Team Approach

Springer

Editors
Juan Duchesne
Tulane School of Medicine
New Orleans
Louisiana
USA

Kenji Inaba
LAC+USC Medical Center
University of Southern California
Los Angeles
California
USA

Mansoor Ali Khan
St Mary's Hospital
Imperial College Healthcare NHS Trust
London
United Kingdom

ISBN 978-3-030-10235-7 ISBN 978-3-319-72607-6 (eBook)
https://doi.org/10.1007/978-3-319-72607-6

Printed on acid-free paper

This Springer imprint is published by the registered company Springer International Publishing AG part of Springer Nature
The registered company address is: Gewerbestrasse 11, 6330 Cham, Switzerland

To my loving wife, Tricia, and all of our kids, Isabella, Esteban, Gabriella, Brook, Samantha and Alix, for always keeping me in check. Thanks to my friend and mentor Norman McSwain for his Tsa-La-Gi leadership and for always reminding us: "what have you done today for the good of mankind…." You will be missed.

Juan C. Duchesne M.D., F.A.C.S., F.C.C.M., F.C.C.P.

To my darling wife, Mehmooda, without whose support I would not have been able to pursue my career in Medicine, never mind Trauma Surgery. To my children, Zain, Mohsin and Zara, who have always provided me with a welcome distraction and unconditional (most of the time) love. And above all, to my mother and father who sacrificed much so that I was never left wanting. And a special thanks to my dear friend the late Colonel Peter Roberts for two decades of priceless mentorship.

Mansoor A. Khan M.B.B.S.(Lond), Ph.D., F.R.C.S., F.E.B.S., F.A.C.S.

To my wife, Susie, and son, Koji, thank you for all of your support.

Kenji Inaba, M.D., F.A.C.S., F.R.C.S.C.

Foreword

Originally coined by the US Navy in reference to techniques for salvaging a ship that had sustained serious damage, the term "damage control" has been adapted to truncating initial surgical procedures on severely injured patients in order to expedite re-establishing a survivable physiological status. After initial temporizing procedures, patients then undergo aggressive correction of their coagulopathy, hypothermia, and acidosis in the intensive care unit before returning to the operating room for the definitive repair of their injuries. This approach has been shown to lead to better-than-expected survival rates for patients with severe trauma. In order to maximize outcomes in this group of patients' damage control encompass not only intra-abdominal interventions but rather all interventions from first contact on the scene by paramedics, different modalities of resuscitation on the field and throughout the hospital and breaking through surgical interventions by different modalities. The book *Damage Control in Trauma Care* describes in detail the history behind the origin of damage control surgery to the most up-to-date advances in research by experts in the field.

New Orleans, LA, USA Juan Duchesne

Contents

1 Origin of the Bogota Bag and Its Application

David V. Feliciano and Oswaldo A. Borraez Gaona

Abstract

The open abdomen is used when the abdominal incision cannot be closed, when an early reoperation is necessary, to prevent an abdominal compartment syndrome, for the treatment of secondary or tertiary peritonitis, for the treatment of omphaloceles in neonates, and for the treatment of missing portions of the abdominal wall. The unique contribution of Oswaldo A. Borraez Gaona, MD, of Bogota, Colombia, was the application of a plastic bag over the open abdomen in injured patients. The bag allows for rapid access for a relaparotomy and covers and protects the viscera until edema and/or infection resolves.

D.V. Feliciano, M.D. (✉)
University of Maryland School of Medicine, Shock TraumaCenter/University of Maryland Medical Center, Baltimore, MD, USA

Emeritus, Division of General Surgery, Indiana University, Indiana University School of Medicine, Indianapolis, IN, USA

O.A. Borraez Gaona, M.D.
National University of Colombia, Colombian Surgical Association, Bogota, Colombia

1.1 Historical Development of the Open Abdomen

1.1.1 Slow Clinical Recognition of the Abdominal Compartment Syndrome

As open abdominal surgery for elective, emergent, and trauma indications progressed in the latter half of the nineteenth century, there was no mention of leaving the abdomen open. This seems surprising as surely some patients in that era had distension of the midgut at completion of operation.

Numerous historical reviews of the abdominal compartment syndrome, however, have documented that the adverse consequences of increased intra-abdominal pressure were recognized in the early twentieth century [1, 2]. In 1911, Emerson's experiments in small animals documented that an increase in intra-abdominal pressure from 27 to 46 cm H_20 led to a respiratory and cardiovascular death [3]. Later studies by Thorington and Schmidt [4] in 1923 and by Overholt [5] in 1931 noted that renal failure was another adverse effect of experimentally induced increases in intra-abdominal pressure. There were subsequent similar laboratory studies [6–9] and an occasional clinical study [10] over the next 50 years. But, clinical relevance was first established at the University of Virginia in the early 1980s. After observations in four patients

J. Duchesne et al. (eds.), *Damage Control in Trauma Care*,
https://doi.org/10.1007/978-3-319-72607-6_1

later reported [11], the authors noted the beneficial effect on renal function by relieving elevated intra-abdominal pressure in mongrel dogs [12]. A similar report on four patients at the University of Maryland occurred at the same time [13]. The analogous clinical situation would be to reopen a recent abdominal incision in a patient with oliguria or anuria in the presence of elevated intra-abdominal pressure—the later named abdominal compartment syndrome.

1.1.2 Inability to Close the Distended Abdomen

The dangers of closing an abdominal incision under tension in military conflicts were first described by W.H. Ogilvie. Ogilvie was first a surgeon in civilian life at Guy's Hospital in London but subsequently became a Major General in the Royal Army Medical Corps in World War II. In the first of several legendary papers in the 1940s, he described the use of retention sutures to buttress a closure of the abdominal wall when the sides of the incision were "3 inches" apart [14]. Also, he commented that "when the gap exceeds three inches, closure by direct suture is usually impossible." Because of his concern about necrosis if skin flaps only were used, he suggested a "dodge" that had been used in two patients. Using a "light canvas or stout cotton cloth sterilized in Vaseline … a double sheet of this is cut rather smaller than the defect in the muscles, and sutured into place with interrupted catgut sutures" [14]. Ogilvie recognized that some open abdomens could still not be closed even after edema of the midgut resolved. In such patients, he suggested a version of the visceral packing technique described at Detroit Receiving Hospital over 50 years later [15, 16]. He took "gauze swabs sterilized in and impregnated with Vaseline" and laid them over the bowel with the edges tucked under the edges of the incision [14]. The sides of the incision were then brought together with "strips of Elastoplast or even with stitches over the Vaseline" [14]. Ogilvie specifically noted that "Vaseline gauze makes an admirable peritoneum" [14]. He further described the use of "pinch grafts," presumably partial-thickness skin grafts, applied to the granulating wound after removal of the Vaseline gauze and delayed repair of the incisional hernia that was left [14].

1.1.3 Open Abdomen Treatment for Secondary or Tertiary Peritonitis

Over the past 110 years, a number of approaches to the patient with secondary or tertiary peritonitis have been described. The first of these was debridement and lavage for acute appendicitis described by J. Price in 1905 [17]. Of historic interest, it was, once again, W. H. Ogilvie who was one of the first surgeons to describe leaving the abdomen open temporarily (1–4 days) when sepsis was present [18].

Postoperative peritoneal lavage for peritoneal sepsis became popular 60 years later and was much discussed in the surgical literature of the 1960s and 1970s [19–22]. At the same time, Hovnanian and Saddawi documented that the dissemination of bacteria associated with debridement and irrigation did not increase mortality [23]. A related operative treatment, radical peritoneal debridement (vigorous debridement of exudate on peritoneal surfaces), had a transient period of popularity in the late 1970s, until a later prospective randomized clinical trial did not confirm the benefits suggested in the original paper [24, 25].

In 1979, Steinberg [26] described leaving the abdomen open postoperatively in patients with "acute generalized suppurative peritonitis." Despite the adverse effects of this approach (fluid losses, persistent inflammation, enteroatmospheric fistulas, etc.), results were encouraging enough so that numerous centers around the world adopted this approach [27–30]. A variation of the open abdomen approach was the use of multiple repeat laparotomies through temporary abdominal wall closures described by Wittmann et al. [31]. Kreis et al. [32] have reviewed comprehensively the results of trials on the available techniques—i.e., open abdomen, multiple planned laparotomies through a temporary abdominal wall closure, and relaparotomy on demand. While the on demand strategy has been associated with shorter stays in the intensive care unit and hospital and, therefore, a lower cost of hospitalization, Kreis et al. concluded that "planned relaparotomy has therefore not lost its indication for selected patients" [32].

1.1.4 Open Abdomen in the Treatment of Omphaloceles

In a landmark article in 1948, the legendary Robert E. Gross from Boston Children's Hospital described a two-stage operative approach (skin closure, then delayed fascial closure) to large omphaloceles [33]. This approach was based on Gross' recognition of the dangers of forced reduction of viscera and primary fascial closure. He stated the following: "In this way it is possible to avoid the devastating effects of a high intra-abdominal pressure which resulted from most of the types of surgical repair which have been previously employed and described in the literature" [33]. It is most interesting that Gross' recognition of the abdominal compartment syndrome in 1948 preceded that in trauma surgery by 35 years.

In the modern era, approximately 85% of infants with omphaloceles have bedside insertion of a preformed silo with a subfascial ring. The extra-abdominal bag is then rolled down each day. When the bag is flush with the skin, the infant is taken to the operating room for removal of the silo, closure of the midline aponeurosis, and, if possible, closure of the skin. The remaining 15% of infants undergo an early operation for the following: [1] omphaloceles too large for a silo, [2] small defects amenable to primary closure, or [3] for ischemia of the midgut in the omphalocele [34].

1.2 Contribution of Oswaldo Borraez, MD, Bogota, Colombia

1.2.1 Oswaldo A. Borraez G. MD

While many surgeons have contributed to the historical development of silos over the open abdomen, Oswaldo A. Borraez G, MD of Bogota, Colombia, is regarded as the modern "father" of the silo or Bogota Bag ("Bolsa de Bogota") for patients with trauma or abdominal sepsis [29, 30, 35–37]. Oswaldo Borraez was born in Cachipay, Cundinamarca, Colombia, on August 18, 1954. He studied medicine at the National University of Colombia from 1972 to 1978 and then completed his "internado" (internship) at the San Juan de Dios Hospital, Bogota (closed in 2001). He completed his obligatory medical service at a hospital near Bogota, studied "university teaching" at the Military University in Bogota, and assisted in surgery at the Misericordia (Children's) Hospital while a medical student and during the above activities from 1976 to 1982. He completed his residency in surgery from 1982 to 1985 at the National University of Colombia, primarily at the San Juan de Dios Hospital. Dr. Borraez's mentors were M.M. Manchola, MD, and E. Bonilla, MD, at the Misericordia Hospital and J. Ospina, MD, at the San Juan de Dios Hospital.

In addition to volunteering at San Juan de Dios Hospital from 1986 to 2001, Dr. Borraez has long practiced general and trauma surgery at the San Blas Hospital (public) in Bogota, where he has served as Chief of Surgery, also. His private practice is based at the Clinica Nueva in the center of Bogota, and he is a Professor of Surgery at the National University of Colombia. He has served as President of both the Colombian Trauma Association and the Colombian Surgery Association and is a seminal figure in surgery in Latin America.

1.2.2 Story of the Bogota Bag

In March, 1984, at the San Juan de Dios Hospital in Bogota, Colombia, Doctor Oswaldo A. Borraez G. was a second year resident in General Surgery. He had to manage a young patient who was crushed by a vehicle when trying to change a tire. The patient was admitted in a state of hypovolemic shock due to hepatic rupture caused by the blunt abdominal trauma. Initially, the patient underwent a right hemi-hepatectomy, with large drains left in situ. The patient subsequently required a repeat laparotomy for rebleeding. A few days later, the patient bled again and underwent another surgical procedure. A few days later, he presented with intra-abdominal sepsis, which led to a fourth operation for debridement and lavage of the abdominal cavity. Due to edema of the midgut, it was impossible to close the abdominal wall. Doctor Borraez decided to cover the exposed abdominal viscera with a plastic intravenous fluid bag. This was fixed to the musculoaponeurotic layers and was the first procedure of its kind in the world [28–32]. To the faculty at San Juan de Dios, this did not seem like a good idea initially (Fig. 1.1).

On the morning after the procedure, Dr. Borraez was called to a meeting with the Chief of Surgery at the University to explain why he had not been able to close the fascia in the abovementioned patient. After a review by the respective professor and the corresponding academic group, it was decided that further procedures were not to be undertaken on the patient. The patient subsequently had peritoneal lavage and reapplication of the plastic sheet. This plastic sheet was removed from the patient when there was satisfactory granulation of the abdominal viscera, which took approximately 6 months.

Two weeks later Doctor Borraez was called to aid the gynecology service in the management of an obese patient with abdominal sepsis of gynecological origin. Due to extensive edema of the midgut, the incision could not be closed. Once again, a plastic bag was used to cover the open abdomen. This patient survived, as well. The plastic silo technique has subsequently been widely accepted throughout the world.

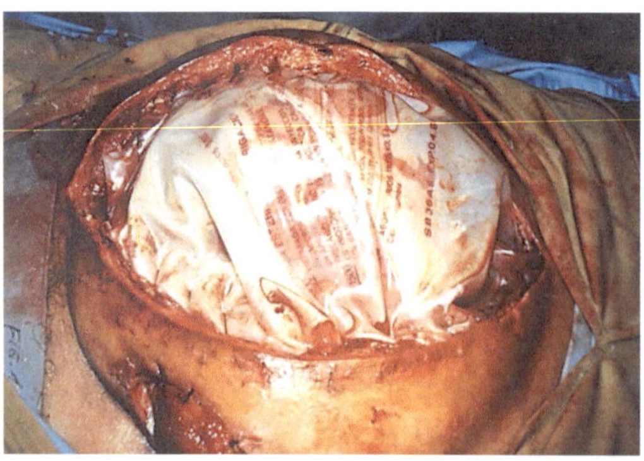

Fig. 1.1 First trauma patient with Bogota bag over open abdomen after laparotomy for blunt hepatic rupture, Hospital San Juan de Dios, Bogota, Colombia (Courtesy of Oswaldo A. Borraez G., MD)

It was Dr. David Feliciano who observed several patients managed with this technique at San Juan de Dios Hospital and then referred to it as the "Bolsa de Bogota." The technique was subsequently renamed the "Borraez bag," by which it is now known in Colombia and throughout the world [36].

In 1994, a decade after having introduced the technique, Dr. Borraez added the placement of a second bag, left free and loose, covering all intra-abdominal organs and below the abdominal wall, while the other bag is placed and fixed to the skin. The purpose of this inner bag was to prevent adhesions and facilitate later closure of the abdominal wall.

After the appearance of this technique, many variants have appeared in different parts of the world, and the basic element is the plastic bag.

1.3 Modern Indications for the Open Abdomen

Many of the indications to leave the midline linea alba open under a bag/silo or vacuum-assist device have been described in the aforementioned historical review.

In patients on the modern Trauma Service (Table 1.1), the inability to close the midline incision due to the risk of creating an abdominal compartment syndrome continues to be a prime indication. The historic reasons that have been felt to contribute to distension of the midgut after major laparotomies for trauma are as follows: [1] resuscitation with crystalloid solutions, [2] failure of the sodium pump in the cell membrane secondary to shock, [3] interstitial edema, [4] reperfusion injury, and [5] postoperative ileus. In the modern era of "damage control resuscitation," infusions of crystalloid solutions are eliminated or

Table 1.1 Indications for open abdomen in trauma patients

• Unable to close midline incision secondary to edema and distension of midgut (and to avoid primary abdominal compartment syndrome)
• Need for reoperation as part of "damage control" sequence
• Loss of continuity or substance of abdominal wall

minimized, and blood component replacement is directed by thromboelastography. Therefore, edema and distension of the midgut as an indication for the open abdomen are much decreased.

The need for a planned reoperation as part of the "damage control" sequence remains a major indication to leave the midline incision open after a first operation [37]. Classical trauma patients in this category include those with the following: [1] perihepatic, extraperitoneal pelvic, or diffuse intra-abdominal packing, [2] disconnected segments of small bowel or stapled off segments of the colon, and [3] presence of an intravascular intraluminal shunt.

The third category of trauma patient in whom an open abdomen would be appropriate would be one with transection of the rectus muscle(s) and/or subcutaneous tissue by a lap seatbelt or loss of the abdominal wall from a close-range shotgun wound. In both groups, extensive debridement of frayed muscle and necrotic subcutaneous tissue and skin may be necessary after a laparotomy. Open packing of the resultant defect over absorbable mesh or temporary rayon cloth is appropriate with definitive closure in 3–6 months [15, 16].

In patients on the Acute Care Surgery Service (Table 1.2), the indications are similar (Table 1.2). Reclosure of the midline incision after a dehiscence or evisceration is always preferred. It is often true, however, that necrosis of the midline linea alba, distention of the midgut, or a concurrent intra-abdominal abscess or fistula prevents reclosure. Once again, such a patient will benefit from the application of a temporary bag/silo and early application of a vacuum-assist device.

As noted in the section on history, some centers continue to perform sequential operations in the open abdomens of patients with secondary or tertiary peritonitis. This practice allows for vigorous cleansing of purulence, debridement of necrotic tissue, and localization of further sites of infection. When intraperitoneal sepsis has been controlled, the patient's bag/silo is switched to a vacuum-assist device.

Table 1.2 Indications for open abdomen in acute care surgery patients

• Failed primary closure (delayed dehiscence or evisceration)
• Secondary or tertiary peritonitis
• Pancreatic abscess or infected necrotic pancreatitis
• Loss of abdominal wall from necrotizing soft tissue infection

Some centers continue to utilize the "chronic open lesser sac drainage" (COLD) technique in preference to repeated percutaneous drains or video-assisted retroperitoneal debridements in a patient with a pancreatic abscess or infected pancreatic necrosis [38]. This open abdomen technique allows for granulation and gradual filling in of the lesser sac as retroperitoneal sepsis resolves.

An occasional necrotizing soft tissue infection results in full-thickness loss of the abdominal wall. The time-honored management of repeated debridements of the abdominal wall should be accompanied by absorbable mesh coverage and compression of the midgut below the musculoaponeurotic wall. The subsequent conversion to a vacuum-assisted device makes little sense in such patients, as there is a fixed loss of tissue.

1.4 Options for Coverage of the Open Abdomen

A comprehensive list of all options for coverage of the open abdomen for one of the indications discussed is beyond the scope of this chapter. Table 1.3 includes historic and current choices.

Table 1.3 Options for coverage of the open abdomen

Temporary silos
Adherent plastic drape
Fabric with zipper sewn in
Genitourinary irrigation bag (Fig. 1.2)
Human cadaveric acellular dermis
"Permanent" prosthesis, especially polytetrafluoroethylene
X-ray cassette bag
Wittmann patch
Temporary soft cover
Absorbable mesh
Parachute silk
Porcine xenograft
Vacuum-assisted closure
Visceral packing

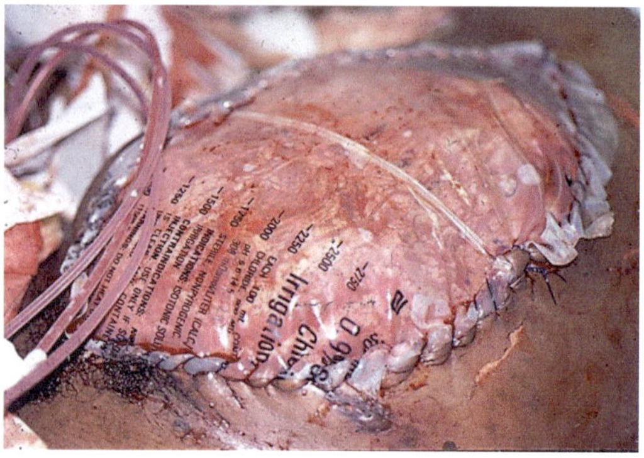

Fig. 1.2 Plastic irrigating bag sewn to the skin edges of the abdominal incision makes an excellent temporary silo. Damage control and alternate wound closures in abdominal trauma (Used with permission. Feliciano DV, Moore EE, Mattox KL. In Feliciano DV, Moore EE, Mattox KL (eds): Trauma. Third Edition. Stanford, CT, Appleton and Large, 1996, pp. 717–32)

References

1. Burch JM, Moore EE, Moore FA, Franciose R. The abdominal compartment syndrome. Surg Clin North Am. 1996;76:833–42.
2. Saggi BH, Sugerman HJ, Ivatury RR, Bloomfield GL. Abdominal compartment syndrome. J Trauma. 1998;45:597–609.
3. Emerson H. Intra-abdominal pressures. Arch Int Med. 1911;7:754–84.
4. Thorington JM, Schmidt CF. A study of urinary output and blood-pressure changes resulting in experimental ascites. Am J Med Sci. 1923;165:880–6.
5. Overhold R. Intraperitoneal pressure. Arch Surg. 1931;22:691–703.
6. Waggoner GW. Studies on intra-abdominal pressure. I. Negative intra-abdominal pressure as a normal condition. Am J Med Sci. 1926;171:697–707.
7. Lecours R. Intra-abdominal pressures. Can Med Assoc J. 1946;55:450–7.
8. Richardson JD, Trinkle JK. Hemodynamic and respiratory alterations with increased intra-abdominal pressure. J Surg Res. 1976;20:401–4.
9. Kashtan J, Green JF, Parsons EQ, Holcroft JW. Hemodynamic effects of increased abdominal pressure. J Surg Res. 1981;30:249–55.
10. Guazzi M, Polese A, Magrini F, Fiorentini C, Olivari CMT. Negative influences of ascites on the cardiac function of cirrhotic patients. Am J Med. 1975;59:165–70.
11. Kron IL, Harman PK, Nolan SP. The measurement of intra-abdominal pressure as a criterion for abdominal re-exploration. Ann Surg. 1984;199:28–30.
12. Harman PK, Kron IL, McLachlan HD, Freedlender AE, Nolan SP. Elevated intra-abdominal pressure and renal function. Ann Surg. 1982;196:594–7.
13. Richards WO, Scovill W, Shen B, Reed W. Acute renal failure associated with increased intra-abdominal pressure. Ann Surg. 1983;197:183–7.
14. Ogilvie WH. The late complications of abdominal war wounds. Lancet. 1940;236:253–6.
15. Saxe JM, Ledgerwood AM, Lucas CE. Management of the difficult abdominal closure. Surg Clin North Am. 1993;73:243–51.
16. Bender JS, Bailey CE, Saxe JM, Ledgerwood AM, Lucas CE. The technique of visceral packing: recommended management of difficult fascial closure in trauma patients. J Trauma. 1994;36:182–5.
17. Price J. Surgical intervention in cases of peritonitis. Proc Philadelphia County Med Soc. 1905;26:92.
18. Ogilvie WH. Surgical lessons of war applied to civil practice. Br Med J. 1945;1(4400):619–23.
19. Schumer W, Lee DK, Jones B. Peritoneal lavage in postoperative therapy of late peritoneal sepsis. Surgery. 1964;55:841–5.
20. McKenna JP, Currie DJ, MacDonald JA, Mahoney LJ, Finlayson DC, Lanskail JC. The use of continuous postoperative peritoneal lavage in the management of diffuse peritonitis. Surg Gynecol Obstet. 1970;130:254–8.
21. Stephen M, Loewenthal J. Generalized infective peritonitis. Surg Gynecol Obstet. 1978;147:231–4.
22. Stephen M, Loewenthal J. Continuing peritoneal lavage in high-risk peritonitis. Surgery. 1979;85:603–6.
23. Hovnanian AP, Saddawi N. An experimental study of the consequences of intraperitoneal irrigation. Surg Gynecol Obstet. 1972;134:575–8.
24. Hudspeth AS. Radical surgical debridement in the treatment of advanced generalized bacterial peritonitis. Arch Surg. 1975;110:1233–6.
25. Polk HC Jr, Fry DE. Radical peritoneal debridement for established peritonitis. The results of a prospective randomized clinical trial. Ann Surg. 1980;192:350–5.
26. Steinberg D. On leaving the peritoneal cavity open in acute generalized suppurative peritonitis. Am J Surg. 1979;137:216–20.
27. Duff JH, Moffat J. Abdominal sepsis managed by leaving abdomen open. Surgery. 1981;90:774–8.
28. Maetani S, Tobe T. Open peritoneal drainage as effective treatment of advanced peritonitis. Surgery. 1981;90:804–9.
29. Gomez A, Aduen J, Fernandez G, de Lattoz J, Castro A, Brutrago F, Alvarez E, Calderon F, Vargas R, Montenegro G. Infection intraabdominal severa. Analisis de 117 cases. Revista Colombiana de Cirugia. 1989;4:77–81.
30. Borraez O. Abdomen aiorto. Utilizacion del polivinilo Cirugia. 2001;16:39–43.
31. Wittmann DH, Aprahamian C, Bergstein JM. Etappenlavage: advanced diffuse peritonitis managed by planned multiple laparotomies utilizing zippers, slide fastener, and Velcro analogue for temporary abdominal closure. World J Surg. 1990;14:218–26.
32. Kreis BE, de Mol van Otterloo AJ, Kreis RW. Open abdomen management: a review of its history and a

proposed management algorithm. Med Sci Monit. 2013;19:524–33.
33. Gross RE. A new method for surgical treatment of large omphaloceles. Surgery. 1948;24:277–92.
34. Rescorla FJ. Personal communication. Indianapolis, Indiana: Chief of Surgery, Riley Children's Hospital of Indiana University; 2017.
35. Abaunza H. Evolucion de la cirugie de algunos organos. Desde sus pioneros hasta los cirujanos actuals. Cirugia. 1996;11:66–74.
36. Feliciano DV, Burch JM. Towel clips, silos, and heroic forms of wound closure. In: Maull KI, Cleveland HC, Feliciano DV, Rice CL, Trunkey DD, Wolferth CC, editors. Advances in trauma and critical care, vol. 6, St. Louis: Mosby-Year Book; 1991.
37. Roberts DJ, Ball CG, Feliciano DV, Moore EE, Ivatury RR, Lucas CE, Fabian TC, Zygun DA, Kirkpatrick AW, Stelfox HT. History of the innovation of damage control for management of trauma patients: 1902-2016. Ann Surg. 2017;265:1034–44.
38. Bouwense SAW, Bollen TL, Fockens P, Besselink MGH. Treatment of local complications. In: Adams DB, Cotton PB, Zyromski NJ, Windsor JA, editors. Pancreatitis: medical and surgical management. West Sussex, UK: Wiley Blackwell; 2017.

2 Applications of Damage Control Surgery in Modern Civilian Trauma Care

Derek J. Roberts

Abstract

Modern trauma damage control (DC) integrates the stages of DC surgery into the process of DC resuscitation. Although widely believed to improve survival when appropriately indicated, there is limited evidence supporting a benefit of DC surgery (and its component DC interventions) in injured patients. Further, the procedure is associated with a number of potentially severe and often resource-intensive complications. Several studies have recently reported data suggesting that a variation exists in the use of DC laparotomy across trauma centers or that the procedure may be overused. These and other studies have also suggested that overutilization of the procedure may be associated with increased morbidity and mortality. Variation in the use of DC surgery between trauma centers may occur because surgeons are frequently uncertain which "operative profile" (i.e., DC or definitive surgery) is best in varying clinical situations. In this chapter, I review the structure, effectiveness, and safety of modern trauma DC; recent studies suggesting variation in and potential harm related to the overuse of DC surgery between trauma centers; and published consensus indications for the use of DC surgery and DC interventions that aim to reduce this variation and guide future research.

2.1 Background

In injured patients receiving traditional, crystalloid-based resuscitation, significant hemorrhage is frequently complicated by development of a "bloody vicious cycle" (a.k.a., "lethal triad") of hypothermia, acidosis, and coagulopathy [1–3]. Resuscitation of hemorrhagic shock also produces ischemia-reperfusion injury of the bowel, which increases intestinal wall permeability, leading to sequestration of fluid in the bowel wall and its supporting mesenteries (i.e., abdominal visceral edema) [1, 4, 5]. This process, when combined with large-volume crystalloid fluid administration, increases intra-abdominal pressure (IAP) and may culminate in post-injury abdominal compartment syndrome (ACS; defined by the Abdominal Compartment Society as a sustained IAP >20 associated with new organ dysfunction/failure) [1, 6–8]. The vicious cycle and ACS have historically been associated with a high risk of death after major injury despite attempts at definitively controlling hemorrhage and preventing and/or treating intra-abdominal hypertension (IAH), respectively [1, 2].

D.J. Roberts, M.D., Ph.D.
Department of Surgery, University of Calgary, Calgary, AB, Canada

J. Duchesne et al. (eds.), *Damage Control in Trauma Care*,
https://doi.org/10.1007/978-3-319-72607-6_2

In an attempt to prevent the onset of and/or limit the effects of the vicious cycle and post-injury ACS, surgeons adopted damage control (DC) laparotomy to manage severely injured civilians in the 1980s/early 1990s [1]. In 1983, Stone et al. reported that "staged" laparotomy [i.e., abbreviated initial laparotomy with planned reoperation after a period of ongoing resuscitation in the intensive care unit (ICU)] was associated with improved survival in injured patients who developed "major coagulopathy" during operation [9]. Rotondo, Schwab, and colleagues subsequently proposed in 1993 that abbreviated trauma laparotomy be termed "damage control" and reported data suggesting that it improved survival in a "maximum injury subset" of patients with abdominal vascular and multiple concomitant abdominal visceral injuries [10]. In 1998 (during the early dispersion and exploration stage of the innovation of trauma DC), during a time when high-volume crystalloid fluid resuscitation (and therefore severe abdominal visceral edema) was common, Ivatury and colleagues advocated for routine temporary abdominal closure (TAC) of the open abdomen (i.e., open abdominal management) after DC to prevent the adverse physiologic consequences of IAH [1, 11]. Finally, beginning largely in the mid-1990s, the DC concept was adapted to rapidly manage visceral and vascular injuries in the neck, chest, and extremities [1].

In contrast to definitive (i.e., single-stage) surgery, DC allows the initial operation for control of exsanguinating hemorrhage and/or gross contamination to be abbreviated using what Feliciano et al. termed "rapid conservative operative techniques" (now also referred to, using the DC lexicon, as "DC interventions") [1, 12, 13]. This approach has long been thought to benefit critically injured patients who are "more likely to die from an uncorrected shock state than from failure to complete organ repairs" [14]. In the abdomen, DC interventions include therapeutic perihepatic packing, closed suction drainage of pancreaticobiliary injuries, rapid intestinal resection without re-anastomosis (leaving the intestinal tract in discontinuity until a later operation), and lateral arteriorrhaphy (e.g., superior mesenteric artery injuries), temporary intravascular shunting (e.g., common iliac artery injuries), and ligation (e.g., infrarenal inferior vena cava injuries) of major abdominal vascular injuries [15]. Abbreviating the index operation during DC theoretically limits further declines in core body temperature and pH and therefore allows for rewarming and correction of metabolic and coagulation disturbances in the ICU [16]. Once physiology is deemed adequately restored, injured patients are returned to the operating room (OR) for additional surgery (e.g., removal of temporary intravascular shunts and performance of vascular repairs or intestinal anastomoses for reestablishment of bowel continuity) and/or primary fascial closure (i.e., fascia-to-fascia closure of the open abdomen within the index hospitalization), often within 6–48 h of initial operation [1, 16].

In this chapter, I review the structure, effectiveness, and safety of modern trauma DC; recent studies suggesting variation in and potential harm related to the overuse of DC surgery between trauma centers; and published consensus indications for the use of DC surgery and DC interventions that aim to reduce this variation and guide future research.

2.2 The Structure of Modern Trauma DC (Integrating the Stages of DC Surgery with the Process of DC Resuscitation)

The stages of DC surgery were initially suggested by Rotondo, Schwab, and colleagues to include DC 1 [immediate operation for control of hemorrhage and contamination using one or more DC interventions followed by temporary closure of the abdomen (or thorax) and transfer to the ICU], DC 2 (resuscitation in the ICU with the goal of correcting hypothermia, acidosis, and coagulopathy), and DC 3 [reoperation for definitive repair of injuries and closure of the abdomen (or thorax)] [1, 16]. This group and others later expanded these stages to include DC 0 [or "damage control ground zero," which includes those interventions performed in the prehospital and immediate in-hospital setting before operation (e.g., prehospital transport/care, rewarming, and initiation of a predesigned massive transfusion protocol)] and DC 4 (abdominal wall reconstruction, frequently using component separation methods and synthetic or biological mesh reinforcement) [17, 18].

DC interventions are rapid, often technically simple procedures that may be used in either the pre- [e.g., balloon catheter tamponade of significant, ongoing hemorrhage from a zone III neck wound in the emergency department (ED)] or intraoperative setting [15]. These interventions are designed to temporarily or sometimes definitively manage exsanguinating hemorrhage, gross contamination, and/or a massive pulmonary air leak in situations where several uncommonly encountered thoracic (e.g., a penetrating, through-and-through pulmonary parenchymal injury that does not involve the hilar structures), abdominal (e.g., devascularization or massive destruction of the pancreas, duodenum, or pancreaticoduodenal complex), pelvic (e.g., severe blunt pelvic trauma with ongoing, massive extraperitoneal hemorrhage), and/or vascular (e.g., significant, ongoing bleeding from a zone I or III penetrating neck injury) injuries are encountered [15, 19–46]. These injuries are characteristic of those that few surgeons have experience treating and therefore are associated with massive hemorrhage, physiological exhaustion (hypothermia, acidosis, and coagulopathy), and a high mortality when attempts are made to manage them definitively (see Table 2.1 for consensus definitions of a number of DC interventions reported in 2015) [15, 19–46].

Table 2.1 Reported descriptions of thoracic, abdominal/pelvic, and vascular damage control interventions reported in 2015

Intervention	Description
Thoracic damage control interventions	
Pneumonorrhaphy [19–21]	After small injured vessels and bronchi within the parenchyma of a superficial pulmonary laceration are selectively ligated, the edges are approximated
Pulmonary tractotomy [19–23]	The lung bridging a pulmonary parenchymal wound is divided using a GIA 55/75 vascular stapler or between two long vascular clamps, and then small injured parenchymal vessels and bronchi lying underneath are selectively ligated
Pulmonary wedge resection [19–21]	A GIA 55/75 or TA 30/60/90 vascular stapler is used to resect a peripheral portion of a pulmonary lobe or segment of the lung
Rapid, simultaneously stapled pneumonectomy [21, 24]	A TA 90/55 vascular stapler is placed across the pulmonary hilar structures and fired, resulting in an en masse simultaneous division of the main stem bronchus and pulmonary vessels
Intraluminal drainage of the proximal esophagus and wide drainage of the pleural space [25, 26]	The esophagus above or at the site of an esophageal injury is drained with a nasogastric tube connected to low suction, while the pleural space is widely drained with thoracostomy tubes
Therapeutic mediastinal and/or pleural space packing [27–29]	Compressive gauze packing is applied to the mediastinal and/or pleural surface to tamponade venous and/or coagulopathic hemorrhage at least until the first reoperation (which frequently occurs within <24–48 h)
Temporary thoracic closure [25–27, 30]	The thoracotomy incision is temporarily closed en masse using a heavy, nonabsorbable, running suture or with towel clips, a patch or silo/Bogotá bag, or a modified Barker's vacuum pack or commercial negative pressure wound therapy device
Abdominal/pelvic damage control interventions	
Therapeutic perihepatic packing	Compressive gauze packing is placed around the liver to tamponade venous and/or coagulopathic hemorrhage from the hepatic parenchyma or surrounding juxtahepatic veins at least until the first reoperation (which frequently occurs within <24–48 h)

(continued)

Table 2.1 (continued)

Intervention	Description
Staged pancreaticoduodenectomy [31–34]	During the index laparotomy, major vascular hemorrhage is controlled; where necessary (sometimes this has already been done by the inciting trauma), the duodenum distal to the pylorus, common bile duct, pancreas distal to the injury, and distal duodenum or jejunum are transected; and the right upper quadrant and peripancreatic space are widely drained (some authors also report use of T- or biliary drainage tubes at this time). Reconstruction (pancreaticojejunostomy, hepaticojejunostomy, and duodenojejunostomy) is delayed until reoperation
Therapeutic renal fossa packing [35]	Compressive gauze packing is applied to the renal fossa to tamponade venous and/or coagulopathic hemorrhage from the kidney at least until the first reoperation (which frequently occurs within <24–48 h)
Bilateral externalized ureteral stenting and diversion [35]	When neither transurethral or suprapubic drainage effectively evacuates urine from the injured bladder, J-stents are passed up each ureteral orifice and then externalized to divert the urinary output of both kidneys until definitive repair of the bladder is possible
Temporary abdominal closure/ open abdominal management	The abdomen is temporarily closed using a Barker's vacuum pack, commercial negative pressure peritoneal therapy device, silo/Bogotá bag, mesh or sheet, or another technique
Extraperitoneal pelvic packing [36–38]	After a 6- to 8-cm midline incision is made extending from the pubic symphysis cephalad (dividing the midline abdominal fascia) and the preperitoneal space is opened using digital dissection (where necessary), laparotomy pads are placed on either side of the bladder, the fascia is closed with a heavy suture, and the skin is closed with staples
Bilateral internal iliac artery ligation [39]	Both internal iliac arteries are ligated using heavy, permanent sutures during laparotomy
Vascular damage control interventions	
Balloon catheter tamponade [40–44]	A Foley, Fogarty, Sengstaken-Blakemore, or improvised balloon catheter (created using a red rubber catheter and Penrose drain) is inserted into a bleeding wound tract. The balloon of the catheter is then inflated with sterile water and repositioned until adequate hemostasis is achieved
Temporary intravascular shunting [45, 46]	After an embolectomy and administration of local intravascular heparinized saline, the defect in the injured artery and/or vein is bridged with a Pruitt-Inahara, Argyle, Javid, or Sundt vascular shunt or with a piece of an intravenous line or nasogastric/chest tube (cut to length such that it overlaps within the vessel by approximately 2 cm and secured into place with a heavy silk tie on either end). The shunt is left in place until at least the first reoperation (which frequently occurs within <24–48 h)

Where *GIA* indicates gastrointestinal anastomosis and *TA*, thoracoabdominal
Table and table legend reproduced with permission from reference [15]. Copyright Wolters Kluwer Health (2015)

In modern civilian trauma care, many surgeons have suggested that DC surgery (or, more specifically, DC 1) should most appropriately be considered one of the first, essential components of the process of DC resuscitation [47]. DC resuscitation is characterized by rapid hemorrhage control (open or endovascular, including the use of DC interventions in the preoperative setting or in the OR during DC 1), permissive hypotension, administration of blood products in a ratio approximating whole blood [i.e., 1:1:1 plasma/platelets/ packed red blood cells (PRBCs)], and minimal use of crystalloid fluids [48–50]. This now internationally adopted resuscitation strategy is initiated in the prehospital setting (a.k.a., during DC 0) and continued through DC stages 1–4. DC resuscitation was developed in order to preemptively treat the lethal triad (including the acute coagulopathy of trauma, which occurs early after injury, is likely caused by the degree of tissue injury after trauma, and is independent of the amount of crystalloid fluids administered to the patient), preserve oxygen-carrying capacity, repair the endothelium, and prevent the adverse physiological consequences of large-volume crystalloid fluid resuscitation [47–50]. In the recently reported PROPPR randomized controlled trial (RCT) comparing a 1:1:1 versus 1:1:2 ratio of plasma/platelets/PRBCs, although 24-h and 30-day mortality was similar between the study groups, more patients in the 1:1:1 group achieved hemostasis, and fewer experienced death due to exsanguination at 24 h [50]. Thus, DC resuscitation with a 1:1:1 ratio of blood products likely has a hemostatic benefit among exsanguinating civilian trauma patients.

2.3 Effectiveness and Safety of DC Surgery in Civilian Trauma Patients

Although widely believed to improve survival when appropriately indicated, there is limited evidence supporting a benefit of DC surgery in injured patients [1, 16]. A Cochrane systematic review on DC laparotomy conducted in 2013 identified few relevant observational studies and no RCTs [16, 51]. Importantly, as the "operative profile" (DC versus definitive surgery) chosen in these seven observational studies was not randomly assigned, their conclusions are inherently limited by confounding by indication. This relatively common limitation of observational treatment studies occurs when other, unmeasured reasons associated with the choice to perform DC surgery and with patient outcome confound the association between DC surgery and outcomes (i.e., those selected for DC are inherently different from those selected for definitive surgery because they were selected to undergo DC surgery for a reason) [52].

Considering the above limitation, Stone et al., Rotondo et al., and Chinnery et al. each reported a large improvement in unadjusted survival when DC or staged laparotomy was used instead of definitive surgery to manage: (1) patients who developed a "major coagulopathy" during laparotomy, (2) hemodynamically unstable patients with combined abdominal vascular and pancreas gunshot injuries, and (3) those who received >10 U PRBCs and had ≥1 major abdominal vascular and ≥2 abdominal visceral injuries, respectively [9, 10, 53, 54]. Further, Rice and colleagues reported that, when compared to only minor deviations, moderate or major deviations from a protocol that suggested the use of DC surgery in patients with a temperature <35 °C, lactate >4 mmol/L (or more than twice the upper limit of normal), or corrected pH <7.3 were independently associated with improved survival [54, 55]. Finally, Asensio et al. reported that implementing a guideline that suggested the use of DC surgery for patients with 1 of 12 different clinical findings/events (transfusion >4 L PRBCs or >5 L PRBCs/whole blood combined; total OR fluid replacement >12 L; OR patient temperature ≤34°C, serum [HCO3-] ≤15 mEq/L, or arterial pH ≤7.2; a thoracic or abdominal vascular injury or complex hepatic injury requiring packing; those requiring ED or OR thoracotomy; or patients that develop intraoperative coagulopathy or dysrhythmias) was associated with a decreased unadjusted odds of infections, an increased unadjusted odds of abdominal wall closure, and a reduced unadjusted length of ICU and hospital stay [54, 56].

As DC surgery became widely adopted worldwide in the 1990s and 2000s, it was increasingly reported to be associated with a number of potentially severe and often resource-intensive complications considered by some (at least initially) to be "diseases of survivorship" [1, 54, 57, 58]. DC surgery and open abdominal management have been reported to be associated with an ~10–25% risk of an intra-abdominal abscess or abscesses, a mean of approximately five reoperations, an ~15% risk of readmission to hospital, and an ~8% risk of subsequent surgical procedures, especially those relating to massive or complex ventral herniae [54, 59–61]. Development of an enteroatmospheric fistula, defined as an enteric fistula in the middle of an open abdomen, occurs in approximately 5% of patients with an open abdominal wound and is considered to be a "surgical nightmare" by international surgical opinion leaders [54, 61, 62]. Defining characteristics include the absence of a fistula tract, the lack of well-vascularized surrounding tissue, a low probability of spontaneous closure, and the spillage of enteric content directly into the peritoneal cavity [8, 54, 62, 63]. These fistulae are difficult to control and may result in repeated episodes of intra-abdominal sepsis, long lengths of ICU and hospital stay, significant costs to the health-care system, and an elevated risk of mortality [54, 64]. Moreover, although many patients can ultimately have their abdomen closed after DC laparotomy, those who cannot are often managed with a "planned ventral hernia," in which a split-thickness skin graft or mobilized native skin flap is used to cover the granulated viscera of the open abdomen, resulting in a massive and complex abdominal wall hernia that may be repaired using a components separation technique in 6–12 months [54, 65]. Possibly because of the above complications, survivors of open abdominal management have been reported to suffer from decreased physical functioning, a reduced quality of life (at least in the short term), and an increased incidence of depression and post-traumatic stress disorder [54, 66–69].

2.4 Variation in and Potential Harm Related to Overuse of DC Surgery Between Trauma Centers

Several authors have recently reported data suggesting that a variation in the use of DC laparotomy may exist across trauma centers or that the procedure may be overused [57, 70]. DC was used in 9% of patients undergoing emergent laparotomy at a level 1 trauma center in the United States in 2008 as compared to a relatively consistent rate of 29–37% in trauma patients at a different American level 1 center between 2004 and 2010 [54, 71, 72]. This variation in the use of DC across trauma centers could relate to increasing use of the procedure for indications other than those that have been previously studied or suggested to be appropriate in the literature [16, 54]. In support of this, one retrospective cohort study reported that one in five patients who received DC laparotomy at a level 1 trauma center between 2004 and 2008 failed to meet at least one of the traditional indications [16, 73]. In this study, only 33% were acidotic, 43% hypothermic, and 48% coagulopathic upon arrival to the ICU from the OR [16, 54, 73].

Variation in rates of use of DC surgery across trauma centers is concerning as accumulating evidence suggests that overutilization of the procedure for inappropriate indications may be associated with increased morbidity and mortality [57, 58, 70, 73–75]. In one retrospective cohort study conducted at a level 1 trauma center between 2005 and 2009, the use of DC instead of definitive laparotomy in trauma patients without severe head injury, a systolic blood pressure (BP) >90 mmHg, and no combined abdominal injuries was independently associated with a three times increased odds of major postoperative complications and a 10-day longer length of hospital stay [16, 75]. Further, in a propensity-matched cohort study conducted at the same trauma center, the use of DC instead of definitive laparotomy (for packing, hemodynamic instability, or intra-abdominal contamination; to facilitate a second look laparotomy, expedite postoperative care/interventions, or prophylax against ACS; or for other/unclear reasons) in injured patients was associated with a 13% increased probability of postoperative ileus, a 4% increased probability of postoperative gastrointestinal bleeding, an 11% increased probability of fascial dehiscence, a 19% increased probability of superficial surgical site infection, and an 18% increased probability of perioperative death [58].

Several other authors and I have therefore suggested that clinical outcomes and health system costs may improve with more selective use of DC surgery, especially given that DC resuscitation may effectively prevent or treat hypothermia, acidosis, and coagulopathy in trauma patients [1, 70]. In support of this, Higa et al. observed that the rate of use of DC decreased from 36 to 9% among trauma patients undergoing emergent laparotomy between 2006 and 2008 despite similar patient demographics and Injury Severity Scale (ISS) scores among the patients managed between these time periods [71]. This decline in the rate of use of DC laparotomy was associated with a significant improvement in primary fascial closure rates (50% in 2006 versus 86% in 2008), perioperative mortality (22% in 2006 versus 13%

in 2008), and total hospital costs ($44,312 in 2006 versus $32,992 in 2008) among patients undergoing emergent trauma laparotomy [54, 71].

2.5 Published Consensus Indications for Use of DC Surgery and DC Interventions in Civilian Trauma Patients

Variation in the use of DC surgery between trauma centers may occur because surgeons are frequently uncertain which operative profile is best in varying clinical situations [15, 70, 76]. This uncertainty is likely exacerbated by the fact that limited data exists on the effectiveness and safety of DC surgery and DC interventions [15, 70, 76]. These procedures are also difficult to study, especially considering the multitude of potential clinical situations that may be encountered by surgeons who (routinely or uncommonly) perform emergent thoracic, abdominal, and/or peripheral vascular operations on injured patients across level 1, 2, and/or 3 trauma centers [15, 70, 76]. Despite this, however, surgeons must decide when to use DC (or specific DC interventions) over definitive surgery (or specific definitive surgical interventions) in their practice [15].

Therefore, the indications for trauma damage control international study group and I initiated a program of research in 2013 to determine the specific clinical situations in which the expected survival benefit of conducting DC surgery (or a specific DC intervention) is likely to exceed the expected risk of negative consequences [15, 16]. We first conducted a scoping review to synthesize the literature on DC surgery and DC interventions, identify a comprehensive list of their reported indications for use, and examine the content and evidence upon these indications were based [15, 54, 77]. An indication was defined as "a clinical finding/scenario that advised use of DC surgery (or a DC intervention) over definitive surgery (or a definitive surgical intervention)" [57]. This study identified 270 published, peer-reviewed articles (58% of which represented original research) that reported 1107 indications for DC surgery and 424 indications for the 16 different DC interventions previously listed in Table 2.1 [54, 77].

We used qualitative research methods to synthesize the above indications into 123 codes representing unique indications for DC surgery and 101 codes representing unique indications for DC interventions [15, 57]. Within these codes, we included summarized or commonly used decision thresholds for reported indications with cutoffs (e.g., temperature or pH <X) [15, 57]. In an expert appropriateness rating study, an international panel of trauma surgery experts ($n = 9$ surgeons) then rated 101 (82.1%) of the coded indications for DC surgery and 78 (77.2%) of the coded indications for DC interventions to be appropriate for use in surgical practice [15, 57].

In 2014, we subsequently surveyed 366 surgeons who treat injured patients in level 1–3 trauma centers in the United States, Canada, Australia, and New Zealand to determine their opinions on the appropriateness of many of the indications rated in the expert appropriateness rating study [70]. In total, 201 (56.0%) of the surveyed surgeons responded [70]. These respondents rated 15 (78.9%) preoperative and 23 (95.8%) intraoperative indications to be appropriate for use in their practices [70]. There was substantial agreement between the opinions of practicing surgeons with different training, experience, and practice settings on the appropriateness of reported candidate indications for the use of DC surgery (Fig. 2.1) [70]. The reduced list of candidate indications for DC surgery that were rated to be appropriate by both experts and practicing surgeons (in both the expert appropriateness rating study and the survey of practicing surgeons) is listed in Table 2.2 [57, 70].

Nearly all agreed that the expected benefits of DC surgery outweighed the expected risks when adults requiring emergent operation were found to have (1) persistent hemodynamic instability (systolic BP <90 mmHg) in the preoperative setting or during operation (or if they were reported to have a successfully resuscitated cardiac arrest during transport to hospital), (2) persistent hypothermia (core body temperature <34 °C) or acidosis (arterial pH <7.2) during operation, or (3) hypothermia, acidosis, and clinical (absence of

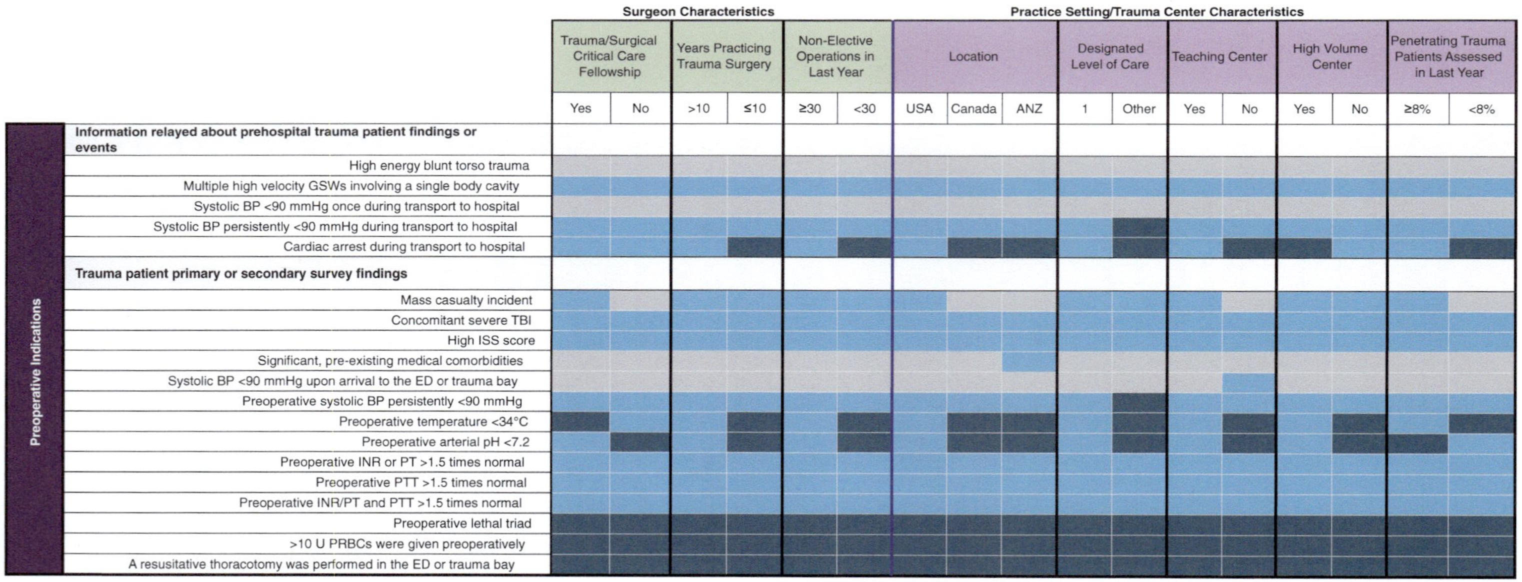

Fig. 2.1 Color map of respondents' appropriateness ratings of published candidate pre- and intraoperative indications for the use of damage control surgery stratified by surgeon- and trauma center-level characteristics, where ANZ indicates Australia and New Zealand (i.e., Australasia); BP, blood pressure; ED, emergency department; GSWs, gunshot wounds; INR, international normalized ratio; ISS, Injury Severity Scale; PT, prothrombin time; and PTT, partial thromboplastin time. Interpolated median values that lied halfway between two integers were rounded upward. Disagreement was defined as at least 33% of respondents rating the indication as 1–2 (significant harm-harm) on the Likert Scale and at least another 33% rating it 4–5 (benefit-significant benefit). Figure and figure legend reproduced with permission from reference [70]

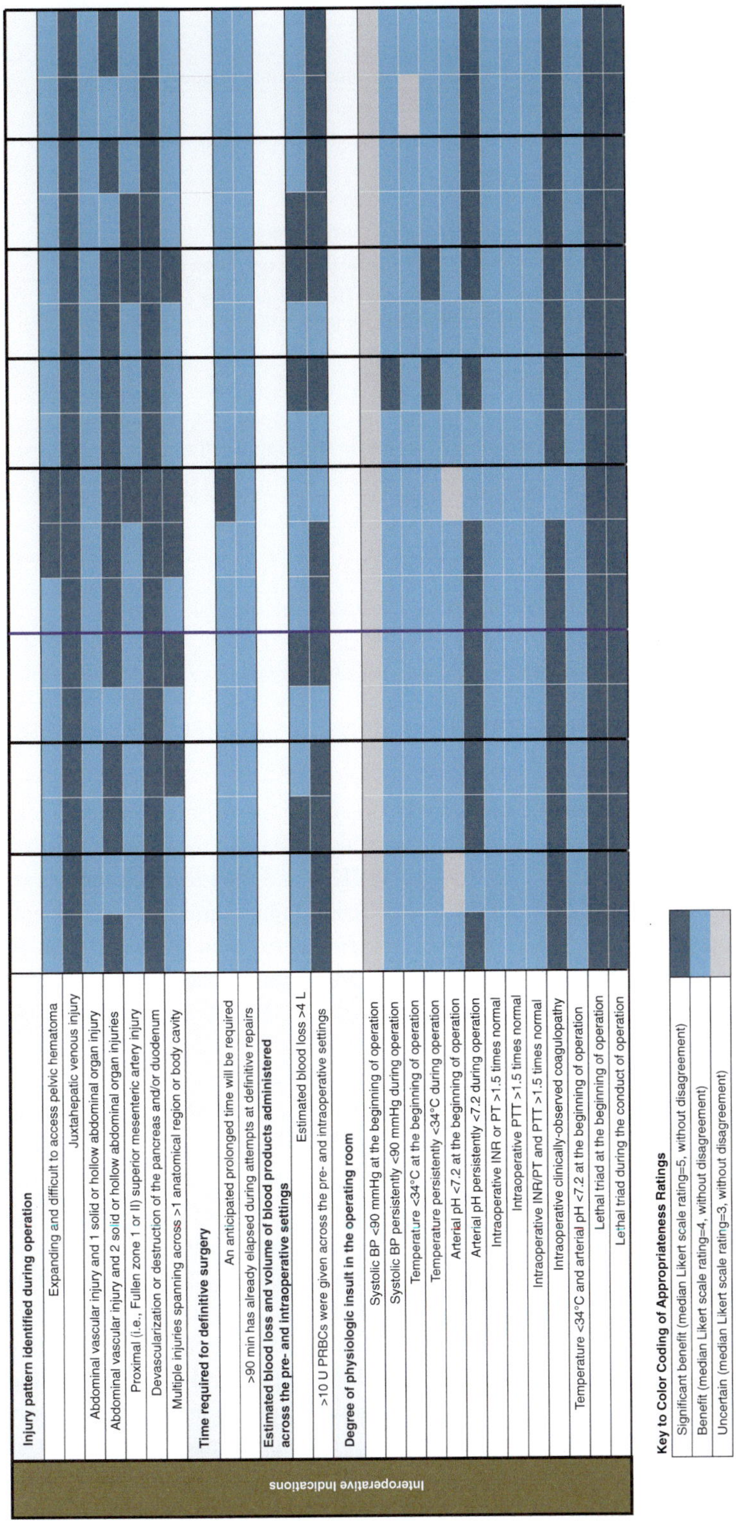

Fig. 2.1 (continued)

Table 2.2 Published candidate indications for the use of damage control surgery in adult civilian trauma patients that were rated to be appropriate by a panel of experts and the majority of practicing surgeons

Indication
Degree of physiologic insult in the pre- or intraoperative settings
• Persistent systolic BP <90 mmHg or a successfully resuscitated cardiac arrest during transport to hospital
• Persistent systolic BP <90 mmHg in the preoperative setting or during operation
• Preoperative core body temperature <34 °C, arterial pH <7.2, or INR/PT >1.5 times normal (with or without a concomitant PTT >1.5 times normal)
• Core body temperature <34 °C and arterial pH <7.2 at the beginning of operation
• Persistent core body temperature < 34 °C or persistent arterial pH <7.2 during operation
• INR/PT and PTT >1.5 times normal or a clinically observed coagulopathy during operation
• Core body temperature <34°, arterial pH <7.2, and laboratory-confirmed (INR/PT and/or PTT >1.5 times normal) or clinically observed coagulopathy in the preoperative setting, at the beginning of operation or during the conduct of operation
Estimated blood loss and amount or type of resuscitation provided
• Estimated blood loss >4 L in the operating room
• >10 U of PRBCs were administered to the patient in the pre- or pre- and intraoperative settings
Injury pattern identified during operation
• An expanding and difficult to access pelvic hematoma
• A juxtahepatic venous injury
• An abdominal vascular injury and at least one major associated abdominal solid or hollow organ injury
• Devascularization or destruction of the pancreas, duodenum, or pancreaticoduodenal complex with involvement of the ampulla/proximal pancreatic duct and/or distal CBD

Where *BP* indicates blood pressure, *CBD* common bile duct, *INR* international normalized ratio, *PT* prothrombin time, and *PTT* partial thromboplastin time
Table and table legend reproduced with permission from reference [70]

visible blood clots during surgery) or laboratory [international normalized ratio (INR)/prothrombin time (PT) or partial thromboplastin time (PTT) >1.5 times normal] coagulopathy in the preoperative setting or during operation [54, 57, 70]. They also agreed that injured patients with physiologic derangements that improve or reverse during resuscitation and operation were candidates for definitive closure of their injured cavity at the end of the index operation [70]. These findings suggest that surgeons likely believe that unless patients present with or develop the entire lethal triad or have hypotension, hypothermia, and/or acidosis that persists during DC resuscitation (including the emergent operation for rapid hemorrhage control), it is likely frequently safe to perform a definitive (instead of DC) operation (provided that the other scenarios listed in Table 2.2 have not been encountered) [70].

Published indications that were independent of patient physiology and assessed to be appropriate by experts and the broader surgical community included an estimated blood loss >4 L, the administration of a massive transfusion (>10 U) of PRBCs, and the identification of one of the four different injury patterns during operation [57, 70]. The assessment of massive blood loss or requirement for massive transfusion as appropriate indications for DC surgery is not surprising as DC surgery has long been used as a strategy to improve the increased morbidity and mortality associated with exsanguination in trauma patients [78–80]. Further, the above injury patterns assessed to appropriately indicate the use of DC are characteristic of those that (1) often result in exsanguination during exposure and attempts at definitive repair (juxtahepatic venous injuries), (2) require urgent transport to the angiography suite for embolization soon after they are discovered intraoperatively (an expanding and difficult to access pelvic hematoma), (3) are complicated by competing management priorities (hemorrhage and contamination) or multifocal hemorrhage (an abdominal vascular injury and at least one major associated abdominal solid or hollow organ injury), or (4) require a pancreaticoduodenectomy (devascularization or destruction of the pancreas, duodenum, or pancreaticoduodenal complex) [70, 81, 82].

Table 2.3 provides a list of the indications for the use of DC interventions that were assessed by the expert panel to be appropriate for use in the ED or OR setting [15]. Interestingly, several of the indications for the use of DC surgery and intraoperative DC interventions were identical or nearly identical [15, 54, 57]. Experts assessed these identical or nearly identical indications to have a similar appropriateness for use in practice

Table 2.3 Indications for the use of thoracic, abdominal/pelvic, and vascular damage control interventions that were rated to be appropriate by a panel of experts[a]

Indication(s) for
Thoracic DC interventions in patients undergoing thoracotomy
Rapid lung-sparing surgery (pneumonorrhaphy, pulmonary tractotomy, and pulmonary wedge resection)
Whenever possible when an emergent thoracotomy is required for thoracic trauma
Pulmonary tractotomy
Through-and-through pulmonary parenchymal injuries that do not involve the hilar structures
Rapid, simultaneously stapled pneumonectomy
An irreparable main bronchus injury and significant hemodynamic instability in the OR
Therapeutic mediastinal and/or pleural space packing
Inability to control bleeding with conventional methods (due to a coagulopathy or for other reasons)
Temporary thoracic closure
Signs of thoracic compartment syndrome develop during attempted thoracic wall closure[b]
Hypothermia, acidosis, and coagulopathy in the OR
Temporary thoracic closure with a silo/Bogotá bag
Signs of thoracic compartment syndrome develop during attempted thoracic wall closure en masse or with towel clips
Abdominal/pelvic DC interventions in patients undergoing laparotomy
Therapeutic perihepatic packing
An expanding or ruptured extensive subcapsular hematoma/hematomata
An extensive bilobar hepatic parenchymal injury
A juxtahepatic venous injury
A AAST grade III–V liver injury and a concomitant severe traumatic brain injury or multiple other concomitant solid and/or hollow abdominal organ injuries
Administration of a large volume of PRBCs preoperatively or across the pre- and intraoperative settings in a patient with a liver injury[c]
A liver injury with hemodynamic instability, hypothermia, acidosis, and/or coagulopathy in the OR
Inability to control hepatic bleeding by conventional methods
To facilitate transfer of a patient from a hospital with little experience with (or resources for) management of major liver injury to a level 1 trauma center
Staged pancreaticoduodenectomy
Devascularization or massive disruption of the pancreas, duodenum, or pancreaticoduodenal complex with involvement of the ampulla/proximal pancreatic duct and/or distal CBD (especially when there is an associated massive hemorrhage from the head of the pancreas/pancreaticoduodenal complex)
Temporary abdominal closure/open abdominal management
Coagulopathy (especially when combined with hypothermia and acidosis) in the OR
Administration of a large volume of crystalloids or PRBCs preoperatively or across the pre- and intraoperative settings
Inability to close the abdominal fascia without tension
Signs of abdominal compartment syndrome develop during attempted abdominal wall closure

(continued)

Table 2.3 (continued)

Indication(s) for
Need for a planned relaparotomy to remove intra-abdominal packs or reassess the extent of bowel viability
Extraperitoneal pelvic packing
Significant hemodynamic instability in the ED in patients with a pelvic fracture where IR is not immediately available
Severe pelvic trauma with massive, ongoing hemorrhage in the OR
Evidence on ongoing massive hemorrhage in patients with a pelvic fracture despite pelvic angioembolization
Vascular DC interventions
Balloon catheter tamponade
Significant, ongoing bleeding from a neck or supraclavicular fossa wound in the ED
Significant, ongoing bleeding from a difficult to access anatomical location or vessel in the OR[d]
Significant, ongoing bleeding from a deep or transfixing hepatic parenchymal wound in the OR
Temporary intravascular shunting
An extremity vascular injury requiring operation and a life-threatening injury in another anatomical location that requires surgery
An extremity or abdominal vascular injury requiring operation and an anticipated prolonged operative time with a suboptimal response to resuscitation
An extremity or abdominal vascular injury requiring operation and hypothermia, acidosis, and coagulopathy in the OR
Presentation of a patient with an extremity or abdominal vascular injury requiring operation during a mass casualty incident or to a hospital with little experience with surgical management of vascular trauma

Where CBD indicates common bile duct; DC, damage control; ED, emergency department; IR, interventional radiology; OR, operating room; and PRBCs, packed red blood cells

Table and table legend reproduced with permission from reference [15]. Copyright Wolters Kluwer Health (2015)

[a]Where hypothermia, acidosis, and coagulopathy have most commonly been defined in the peer-reviewed literature as a temperature <34, pH <7.2, and a PT or PTT >1.5 times normal and the absence of visible blood clots during operation/diffuse oozing from all injured tissues [57]

[b]Suggested signs of thoracic compartment syndrome in this setting have been reported to include sudden cardiopulmonary failure, hemodynamic instability, or increased airway pressures (with resultant difficulty with ventilation)

[c]Where a large volume of PRBCs was most often defined in the literature as >10 or >12.5 units

[d]Difficult to access anatomical locations have been reported to include the head, zone III of the neck, the angle of the mandible, and the trunk while difficult to access vessels have been reported to include the carotid artery behind the pharynx; the carotid artery or internal jugular vein at the base of the skull; the internal maxillary artery; the second, third, and fourth portions of the vertebral artery; or the distal branches of the internal iliac artery in the pelvis

[15, 54, 57]. Thus, surgeons may believe that in certain intraoperative circumstances, one or more specific DC interventions should be preferentially performed when patients are selected to undergo DC surgery [54]. These include extraperitoneal pelvic packing (severe pelvic trauma and an expanding and difficult to access pelvic hematoma or massive, ongoing hemorrhage in the OR), therapeutic perihepatic packing (a juxtahepatic venous injury), and staged pancreaticoduodenectomy (devascularization of massive disruption of the pancreas, duodenum, or pancreaticoduodenal complex) [15, 54, 57, 70]. Finally, the expert panel suggested that DC surgery and TAC/open abdominal management were appropriate when patients have been administered a large volume of crystalloid fluids and/or PRBCs, when the abdominal wall is unable to be closed without tension at the conclusion of laparotomy, or when signs of post-injury ACS develop during attempted abdominal wall closure [15, 54, 57].

The above indications may be used as a type of consensus opinion to guide surgical practice in the current era of DC resuscitation [70]. They may also be used to educate surgical trainees and surgeons on the appropriate use of DC surgery and DC interventions in practice, to guide trauma center quality improvement practices regarding choice of operative profile (through morbidity and mortality rounds, audit and feedback, and other mechanisms), and to design future (adjusted/propensity-matched) prospective observational and experimental studies focused on examining outcomes between patients treated with DC (or a specific DC intervention) versus definitive surgery (or a specific definitive surgical intervention) [54].

2.6 Summary

Modern trauma DC integrates the stages of DC surgery into the process of DC resuscitation. Although widely believed to improve survival when appropriately indicated, there is limited evidence supporting a benefit of DC surgery in injured patients [1, 16]. Further, the procedure is associated with a number of potentially severe and often resource-intensive complications [1, 57, 58]. Several studies have recently reported data suggesting that a variation exists in the use of DC laparotomy across trauma centers or that the procedure may be overused [57, 70]. These and other studies have also suggested that overutilization of the procedure may be associated with increased morbidity and mortality [57, 58, 70, 73–75]. The list of indications identified as being appropriate by both experts and practicing surgeons described in this chapter may be used to guide practice and reduce variation in the use of DC surgery until results of appropriately designed prospective studies become available in the future [54].

Disclosure I have no conflicts of interest to declare.

References

1. Roberts DJ, Ball CG, Feliciano DV, Moore EE, Ivatury RR, Lucas CE, et al. History of the innovation of damage control for management of trauma patients: 1902-2016. Ann Surg. 2017;265(5):1034–44.
2. Elerding SC, Aragon GE, Moore EE. Fatal hepatic hemorrhage after trauma. Am J Surg. 1979;138(6):883–8.
3. Kashuk JL, Moore EE, Millikan JS, Moore JB. Major abdominal vascular trauma--a unified approach. J Trauma. 1982;22(8):672–9.
4. Malbrain ML, Vidts W, Ravyts M, De Laet I, De Waele J. Acute intestinal distress syndrome: the importance of intra-abdominal pressure. Minerva Anestesiol. 2008;74(11):657–73.
5. Malbrain ML, De Laet I. It's all in the gut: introducing the concept of acute bowel injury and acute intestinal distress syndrome. Crit Care Med. 2009;37(1):365–6.
6. Burch JM, Moore EE, Moore FA, Franciose R. The abdominal compartment syndrome. Surg Clin N Am. 1996;76(4):833–42.
7. Meldrum DR, Moore FA, Moore EE, Franciose RJ, Sauaia A, Burch JM. Prospective characterization and selective management of the abdominal compartment syndrome. Am J Surg. 1997;174(6):667–72. discussion 72-3
8. Kirkpatrick AW, Roberts DJ, De Waele J, Jaeschke R, Malbrain ML, De Keulenaer B, et al. Intra-abdominal hypertension and the abdominal compartment syndrome: updated consensus definitions and clinical practice guidelines from the world Society of the Abdominal Compartment Syndrome. Intensive Care Med. 2013;39(7):1190–206.
9. Stone HH, Strom PR, Mullins RJ. Management of the major coagulopathy with onset during laparotomy. Ann Surg. 1983;197(5):532–5.
10. Rotondo MF, Schwab CW, McGonigal MD, Phillips GR 3rd, Fruchterman TM, Kauder DR, et al. 'Damage control': an approach for improved survival in exsanguinating penetrating abdominal injury. J Trauma. 1993;35(3):375–82. discussion 82-3
11. Ivatury RR, Porter JM, Simon RJ, Islam S, John R, Stahl WM. Intra-abdominal hypertension after life-threatening penetrating abdominal trauma: prophylaxis, incidence, and clinical relevance to gastric mucosal pH and abdominal compartment syndrome. J Trauma. 1998;44(6):1016–21. discussion 21-3
12. Feliciano DV, Burch JM, Spjut-Patrinely V, Mattox KL, Jordan GL Jr. Abdominal gunshot wounds. An urban trauma center's experience with 300 consecutive patients. Ann Surg. 1988;208(3):362–70.
13. Rotondo MF, Zonies DH. The damage control sequence and underlying logic. Surg Clin N Am. 1997;77(4):761–77.
14. Ball CG. Damage control surgery. Curr Opin Crit Care. 2015;21(6):538–43.
15. Roberts DJ, Bobrovitz N, Zygun DA, Ball CG, Kirkpatrick AW, Faris PD, et al. Indications for use of thoracic, abdominal, pelvic, and vascular damage control interventions in trauma patients: a content analysis and expert appropriateness rating study. J Trauma Acute Care Surg. 2015;79(4):568–79.
16. Roberts DJ, Zygun DA, Kirkpatrick AW, Ball CG, Faris PD, Bobrovitz N, et al. A protocol for a scoping and qualitative study to identify and evaluate indications for damage control surgery and damage control interventions in civilian trauma patients. BMJ Open. 2014;4(7):e005634.

17. Johnson JW, Gracias VH, Schwab CW, Reilly PM, Kauder DR, Shapiro MB, et al. Evolution in damage control for exsanguinating penetrating abdominal injury. J Trauma. 2001;51(2):261–9. discussion 9-71
18. Ramirez OM, Ruas E, Dellon AL. "Components separation" method for closure of abdominal-wall defects: an anatomic and clinical study. Plast Reconstr Surg. 1990;86(3):519–26.
19. Petrone P, Asensio JA. Surgical management of penetrating pulmonary injuries. Scand J Trauma Resusc Emerg Med. 2009;17:8.
20. Trauma. 7th ed. China: McGraw Hill Companies Inc.; 2013.
21. Asensio JA, Mazzini FN, Perez-Alonso AJ, Petrone P, Ceballos J, Karsidag T, et al. Pulmonary injuries. In: Cioffi WG, Asensio JA, Adams CA, Biffl WL, Connolly MD, Jurkovich GJ, editors. Atlas of trauma/emergency surgical techniques. Philadelphia, PA: Elsevier Saunders; 2014. p. 93–104.
22. Wall MJ Jr, Hirshberg A, Mattox KL. Pulmonary tractotomy with selective vascular ligation for penetrating injuries to the lung. Am J Surg. 1994;168(6):665–9.
23. Asensio JA, Demetriades D, Berne JD, Velmahos G, Cornwell EE 3rd, Murray J, et al. Stapled pulmonary tractotomy: a rapid way to control hemorrhage in penetrating pulmonary injuries. J Am Coll Surg. 1997;185(5):486–7.
24. Wagner JW, Obeid FN, Karmy-Jones RC, Casey GD, Sorensen VJ, Horst HM. Trauma pneumonectomy revisited: the role of simultaneously stapled pneumonectomy. J Trauma. 1996;40(4):590–4.
25. Chovanes J, Cannon JW, Nunez TC. The evolution of damage control surgery. Surg Clin N Am. 2012;92(4):859–75. vii-viii
26. Rotondo MF, Bard MR. Damage control surgery for thoracic injuries. Injury. 2004;35(7):649–54.
27. Caceres M, Buechter KJ, Tillou A, Shih JA, Liu D, Steeb G. Thoracic packing for uncontrolled bleeding in penetrating thoracic injuries. South Med J. 2004;97(7):637–41.
28. Moriwaki Y, Toyoda H, Harunari N, Iwashita M, Kosuge T, Arata S, et al. Gauze packing as damage control for uncontrollable haemorrhage in severe thoracic trauma. Ann R Coll Surg Engl. 2013;95(1):20–5.
29. Vargo DJ, Battistella FD. Abbreviated thoracotomy and temporary chest closure: an application of damage control after thoracic trauma. Arch Surg. 2001;136(1):21–4.
30. Rosenblatt MS, Aldridge SC, Millham FH, Woodson J, Hirsch EF. Temporary thoracotomy wound closure following penetrating thoracic aorta injury. Military Med. 1993;158(1):58–9.
31. Eastlick L, Fogler RJ, Shaftan GW. Pancreaticoduodenectomy for trauma: delayed reconstruction: a case report. J Trauma. 1990;30(4):503–5.
32. Carrillo C, Fogler RJ, Shaftan GW. Delayed gastrointestinal reconstruction following massive abdominal trauma. J Trauma. 1993;34(2):233–5.
33. Koniaris LG, Mandal AK, Genuit T, Cameron JL. Two-stage trauma pancreaticoduodenectomy: delay facilitates anastomotic reconstruction. J Gastrointest Surg. 2000;4(4):366–9.
34. Ivatury RR, Nassoura ZE, Simon RJ, Rodriguez A. Complex duodenal injuries. Surg Clin N Am. 1996;76(4):797–812.
35. Coburn M. Damage control for urological injuries. Surg Clin N Am. 1997;77(4):821–34.
36. Ertel W, Keel M, Eid K, Platz A, Trentz O. Control of severe hemorrhage using C-clamp and pelvic packing in multiply injured patients with pelvic ring disruption. J Orthop Trauma. 2001;15(7):468–74.
37. Smith WR, Moore EE, Osborn P, Agudelo JF, Morgan SJ, Parekh AA, et al. Retroperitoneal packing as a resuscitation technique for hemodynamically unstable patients with pelvic fractures: report of two representative cases and a description of technique. J Trauma. 2005;59(6):1510–4.
38. Cothren CC, Osborn PM, Moore EE, Morgan SJ, Johnson JL, Smith WR. Preperitonal pelvic packing for hemodynamically unstable pelvic fractures: a paradigm shift. J Trauma. 2007;62(4):834–9. discussion 9-42
39. DuBose J, Inaba K, Barmparas G, Teixeira PG, Schnuriger B, Talving P, et al. Bilateral internal iliac artery ligation as a damage control approach in massive retroperitoneal bleeding after pelvic fracture. J Trauma. 2010;69(6):1507–14.
40. Morimoto RY, Birolini D, Junqueira AR Jr, Poggetti R, Horita LT. Balloon tamponade for transfixing lesions of the liver. Surg Gynecol Obstet. 1987;164(1):87–8.
41. Poggetti RS, Moore EE, Moore FA, Mitchell MB, Read RA. Balloon tamponade for bilobar transfixing hepatic gunshot wounds. J Trauma. 1992;33(5):694–7.
42. Feliciano DV, Burch JM, Mattox KL, Bitondo CG, Fields G. Balloon catheter tamponade in cardiovascular wounds. Am J Surg. 1990;160(6):583–7.
43. Gilroy D, Lakhoo M, Charalambides D, Demetriades D. Control of life-threatening haemorrhage from the neck: a new indication for balloon tamponade. Injury. 1992;23(8):557–9.
44. Ball CG, Wyrzykowski AD, Nicholas JM, Rozycki GS, Feliciano DVA. Decade's experience with balloon catheter tamponade for the emergency control of hemorrhage. J Trauma. 2011;70(2):330–3.
45. Ding W, Wu X, Li J. Temporary intravascular shunts used as a damage control surgery adjunct in complex vascular injury: collective review. Injury. 2008;39(9):970–7.
46. Subramanian A, Vercruysse G, Dente C, Wyrzykowski A, King E, Feliciano DV. A decade's experience with temporary intravascular shunts at a civilian level I trauma center. J Trauma. 2008;65(2):316–24. discussion 24-6
47. Bogert JN, Harvin JA, Cotton BA. Damage control resuscitation. J Intensive Care Med. 2014.
48. Hess JR, Holcomb JB, Hoyt DB. Damage control resuscitation: the need for specific blood products to treat the coagulopathy of trauma. Transfusion. 2006;46(5):685–6.
49. Holcomb JB, Jenkins D, Rhee P, Johannigman J, Mahoney P, Mehta S, et al. Damage control resuscitation: directly addressing the early coagulopathy of trauma. J Trauma. 2007;62(2):307–10.
50. Holcomb JB, Tilley BC, Baraniuk S, Fox EE, Wade CE, Podbielski JM, et al. Transfusion of plasma,

platelets, and red blood cells in a 1:1:1 vs a 1:1:2 ratio and mortality in patients with severe trauma: the PROPPR randomized clinical trial. JAMA. 2015;313(5):471–82.
51. Cirocchi R, Montedori A, Farinella E, Bonacini I, Tagliabue L, Abraha I. Damage control surgery for abdominal trauma. Cochrane Database Syst Rev. 2013;28(3):CD007438.
52. Sox HC, Goodman SN. The methods of comparative effectiveness research. Annu Rev Public Health. 2012;33:425–45.
53. Chinnery GE, Krige JE, Kotze UK, Navsaria P, Nicol A. Surgical management and outcome of civilian gunshot injuries to the pancreas. Br J Surg. 2012;99(Suppl 1):140–8.
54. Roberts DJ. Identification and evaluation of the indications for use of damage control surgery and damage control interventions in civilian trauma patients: Doctor of Philosophy (Specialization in Epidemiology) Thesis. Department of Community Health Sciences, University of Calgary; 2015. P. 402.
55. Rice TW, Morris S, Tortella BJ, Wheeler AP, Christensen MC. Deviations from evidence-based clinical management guidelines increase mortality in critically injured trauma patients*. Crit Care Med. 2012;40(3):778–86.
56. Asensio JA, McDuffie L, Petrone P, Roldan G, Forno W, Gambaro E, et al. Reliable variables in the exsanguinated patient which indicate damage control and predict outcome. Am J Surg. 2001;182(6):743–51.
57. Roberts DJ, Bobrovitz N, Zygun DA, Ball CG, Kirkpatrick AW, Faris PD, et al. Indications for use of damage control surgery in civilian trauma patients: a content analysis and expert appropriateness rating study. Ann Surg. 2016;263(5):1018–27.
58. Harvin JA, Wray CJ, Steward J, Lawless RA, MvcNutt MK, Love JD, et al. Control the damage: morbidity and mortality after emergent trauma laparotomy. Am J Surg. 2016;212(1):34–9.
59. Miller RS, Morris JA Jr, Diaz JJ Jr, Herring MB, May AK. Complications after 344 damage-control open celiotomies. J Trauma. 2005;59(6):1365–71. discussion 71-4
60. Montalvo JA, Acosta JA, Rodriguez P, Alejandro K, Sarraga A. Surgical complications and causes of death in trauma patients that require temporary abdominal closure. Am Surg. 2005;71(3):219–24.
61. Dubose JJ, Scalea TM, Holcomb JB, Shrestha B, Okoye O, Inaba K, et al. Open abdominal management after damage-control laparotomy for trauma: a prospective observational American Association for the Surgery of Trauma multicenter study. J Trauma Acute Care Surg. 2013;74(1):113–20. discussion 1120-2
62. Di Saverio S, Tarasconi A, Inaba K, Navsaria P, Coccolini F, Navarro DC, et al. Open abdomen with concomitant enteroatmospheric fistula: attempt to rationalize the approach to a surgical nightmare and proposal of a clinical algorithm. J Am Coll Surg. 2015;220(3):e23–33.
63. Bjorck M, Kirkpatrick AW, Cheatham M, Kaplan M, Leppaniemi A, De Waele JJ. Amended classification of the open abdomen. Scand J Surg. 2016;105(1):5–10.
64. Demetriades D, Salim A. Management of the open abdomen. Surg Clin N Am. 2014;94(1):131–53.
65. Fabian TC, Croce MA, Pritchard FE, Minard G, Hickerson WL, Howell RL, et al. Planned ventral hernia. Staged management for acute abdominal wall defects. Ann Surg. 1994;219(6):643–50. discussion 51-3
66. Zarzaur BL, DiCocco JM, Shahan CP, Emmett K, Magnotti LJ, Croce MA, et al. Quality of life after abdominal wall reconstruction following open abdomen. J Trauma. 2011;70(2):285–91.
67. Codner PA, Brasel KJ, Deroon-Cassini TA. Staged abdominal repairs reduce long-term quality of life. Injury. 2012;43(9):1513–6.
68. Cheatham ML, Safcsak K, Llerena LE, Morrow CE Jr, Block EF. Long-term physical, mental, and functional consequences of abdominal decompression. J Trauma. 2004;56(2):237–41. discussion 41-2
69. Cheatham ML, Safcsak K. Longterm impact of abdominal decompression: a prospective comparative analysis. J Am Coll Surg. 2008;207(4):573–9.
70. Roberts DJ, Zygun DA, Faris PD, Ball CG, Kirkpatrick AW, Stelfox HT. Opinions of practicing surgeons on the appropriateness of published indications for use of damage control surgery in trauma patients: an international cross-sectional survey. J Am Coll Surg. 2016;223(3):515–29.
71. Higa G, Friese R, O'Keeffe T, Wynne J, Bowlby P, Ziemba M, et al. Damage control laparotomy: a vital tool once overused. J Trauma. 2010;69(1):53–9.
72. Cotton BA, Reddy N, Hatch QM, LeFebvre E, Wade CE, Kozar RA, et al. Damage control resuscitation is associated with a reduction in resuscitation volumes and improvement in survival in 390 damage control laparotomy patients. Ann Surg. 2011;254(4):598–605.
73. Hatch QM, Osterhout LM, Podbielski J, Kozar RA, Wade CE, Holcomb JB, et al. Impact of closure at the first take back: complication burden and potential overutilization of damage control laparotomy. J Trauma. 2011;71(6):1503–11.
74. Hatch QM, Osterhout LM, Ashraf A, Podbielski J, Kozar RA, Wade CE, et al. Current use of damage-control laparotomy, closure rates, and predictors of early fascial closure at the first take-back. J Trauma. 2011;70(6):1429–36.
75. Martin MJ, Hatch Q, Cotton B, Holcomb J. The use of temporary abdominal closure in low-risk trauma patients: helpful or harmful? J Trauma Acute Care Surg. 2012;72(3):601–6. discussion 6-8
76. Birkmeyer JD, Reames BN, McCulloch P, Carr AJ, Campbell WB, Wennberg JE. Understanding of regional variation in the use of surgery. Lancet. 2013;382(9898):1121–9.
77. Roberts DJ, Bobrovitz N, Zygun DA, Ball CG, Kirkpatrick AW, Faris PD, et al. Indications for use of damage control surgery and damage control interventions in civilian trauma patients: a scoping review. J Trauma Acute Care Surg. 2015;78(6):1187–96.
78. Wade CE, del Junco DJ, Holcomb JB, Holcomb JB, Wade CE, Brasel KJ, et al. Variations between level

I trauma centers in 24-hour mortality in severely injured patients requiring a massive transfusion. J Trauma. 2011;71(2 Suppl 3):S389–93.

79. Rahbar E, Fox EE, del Junco DJ, Harvin JA, Holcomb JB, Wade CE, et al. Early resuscitation intensity as a surrogate for bleeding severity and early mortality in the PROMMTT study. J Trauma Acute Care Surg. 2013;75(1 Suppl 1):S16–23.
80. Asensio JA, Petrone P, O'Shanahan G, Kuncir EJ. Managing exsanguination: what we know about damage control/bailout is not enough. Proc (Bayl Univ Med Cent). 2003;16(3):294–6.
81. Buckman RF Jr, Miraliakbari R, Badellino MM. Juxtahepatic venous injuries: a critical review of reported management strategies. J Trauma. 2000;48(5):978–84.
82. Asensio JA, Petrone P, Roldan G, Kuncir E, Demetriades D. Pancreaticoduodenectomy: a rare procedure for the management of complex pancreaticoduodenal injuries. J Am Coll Surg. 2003;197(6):937–42.

Damage Control Surgery: Military

3

Carlos Rodriguez and Peter Rhee

Abstract

The term "damage control" is rooted in Navy history as the way to approach shipboard battle damage. Essentially, it applied to quick measures aimed at stopping flood waters from rushing in and sinking a ship. In surgery, the term has come to mean application of expedient approaches to stemming exsanguinating hemorrhage and controlling contamination, in the physiologically deranged patient, to the point where resuscitation can occur. Trauma surgery typically has four stages. First is hemorrhage control, second is contamination control, third is evaluation or diagnosis, and fourth is reconstruction. Damage control surgery mandates the first two stages but defers the third and fourth stages till a more appropriate time and place. In civilian damage control, it was originally developed as a temporizing measure that provides time for restoration of normal physiology and, later, normal anatomy. In this chapter, we look to apply damage control surgery methods to the combat trauma environment. In this setting, the logistics are often completely different than in civilian trauma centers and are often done not for physiology restoration but due to the logistics and resources of the combat environment.

C. Rodriguez, M.D., D.O., M.B.A., F.A.C.S.
Medical Corps, US Navy, Washington, DC, USA

Uniformed Services University of the Health Sciences, Walter Reed National Military Medical Center, Bethesda, MD, USA

P. Rhee, M.D., M.P.H., F.A.C.S., F.C.C.M. (✉)
Grady Memorial Hospital, Atlanta, GA, USA

USUHS, Emory, Morehouse, Atlanta, GA, USA
e-mail: prhee@gmh.edu

In the recent wars in Iraq and Afghanistan, most of combat injuries occurred from improvised explosive devices (IED). Closer examination of the combat-related deaths shows that approximately half are due to bullets and half were due to explosions [1]. The injuries from bullets were very different than civilian penetrating trauma as the clear majority are from high-velocity weapons rather than low-velocity weapons such as handguns which are typical in civilian trauma. The injuries from explosions are also unique to combat. It presents with a combination of blast injury with penetrating injuries from the secondary blast trauma with fragmentation penetrating the body. Primary blast injury is typically defined as the injury due to the blast over pressure, secondary blast injury is injury from fragmentation injury, and tertiary blast injury is from the body being thrown into objects [2]. Quaternary are the other injuries from vectors such as chemical,

J. Duchesne et al. (eds.), *Damage Control in Trauma Care*,
https://doi.org/10.1007/978-3-319-72607-6_3

biological, radiologic, radiation, toxic inhalation, asphyxiation (carbon monoxide, cyanide) dust, or exacerbation of chronic illness. With an injury mechanism being the combination of blunt and penetrating forces imparted to the victim, IEDs create the pan-ultimate poly-trauma injuries. However, injury patterns are fairly predictable and are dependent upon size of blast, distance from detonation point, composition of explosive (e.g., metal casing, ball bearings packed around explosive, etc.), and presence of properly worn body armor [3, 4].

In blast events, extremities are the most common site of injury, and uncontrolled hemorrhage is the most common cause of potentially survivable death [1, 5]. This has been the experience with the US casualties as they are required to wear body armor. However opposing forces or incidental casualties often do not wear body armor. With uncontrolled hemorrhage being lethal, its control has replaced airway as being the first step in approaching the combat trauma patients [6]. In civilian trauma, the access to the trauma center is quick. There are urgent airway issues. However, in the combat setting, the priorities are different. Self, buddy, or first aid is quick but is often care under fire. In this setting, airway is very difficult to manage and is often unsalvageable due to circumstances and resources. For example, it takes more than one other personnel to adequately manage the airway if a casualty requires it, and when under fire, the priority is to sustain and remain engaged if possible [7]. Tactical combat casualty care is when imminent danger from being under fire has ceased. During this stage, airway control by buddy or medic aid is difficult and often futile. Thus, the attention has really focused on hemorrhage control as data continues to confirm that the primary possibly preventable cause of death remains uncontrolled hemorrhage [1, 7]. Understanding damage control principles aimed at stemming exsanguinating hemorrhage is a vital tool for any deploying surgeon.

The extent of damage control provided by medical providers is limited by available resources. In far forward combat trauma settings, all that may be available for damage control is what the unit's medic is carrying or what is contained in the Wounded Warrior's Individual First Aid Kit (IFAK).

As the Wounded Warrior progresses through echelons of care from point of injury back to the States, medical resources become more robust and more sophisticated—where definitive surgical intervention may be undertaken. Here, we discuss surgical care of the combat casualty from point of injury through the various roles or levels of care in the combat setting. In contrast to civilian trauma, the numbering system is different. For example, a level I trauma center refers to the care received at the highest level. In the US military system, Role 1 or level 1 refers typically to care at the level of the battalion aid station. Thus, it is not forward care meaning in the firefight or in the field. Aid stations typically are in garrison areas and are somewhat remote to the firefight. There the highest level or resource is typically a physician assistant or a general medical officer who has completed 1 year of postgraduate training. It can be experienced professional physicians such as family practice or medicine but rarely do they have a surgeon [8, 9]. In the Role 2 or level 2 situation, it typically refers to a site with very remote capabilities and a skeleton surgical crew. It has anesthesia capabilities and one or two general surgeons and typically no specialist surgeons. On occasion, it may have one orthopedic surgeon available. These facilities are known as forward resuscitative surgery (FRS) units by the Army or the forward resuscitative surgery suite (FRSS) by the Navy. The operating room is not state of the art but rather in a tent or makeshift area. Sterility is not possible in these areas and being clean is the most one can ask for [10]. Role 3 or level 3 in the military refers to a hospital with numerous surgeons and subspecialty surgical capabilities. These facilities are known as Combat Support Hospital (CSH) in the Army and Field Hospitals by the Navy [11, 12]. There are typically in large military bases. Role 4 or level 4 is a fixed hospital such as the hospital in Landstuhl Germany. Patients were typically transported from the point of injury to either a Role 1 or 2 and then to Role 3 and then to Role 4 during the war in Iraq and Afghanistan. From the Role 4 facility, the casualty is transferred to a Role 5 facility which is in the Continental United States (CONUS) which has rehabilitation capability.

As Wounded Warriors pass through the echelons of care, it is important to understand that during movement from hospital to hospital, patients will not always have access to surgical care. Evacuation times from Role 2 to Role 3 will vary depending on combat theater. In some cases, these times exceed an hour. It is imperative to ensure patients are hemostatic prior evacuation.

3.1 Role 1/Buddy Care: C, A, B, C

Essentially, Role 1 care is self-care, buddy care, or care rendered at the Battalion Aid Station. There are no surgeons at Role 1 facilities. Goals are simple and akin to ATLS—stop catastrophic hemorrhage as quickly as possible, stabilize airway and breathing, and begin resuscitation as necessary. There is no holding capacity or operative capability associated with echelon 1 care. In fact, the overarching principle is to transport combat trauma patients to hospital-level care (Role 2 or 3) within the "golden hour" of injury [13].

In any bleeding scenario, the goal is to quickly and expediently control hemorrhage. The first step to hemorrhage control is direct pressure. Self- and buddy care are conducted in the field with supplies found in the Individual First Aid Kit (IFAK). Over the years, IFAK contents have changed to include field dressings (cotton cravat bandages), hemostatic dressings, and tourniquets. In situations where bleeding is minor, many times direct pressure is all that is needed. Wrapping of extremities with compression dressings are ideal. Ace wrap are typically available and will stop both soft tissue and some vascular bleeding. As wound complexity and size increase, other solutions exist. There are special dressings impregnated with hemostatic agents such as kaolin, in "combat gauze" which are in most IFAK. These dressings are considered temporary and are used to augment pressure dressings [14].

One of the most significant policy shifts during the wars in Iraq and Afghanistan has been the widespread adoption of controlling catastrophic hemorrhage by placing combat tourniquets in the field—at the time of injury. Adoption of this practice began in late 2002. In early 2008, Beekley et al. published their findings that tourniquets (perhaps, more specifically, catastrophic hemorrhage control) were simply saving lives [15]. Eastridge further cemented the practice in 2012 when he showed [2] that death rate from uncontrolled extremity hemorrhage dropped from 23.3 deaths per year to 3.5 deaths per year before and after widespread tourniquet dissemination, respectively.

The Tactical Combat Casualty Care Committee (TCCC committee) was started in 2001. The major principle of care that they formed was that there were various levels of care and capability during combat. The care under fire is different than tactical care which is when the firefight is over. Then the care during transport called casualty care was also different as the environment and resources are different. During care under fire, it is taught that it is preferable to control bleeding with a tourniquet than direct pressure. Applying direct pressure requires either a second pair or hands or means that the soldier has to stop fighting to administer pressure. Thus, to keep as many combatants in the firefight as possible, tourniquets are the first line of therapy. During tactical care, tourniquets are to be released to see if direct pressure will control bleeding. In scenarios when direct pressure does not control bleeding or is not tactically possible, then tourniquets are reapplied [16]. Many tourniquets have been developed and tested, but the favored device is called Combat Application Tourniquets (CAT). Should a single CAT not be sufficient to stop bleeding, a second tourniquet may be applied more proximal than the first [16]. The tourniquets fell out of favor after the Vietnam War due to real and potential problems from the tourniquets, but during the war in Iraq and Afghanistan, the benefit far outweighed the complications [15]. Training is the key to the use of tourniquets. In the civilian sector, the current trend is overuse and misuse, but during bombing scenarios or mass shooting, the use is currently advocated.

While makeshift tourniquets may be used out of necessity, they typically are ineffective in cessation of catastrophic hemorrhage [17]. Should a makeshift tourniquet be necessary, it should be constructed with a strap and windlass [18]. Improperly applied (or constructed) tourniquets may just impede venous return (aka venous tourniquets) and will increase bleeding [19]. Typically the effective tourniquet is extremely painful and over prolonged periods it is unbearable. Data from the Boston Marathon bombing in 2013 showed that of the 46 tourniquets placed, only 1 was effective in stopping arterial bleeding. Again availability of effective tourniquets as well as proper training is required. Again the application of an effective tourniquet on an already injured extremity that will stop arterial bleeding is extremely painful.

CAT tourniquets control extremity hemorrhage well. However, they are difficult, if not impossible, to apply in cases of junctional hemorrhage. In fact, junctional hemorrhage may occur in locations too proximal for even direct pressure. It is reported that 4.6% of all deaths in the recent wars in Iraq and Afghanistan were from junctional hemorrhage and that 20% of all combat casualties with "potentially survivable" injuries died because of junctional hemorrhage [1].

Specialty tourniquets have been developed to combat this problem. Currently, there are four [3] commercially available junctional tourniquets—the Combat Ready Clamp (CRoC), the Junctional Emergency Treatment Tool (JETT), the SAM Junctional Tourniquet (SJT), and the Abdominal Aortic Tourniquet (AAT). Many of these tourniquets have been fielded and used successfully in the care of combat trauma patients [20, 21].

The JETT and SAM tourniquets also provide compression of the pelvis if necessary in cases where pelvic instability is a concern. These tourniquets can also be used where upper extremity junctional hemorrhage is occurring.

Once hemorrhage is controlled, resuscitation begins [16]. If patient is mentating and has a radial pulse, no fluids are indicated [16]. This is because the availability of blood in the field is not available. Although IV access should always be obtained as soon as possible fluids other than blood products will cause harm through increased bleeding and toxicity and thus is not needed. If unattainable, resuscitation is begun through placement of intraosseous catheters with the tibia, humeral head, sternum, and iliac crest as suitable sites [16]. IV access is always preferred, but due to lack of experience and capability, the use of interosseous devices is rapidly increasing. Per the Tactical Combat Casualty Care guidelines, low-volume, low-pressure resuscitation is preferred with fresh whole blood being the fluid of choice. Obviously fresh whole blood is always available depending on how far forward you are. During the Iraq War, fresh whole blood was routinely available in the Role 2 facilities. If component therapy is used, a ratio of 1:1 plasma to red blood cells is preferred; otherwise, Hextend should be used. Hextend however has a maximal dose of 1 L as hemodilution with this fluid will undoubtedly create coagulopathy although it will increase blood pressure [16]. Goals of resuscitation depend on physiologic condition of patient—if no traumatic brain injury (TBI), resuscitate to palpable radial pulse or SBP of 80–90 mmHg. If TBI is suspected, resuscitate to SBP of at least 90 mmHg. The adoption of this new parameter is called permissive hypotension [22]. This decreases the toxicities of non-blood product fluids, and it has been shown that survival is not worsened by the lower blood pressure and in many studies been shown to improve survival. The damage control resuscitation has many points. The first is the adoption of permissive hypotension, and the second is the minimalization of artificial crystalloids and colloids, the onetime use of hypertonic saline as it increases perfusion with less deleterious effects of crystalloids, the use of blood products aggressively and early in the resuscitation phase, and the use of drugs such as tranexamic acid (TXA), prothrombin concentrates (PCC), or even factor VIIa. Ideally the use of fresh whole blood is the best resuscitation methodology found in theater [23–28].

In addition to low-volume, low-pressure resuscitation, pain control and prevention of hypothermia should be considered when transferring from a casualty no matter what level. The transport from one role facility to another is almost always via air, and most air transport is not heated in the cargo area if it is a rotary wing aircraft. Prevention of hypothermia is critical [29, 30]. In addition to pain resulting from trauma, awake patients, with properly applied tourniquets, may develop significant amounts of pain secondary to compression and ischemia within 15 min of tourniquet application. In patients NOT in hemorrhagic shock or NOT at risk to develop hemorrhagic shock, 800 μg transbuccal fentanyl lozenges are used. For those patients in hemorrhagic shock or at risk of developing hemorrhagic shock, ketamine 50 mg intramuscular/intranasally or 20 mg slow intravenous/interosseous infusion is recommended. One caution is that the use of ketamine while preserving or minimizing circulatory compromise or having minimal effect on respiratory drive will cause disassociation and hallucination in the casualty and this can sometimes be problematic during transport [16, 31].

For those patients presenting in hemorrhagic shock, one or more major extremity amputations (i.e., proximal to ankle or wrist), or other evidence of severe bleeding, 1 g of IV TXA should be administered within 3 h of injury [24, 27].

For patients with thoracic trauma causing hemodynamic lability, decompression, via large bore IV catheters in the midclavicular line at the level of the second rib, is classically described as being a lifesaving intervention [16]. Again the stressing point is that if there is evidence of thoracic trauma and tension pneumothorax is suspected AND is causing hypotension, then and only then should the thoracic decompression occur. It is not indicated for decreased breath sounds or low pulse oximeter readings if the patient does not have hypotension. The use of large needle decompression can relieve pressure if the patient has a tension pneumothorax but will create injury to the lung and create pneumothorax which can be life-threatening if it is placed in a patient that does not have physiologic tension pneumothorax. The recent studies have shown these catheters can easily bend to the point where the lumen is no longer patent—rendering them ineffective—or do not enter the chest in the majority of the time [32, 33]. Again, training is the key [16].

So-called sucking chest wounds or open chest wall injuries where air preferentially enters into the pleural space through the injury vice into the lungs via the trachea are treated with three-sided, nonocclusive dressings that do not allow air to enter the pleural space via the chest wall defect but do allow air to escape when over pressurization in the pleural space occurs. Sucking chest wounds are very rare in civilian trauma, but due to the high-velocity weapons used in combat, they are much more common than in civilian trauma. The incidence of sucking chest wounds from explosives is also rare [16, 34].

In either case, if tube thoracostomy is available, it should be placed and connected to suction prior to transportation. Once placed, all chest wall dressings should be made totally occlusive.

Patients are evacuated expeditiously to Role 2 or 3 facilities with the goal of reaching surgical care within the "golden hour" of being injured [35]. While early rapid transport is always desired, it is important to realize that the physiology of exsanguination or death due to airway or breathing is almost always in the first 15 min which is termed the platinum 15 min.

3.2 Role 2 or 3: Surgical Stabilization

In combat trauma, the goal is to arrive to surgical care as soon as feasible. Time costs lives. Definitive surgical care saves lives [13]. Once patients arrive at surgical hospitals, the patients are triaged. Battlefield tourniquets are rechecked and are replaced with more efficacious pneumatic tourniquets when necessary. In penetrating trauma at the Role 2 level, the priorities are different. It is often backward: E, D, C, B, A. Exposure of the patient to determine possible injuries, the Disability is done in 3 s with a quick look-see. If they are moving arms and legs, that is critical information. If the patient has a Breathing problem and has made it to the Role 2 alive, it can usually wait a few minutes more. The same applies for the Airway. If they have made it to a Role 2 facility with an airway issue, the chances of that patient dying from an airway issue right in front of you are minimal. Ignoring obvious bleeding while halting exposure and control of the bleeding while assessing the airway and breathing is a civilian mistake done in the battlefield. Identification of bleeding sources and its control are paramount. If patients are not actively bleeding, primary survey adjuncts may be performed expeditiously by the combat trauma team [36]. IV access is ensured and is also critical. There is nothing that can replace a medic or nurse that can obtain large bore IV access in a hypotensive patient. This cannot be stressed enough. Central venous access is very often required as extremities may not be an option in blast injuries. Training and experience in obtaining central venous access in urgent scenarios in hypotensive patient is a prerequisite before deployment and will otherwise cost lives. Operative plans are developed. Combat trauma patients injured by blasts are truly poly-trauma patients and frequently have injuries in multiple regions of the body. Whenever possible, operative teams should work in parallel to minimize time under general anesthesia (e.g., debridement of lower extremities simultaneously with abdominal exploration). Of note in Afghanistan, surgeons in the field routinely performed an exploratory celiotomy to obtain vascular control at the iliac level as they found this to be the fastest approach while they were trying to get hemorrhage control of causalities that had high above-knee blast injuries [37]. In contrast to the Vietnam War and the war in Afghanistan with the Soviet Union, the blast injuries in the recent wars have been very different. The blast injuries with the former wars were that it was due to antipersonnel land mines which would create below-knee amputations and rarely caused exsanguination from the mines that injured the foot and lower leg. The blast injuries in dismounted patrols during the recent wars are different as they used improvised explosive devices which were buried and were of enormous more energy causing triple amputations and death from exsanguination. The legs were often already amputated above the knee, and the lower arm that was holding the firearm was also injured and amputated. The blast injuries of this most recent war were vastly different than previous wars. In addition the use of body armor protected vital organs so they survived the blast injuries but suffered triple amputations. These triple amputations were more common in the later phases in Afghanistan compared to the early experience in Iraq. This happened as the US military fortified their vehicles and thus the enemy would then in turn build more powerful explosive devices [38, 39].

The differences between a Role 2 and Role 3 are large. It has different location and resources. Role 2s are typically mobile and austere. By design, they are made of tents and move from point to point in support of the main battle lines. Occasionally, they are set up in buildings of opportunity or may have developed a more permanent footprint secondary to longevity in same location (as was seen with many Role 2s in Afghanistan). Nevertheless, resources are such that they can operate for 24 h without resupply. Usually, surgical assets at Role 2s are filled by general and orthopedic surgeons. They do not have CT scans, interventional radiology, or surgical specialists. At the most, they have ultrasound and portable digital x-ray. They have limited blood supply. The operating theaters are not really sterile. Airflow is often uncontrolled and fine dirt and dust is ubiquitous. They do have the ability to obtain fresh whole blood via the walking blood bank as the medical facility is typically in a base. If extremely far forward during an invasion, most all of the soldiers are forward, and thus walking blood bank is not feasible. Most all Role 2 facilities that had fresh walking blood bank had thousands of soldiers, and those who did not have a combat role were able to donate.

Role 3s, however, are hardened structures—brick and mortar. In addition to general and orthopedic surgeons, they may have neurosurgeons, vascular surgeons, radiologists (some with interventional capabilities), and blood banking officers. CT scans are present. Occasionally, there may be an MRI. Some Role 3s can collect their own apheresis platelets and provide extracorporeal membrane oxygenation and renal replacement therapy. By doctrine, hold time at Role 3s is 24–72 h.

Surgical damage control options are dependent upon facility type—Role 2 or 3.

3.3 Role 2

Once a combat trauma patient arrives to a Role 2 facility, patients are taken to the operating room to obtain surgical control of their bleeding, to clean/decontaminate wounds, and to repair/stabilize injuries. If the number of casualties is low, experience has shown that the casualty should be directly taken into the operating room as almost all combat casualties will need some sort of surgery. They all have wounds. Occasionally there are blunt motor vehicle injuries or falls but this is not the norm. For the patients with open bleeding wounds, the casualty can bypass the resuscitation area and be taken directly to the OR for assessment and treatment. If surgical treatment is not needed and resuscitation has begun, the casualty can be then transferred out of the operating room. It is not mandated that all casualties go to the resuscitation area first. In cases of multiple and numerous casualties, the obvious casualty that needs emergent surgical treatment is taken directly into the operating room, and all the rest can be triaged and resuscitated in the resuscitation area first. It depends highly on the scenario. In the Role 2 setting, adjuncts to the primary survey include X-ray, FAST exam, and diagnostic peritoneal lavage/aspiration. Wounds are rarely closed during the initial surgical evaluation. Hemorrhage control is a must.

3.4 Extremity Trauma

Goals: control surgical bleeding, debride nonviable tissue, preserve length

Patients who arrive with tourniquets in place should be taken directly to the operating room for wound exploration and definitive surgical control of bleeding. In the operating room, an assessment of the extremity should be made to determine its viability and if amputation should be performed. Prior to removing the combat tourniquet, either pneumatic or surgical control of vessels proximal to the injury must be obtained if possible. With injuries not involving junctional vessels, pneumatic tourniquets are preferred as they provide a completely hemostatic environment with which to work. If unable to place a pneumatic tourniquet, direct cutdown to the common femoral artery should occur.

For circumstances where lower extremity injuries extend up into the groin (i.e., junctional hemorrhage) or proximity is such that femoral artery cutdown is not possible, surgical control of the iliac vessels should be considered. To ensure adequate cessation of lower extremity inflow, either the external iliac artery or the combination of common iliac and internal iliac arteries needs to be controlled. Again, some of the European surgical facilities chose to routinely get proximal control in the external iliac level. The US casualties with body armor did not typically have intra-abdominal injuries, but civilian or combatant enemy soldiers did not have body armor and they did have torso injuries.

Proximal lower extremity injury is associated with large volume transfusion and is known to be directly associated with delayed wound healing and increased infectious complications [37, 40]. In 2014, Hathaway et al. described increased complications associated with exploratory laparotomy performed for the sole purpose of proximal control when compared to patients who underwent laparotomy for intra-abdominal injuries. Therefore, a graduated approach is recommended at controlling the iliac vessels [37, 41].

First line should be an extraperitoneal approach through a transplant or "hockey stick" incision. The incision is made lateral to the rectus, 2 cm cephalad, and parallel to the inguinal ligament. The incision is brought laterally toward the ASIS and then curved cephalad. To enter the pre-peritoneal space, dissection is carried out down through the external oblique aproneurosis, and the internal oblique, transversus muscle, and transversalis fascia are opened. Once this is accomplished, pre-peritoneal fat will be visible. The fat is separated bluntly from the peritoneum. The external iliac artery (EIA) should be visible at the bottom of the dissection with the external iliac vein being posterior and medial. Should the ureter be encountered first, dissection was carried out too cephalad. Follow the ureter's anterior border in a caudal fashion. The common iliac artery bifurcates at the point where the ureter crosses over the artery. Control of just the external iliac artery or the common iliac artery *and* the internal iliac artery (prevents pelvic collaterals from providing blood to the lower extremity) is needed to provide sufficient inflow control of blood to the lower extremity. Performing this for the first time in theater is not advisable, and at the minimum, a cadaver training should be done by the deploying surgeon, especially if they are not trauma trained and do this routinely [41, 42]. Advanced Surgical Exposures in Trauma (ASSET) is a course offered by the American College of Surgeons and teaches this exposure.

Deploying surgeons might not be familiar with the EIA retroperitoneal exposure. If that is the case, approaching the iliac vessels via laparotomy is recommended. Other less invasive approaches such as the use of resuscitative endovascular balloon occlusion of the aorta (REBOA) may be appropriate [43–45]. While REBOA indications currently do not include proximal control for lower extremity injury, the newer, smaller 7 Fr catheters placed via Seldinger technique may prove faster and less morbid than surgical control. This technique is very useful but still needs to be further tested and documented for its efficacy.

For upper extremity injuries, inflow that is not conducive to tourniquet is managed by surgical control of the axillary artery. In this situation, the axillary artery is best approached with a supine patient via transverse incision cephalad and lateral to the nipple approximately 2 cm below the clavicle. The incision is carried down to the pectoralis major where these muscle fibers are split exposing the pectoralis minor. The fibers of the pectoralis minor are cut thereby exposing the axillary artery for surgical control [42, 46]. Again this can be easy for those who do this routinely, but if never done before, it can be time-consuming.

Once proper control over arterial inflow is obtained, surgeons may proceed with obtaining surgical control of bleeding vessels within the extremity. If the injury is to the subclavian vessels, direct cutdown is an option, but the best and fastest way to get proximal control of the subclavian vessels is through the lateral chest. If the lung is retracted downward, then on the left side the subclavian vessel is clearly visible, and one needs to only open the parietal pleura over the vessel to get control. On the right side, it is not always so obvious as it has more fat around the vessel [46, 47]. Once proximal control has been obtained, shunting the artery is the first maneuver for best outcome. Once the shunt is placed, go distal to control hemorrhage of the now bleeding vessels.

Many of the extremity wounds seen in combat trauma are impregnated with dirt and other organic debris from the blast (picture). While extensive debridement is the gold standard when it comes to infection prevention, time in the OR at a Role 2 facility may be limited as resources are finite and open OR tables are necessary to allow the fighting to continue. If time and resources permit, debridement should be performed sharply with the goal to remove only clearly obvious necrotic tissue and organic debris. Irrigation should be gravity delivered as opposed to pulse lavage. Pulse lavage may be good for bones, but for soft tissue, it will imbed the dirt and debris into the soft tissue and adventitia. Some literatures suggest that pulse lavage actually forces organic debris deeper into tissue and can cause bacterial loads to rebound causing antibiotic-resistant bacterial infections [48].

Decisions need to be made regarding amputation. While there is only one lead surgeon, it is suggested that lead surgeon discuss amputation levels with colleagues. Preserving length leads to improved functional outcomes. Reconstructive surgeons at Role 5 hospitals have moved free flaps to provide soft tissue coverage to keep amputation levels below knee. Extremity length preservation should be in the forefront of the frontline surgeons' mind. At the Role 2 facility, only obviously clear completion amputations need to be done to gain hemorrhage control. Transporting the patient with extremities that may or may not need amputation later is not a problem. Staged damage control surgery is the most beneficial for extremity injuries.

Fractures should be treated by splint or external fixators. No intramedullary rods or ORIF plates and screws should be placed.

Vascular injuries, whenever possible, should be primarily repaired or shunted. Interposition grafting is best done in a controlled Role 3 environment with autologous vein unless it is a single casualty and the surgeon has vascular trauma experience.

The liberal use of fasciotomies is encouraged whenever extremity injuries are present—especially in the setting of large extremity venous injuries requiring ligation. Whenever possible, the popliteal vein should be repaired or shunted. Ligation of this vein is almost always associated with amputation. Should this vein be injured or ligated, lower leg fasciotomies should be performed [49, 50].

When performing lower leg fasciotomies, it should be done through two incisions—medial and lateral. For those surgeons unfamiliar with this procedure, pre-deployment training should include the Advanced Surgical Skills for Exposure in Trauma (ASSET) course. ASSET covers fasciotomies in detail. Nevertheless, care must be taken to ensure all four compartments are thoroughly opened and decompressed—the deep posterior compartment is frequently missed [50].

All large open wounds should be covered with negative pressure therapy sponges or with gauze and lightly wrapped with Kerlix or elastic dressings.

3.5 Pelvis/Perineal Injuries

For those injured by blast who are near the explosion, pelvis and perineal injuries are common. It is useful if the history of the explosion can be obtained. Did it come from the ground or did it come from the side? If patients arrive to the Role 2 with a pelvic binder in place, after finishing the primary survey, plain films of the pelvis should be performed with and without binder in place to look for evidence of unstable pelvic fracture. If the patient has an unstable pelvic fracture and evidence of ongoing bleeding, one option is for the patient to be taken to the OR for pre-peritoneal pelvic packing with or without internal iliac artery clipping with surgical clips along with simultaneous placement of a pelvic external fixator. The pelvic binder is typically easier and just as effective as placing a pelvic external fixator for the non-trauma-trained general surgeon. The use of the binder should also be done being mindful of the transport time. Most Role 2 facilities are within an hour transport. If long transport is required, the binder being on for several hours does have consequences that must be taken into consideration.

When performing pre-peritoneal packing a lower midline incision is made to the pubic symphasis. Dissection is carried out down to the posterior rectus fascia. The fascia is incised, vertically, in the midline enough to easily pass the operating surgeons' hands. A large Richardson retractor is placed on the patient's right side, hematoma is evacuated, and three folded laparotomy pads are placed. The process is repeated on the left. The midline fascia is closed with running suture while the orthopedic surgeons place the external fixator crossbar [51]. The pre-peritoneal packing is controverisal in civilan literature but recently the Denver experience is positive and describes the procedure in detail. When performing packing, the ligation of the internal iliac artery unilateral or bilateral can be considered if the pelvic fracture is the predominant cause of exsanguination. This is done by identifying the external iliac artery and following it cephalad until the branching downward internal iliac artery is identified. Complete control of this artery is not needed. Placing a large clip on this artery is akin to interventional radiology embolizing the internal iliac arteries.

3.6 Perineal Injuries/ Genitourinary Injuries

Perineal injuries can be divided into those involving the genitourinary (GU) system and those that do not. For those that do not, hemostasis, debridement, irrigation, and packing should govern — therapy. Some patients may eventually require fecal stream diversion (from destructive rectal injuries). This is not always needed at the Role 2 facility. Should an exploratory laparotomy not be indicated at the Role 2, diversion should be performed at the Role 3 as opening an uninjured anatomical compartment should be performed in as controlled environment as possible.

GU injuries should be addressed to a limited extent. In the absences of an expanding hematoma, scrotal injuries should be observed at the Role 2. Testicular injuries, if identified, should be initially managed with lightly wrapped, moistened gauze. When there is concern for urethral injury, a suprapubic tube is always helpful and rarely harmful. Urethral injuries should be addressed with sterile dressing and placement of external bladder drainage system. If defect is in the bulbar urethra, an attempt at Foley catheterization may take place. Alternatively, should the surgeon be unable to pass a catheter, suprapubic drainage is recommended—either by direct cutdown or percutaneously under ultrasound guidance [52].

3.7 Abdominal Injuries

With the development and ubiquitous use of body armor, abdominal injuries from battlefield blast wounds have declined [53]. However, there are other circumstances—such as mounted IED blasts, rocket-propelled grenades (RPG), mortar, and suicide IED blasts—where injuries can easily occur. For the civilian and enemy combatants, torso injury is still common. Nevertheless, abdominal examination is important. Peritoneal signs in either blunt or penetrating trauma, with or without hypotension are indications for prompt exploration.

As most Role 2 facilities do not have a CT scan, nonoperative management of penetrating abdominal trauma should be approached with extreme caution, and exploration should strongly be considered in all cases. The issue is one of space and evacuation. By doctrine, hold time at Role 2s is <24 h and bed space is at a premium. Depending on the battle space and rhythm, evacuation times from Role 2 to Role 3 may be hours; however, given the proximity of the Role 2 to the battlefront, it is important to keep beds available for those newly injured. Extended periods of observation may not be a luxury. Again, hemorrhage control and contamination control are minimum. However, depending on the scenario, it should also not be the default. If there is time and resources, completion with diagnosis and reconstruction is preferred. Reconstructing bowel at the first operation is always preferred in contrast to stapling off bowel to be connected back at a later time. After prolonged periods of complete bowel obstruction and bowel edema, the reconstruction of the gastrointestinal tract is more difficult later than earlier.

In the absence of hypotension, blunt abdominal trauma can be even more challenging. FAST exams and diagnostic peritoneal lavages (or aspirations) are adjuncts to the primary survey that are important to master. If either is positive, even in a hemodynamically normal patient, for logistic reasons/evacuation times discussed above, strong consideration should be made to perform abdominal exploration [54]. There are no surgical interventions available in the back of a medical evacuation helicopter or fixed wing aircraft. Missing or delaying injuries is relatively worse than nontherapeutic explorations.

Whatever the indications are for Role 2 laparotomy, goals are the same—to stop hemorrhage, control contamination, identify injuries, and reconstruct if possible [55]. Some objective indications would be:

1. Acidosis (pH < 7.25)
2. Hypothermia ($T < 34$ °C)
3. Shock on presentation (SBP < 70 mmHg)
4. Massive transfusion
5. Multiple, extra-abdominal life-threatening injuries
6. Mass casualties
7. Limited resources

The abdomen should be entered via midline incision. Communication with anesthesia is paramount when opening peritoneum as any tamponade effect will be lost. Four-quadrant packing of the abdomen is then performed not for the once thought purpose of controlling hemorrhage but to better evacuate the abdomen from the bleeding so the source of bleeding can be identified. In civilian blunt trauma laparotomy, the four-quadrant packing was thought to help with the hemorrhage control. However, in blunt trauma, there are no bleeding organs in the left and right lower quadrants. In penetrating trauma, the bleeding sources causing death are more central than peripheral. Fast and early hemorrhage control saves lives. The customary method of four-quadrant packing and letting anesthesia catch up is a myth when we used to perform exploratory laparotomy for solid organ bleeding that usually stops bleeding spontaneously. The packs are removed as quickly as possible because the first and foremost goal is to identify the bleeding and control it. It is difficult to do that under blood. Don't waste time controlling bleeding.

Solid organs should be assessed. Injury to the spleen should prompt splenectomy. Liver injuries should be addressed with liver stitches (with or without omental/falciform ligament flap) and hemostatic packing. It is preferred to keep the laparotomy pads folded in squares when performing hemostatic packing of the liver—two lap pads anterior on left lobe, four pads anterior of right lobe, one pad in gallbladder fossa, and one pad between left lobe and stomach. This provides predictable tamponade across the entire liver. Care must be taken not to place too much pressure on the inferior vena cava when packing the liver as it can decrease preload causing the patient to become hypotensive. Good communication with anesthesia is essential. A good example of this type of packing is found in the Advanced Trauma Operative Management (ATOM) course. Packing may control venous bleeding but will not control arterial bleeding adequately.

Injuries to hollow organs should be quickly controlled with clamps, primary repair, or resection with stapling devices. Bowel should be run from ligament of Treitz to ileocecal valve and from cecum to peritoneal reflection. Should resection of destructive injury be necessary, a nonanatomic resection (i.e., resection not governed by anatomic blood supply) is acceptable. Perform anastomosis if possible at the first operation, but if the scenario and resources do not allow it, then controlling contamination may have to suffice. The third and fourth stage of trauma laparotomy may have to be deferred to the colleagues at the Role 3 facility.

3.8 Retroperitoneal Injuries

The retroperitoneum is broken down into three zones—1, 2, and 3 (picture):

1. Zone 1 (medial)—aorta, inferior vena cava, pancreas, duodenum, common iliac arteries, and common iliac veins
2. Zone 2 (lateral)—right and left kidneys and ureters, gonadal vessels (left drains into renal vein, right drains into IVC)
3. Zone 3 (pelvis)—internal and external iliac arteries and veins, distal ureters, and rectum

Exploration of these zones is based upon mechanism and presence of hematomas.

	Blunt	Penetrating
Zone 1	Explore	Explore
Zone 2	Explore, if expanding hematoma	Explore
Zone 3	Explore, if expanding hematoma	Explore

Exposure of the retroperitoneum is performed by right or left medial visceral rotation. In some cases, both right and left sides need to be explored. The words of wisdom states that for zone I, it highly depends on the mechanism. For blunt trauma, it is very rare to have vascular injury in zone I causing the hematoma but is typically from blunt spinal fracture. If the patient has blunt injury and mild hematoma over the fracture site, exploring this will cause more bleeding than desired or controlled. For zone II, if renal vasculature is suspected in blunt trauma, then explore to perform nephrectomy. If penetrating trauma, explore to determine collection system injury. However, in the Role 2 scenario, this can be delayed till later depending on the scenario. If the ureter is injured, then primary repair or cannulation and externalization may be warranted.

To expose the left retroperitoneum, incision is made at the white line of Toldt, and dissection is carried out medially. Dissection medially can be carried out either with electrocautery, blunt dissection, or a combination of both. The spleen, pancreas, and left kidney are mobilized. This mobilization should give easy access to the renal hilum. Dissection is carried out medially until the aorta is reached. Aortic and common iliac artery injuries should be repaired primarily or shunted. Interposition grafting should generally not be attempted in a Role 2 setting.

To expose the right retroperitoneum, incision is made at the white line of Toldt and dissection is carried out medially—with either electrocautery, blunt dissection, or a combination of both. The duodenum is kocherized and the right kidney is mobilized. Dissection is carried out to the vena cava. Vena cava injuries should be repaired. The infrarenal vena cava may be ligated, if necessary, in the damage control setting. However, ligation is associated with significant morbidity and mortality rates upward of 70% [56].

Sullivan et al. reported outcomes on 51 patients with infrarenal vena cava injuries. Long-term survival rates were 79.3% (23/29) for those undergoing repair and only 40.9% (9/22) who underwent ligation. Of the early survivors whose vena cava was ligated, 10 of 13 underwent immediate, bilateral below-knee fasciotomies. None of the other three required fasciotomies leading the authors to argue for selective fasciotomies based on physical exam/physiologic course [56]. However, in the combat setting, fasciotomies are recommended due to lack of surgical access during potential long evacuation times.

Iliac veins should undergo primary repair, if possible, else ligated. Ligating common iliac veins is associated with increased venous resistance in the affected limb. Similarly to infrarenal IVC injuries, below-knee fasciotomies should be made. However, in the case of iliac vein ligation, fasciotomy only need be performed on the injury's ipsilateral side [49].

3.9 Urinary Tract Injuries

In the setting of damage control, the goal of hemorrhage control is to allow the patient to be resuscitated in order to restore normal physiology, not necessarily normal anatomy. When the kidneys are injured, decision must be made if resection (partial or total) or simple repair is necessary. Principles of renal repair are to ensure the collecting system is approximated with absorbable suture and the renal parenchyma is approximated with hemostatic, bolstered, absorbable sutures. In the forward scenario, nephrectomy has great results, and in dire straights, if the bleeding is controlled, drainage and delayed diagnosis and reconstruction is an option.

Ureteral injuries are approached based on the severity AND location of injury. Contusions are generally treated with stenting. Since trans-cystic ureteral stenting is not likely to be available at the Role 2, ureteral contusion should be well documented in the patient's operative note (and, perhaps, area in question marked with a suture). Prophylactic drains can always be placed with minimal consequence. Ureteral pelvic junction injuries should undergo stenting and primary repair. If not available or unable to perform based on time constraints, a drain should be placed near the injury to allow for some control of urine production. A reimplantation of the injured ureter to another site on the dome of the bladder by tunneling a short portion of the ureter before entering the bladder. A transected ureter should be repaired in a tension-free, spatulated manner over a stent. If inadequate length remains or if stenting is not possible, a pediatric feeding tube can be placed into the ureter and then externalized via a small flank incision. If externalizing the ureter with a tube is not possible, then again placing a drain nearby may have to suffice. Ureteral debridement should be kept to a minimum in order to preserve as much length as possible [52].

Penetrating bladder injuries are treated with exploration which often necessitates the opening of the dome of the bladder followed by a two-layer closure. Then an inner layer should always be performed with an absorbable suture. With penetrating injury to the bladder, it should always be assumed that there are two injuries and not just one. Both suprapubic and transurethral catheters should be placed to minimize effect blood clots may have on bladder drainage. Blunt injury to the bladder will occur typically in three areas almost always with a pelvic fracture. It is extremely rare to have a blunt bladder injury without a pelvic fracture. The site of injury is at the fracture site and is due to the bony penetration into the bladder on the side of the bladder and the dome of the bladder due to overpressure on a full bladder, and this may be intraperitoneal. The third place is at the neck of the bladder and fortunately this is rare [52].

3.10 Transpelvic Injuries (Combined GU/GI Injuries)

There is one very specific injury pattern that should be discussed—penetrating transpelvic wounds. There will be patients who sustain these wounds from blasts or from gunshots. Some patients will be in extremis secondary to vascular injuries. Those without vascular injuries may not present in extremis but may show signs of injury by either blood on digital rectal exam or by bloody urine without evidence of injury to the proximal or distal urinary tract. Sometimes, the transpelvic projectile will pass between the bladder and rectum—injuring both.

When exploring the bladder, especially when a posterior/inferior injury is suspected, it is acceptable to open the dome of the bladder in the midline (to avoid injuring the ureteral-pelvic junction). The midline incision may be carried posteriorly and inferiorly without much morbidity and should be carried out to the extent necessary to examine the entire bladder. Additionally, the bladder may be filled with saline to look for additional injuries prior to closure. The bladder injury should be debrided and closed in layers with both suprapubic and transurethral catheters present for decompression.

In the event of a combination rectal/bladder injury, the rectal injury should be oversewn with the fecal stream proximally diverted. If unable to oversew the rectum, proximal fecal stream diversion should still be performed and pelvic drains should be left. This is not the time for low anterior resection to occur.

3.11 Closing the Abdomen

Civilian laparotomy in the damage control setting is intended to allow for restoration of normal physiology in the setting of devastating trauma. A second look is planned. In the setting of damage control at a Role 2, resources (i.e., access to blood products, advanced surgical equipment, surgical specialists, etc.) are limited. Therefore, temporary abdominal fascial closure should be employed if the surgery cannot be completed. Often the Role 3 will want to perform another laparotomy if the communication between the sending and receiving site is not optimal. While there was a trend toward performing damage control laparotomy in civilian sector, it has now being reserved for only absolutely necessary case as the consequences of the open abdomen can be severe [57]. In the combat setting, again the setting, number of casualties, and lack of resources may deem the need for abbreviated laparotomy. Closing the skin over packs or VAC sponges is desirable in that it helps maintain fluid losses and hypothermia to the intestines which does not like exteriorization and can lead to enterocutaneous fistulas. Closing the skin only also helps maintain some stretch to the abdominal wall, and some intra-abdominal pressure will aid minor venous bleeding to stop.

There are several techniques to use, but all have the same general principles—a nonadherent, fenestrated barrier between the bowel and absorptive dressings coupled with an airtight fluid management system. One technique uses a large plastic barrier (e.g., sterile 3 L bag of saline), the surgeon fenestrates with scissors and places under the fascia to the lateral gutters, gauze dressings are placed over the plastic barrier, and two large bore nasogastric tubes are then placed within the gauze dressings (connected to suction). The closure is completed by placing an adhesive, airtight covering. Vacuum-assisted devices are now ubiquitous in theater and are advisable if available.

3.12 Damage Control in the Chest

As of 2012 in the most recent wars in Iraq and Afghanistan, 7570 combat trauma casualties sustained thoracic trauma for an incident of just over 10.0%. While pulmonary contusions (46.4%) and pneumothoraces (39.5%) accounted for a vast majority of thoracic injuries, their respective mortality rates of 7.0 and 9.89% were much less than the frequent injuries of lacerations (0.78%), thoracic vascular injuries (0.38%), flail chests (0.27%), and cardiac injuries (0.24%) who had associated mortality rates of 14.2, 19.9, 19.9, and 13.3%, respectively [58]. Understanding damage control principles of these, relatively infrequent, yet highly lethal injuries, is vitally important.

Inspection, auscultation, x-ray, and ultrasound are the only noninvasive techniques available for thoracic evaluation in the Role 2 setting, and all play crucial roles in determining direction of surgical therapy. In the Role 3 setting, there have been, as previously stated, numerous subspecialists and CT scans. The cost and radiation have not been much of a problem in the combat casualties, and CT has been used routinely and often. It has been of tremendous assistance in diagnosis and management.

Patients with chest trauma may arrive to the Role 2 with a chest that has undergone needle decompression, a chest wall defect that has been covered with a three-sided nonocclusive dressing, or a pleural space that has received a thoracostomy tube. If a thoracostomy tube is not present and chest trauma is confirmed, rapid assessment of the patient's breathing with thoracostomy tube placement is essential. As taught in advanced trauma life support (ATLS), most thoracic injuries can be temporized via insertion of a thoracostomy tube. The use of small bore chest tubes has been shown that they are just as effective as large bore chest tubes in terms of air, fluid, and blood drainage [59]. The simple advice is that if the air, fluid, or blood can be easily accessed with a needle with or without the use of ultrasound or CT, then using the Seldinger technique to place a small bore tube is acceptable. If empiric placement of chest tubes is required, it is always better and safer to do it after exploration with a finger. After the pleural space has been entered, again the size of the tube does not seem to matter, and thus the only recommendation is to avoid extremely large chest tubes.

If large volumes of blood are evacuated from the chest with thoracostomy tube placement (i.e., >1500 cc within 1 h of tube placement or if >200 cc/h over 3–4 h), patients should proceed to the OR for thoracic exploration. Once the patient is brought into the operating theater, it is not a mandate that the patient undergo a thoracotomy. It should be kept in mind that thoracotomy is only required in 2% of blunt trauma patients and 5% of penetrating trauma patients. In the vast majority of the time, chest drainage with tube thoracostomy is all that is required for thoracic trauma. The lung is a low-pressure system that is high in tissue factor and most bleeding will stop spontaneously. If the patient has hilar injury tract or if the chest wall bleeding is severe enough, on occasion thoracotomy is needed. It should also be kept in mind that when assessing the volume of blood collected from a thoracostomy tube, it may be very helpful when the question of how much has bled and how much is continuing to bleed has been resolved. In a patient who is hemodynamically stable or normal the blood that has been collected and be reinfused and if the bleeding has slowed or stopped thoracotomy may not always be needed. However, if the patient is unstable or abnormal, it is not always necessary to wait if the bleeding seems to be from an arterial source. Keen judgment is always irreplaceable. The goals of thoracic damage control surgery are to control hemorrhage, since, in the absence of diaphragmatic laceration/herniation (transdiaphragmatic injury), contamination is highly unlikely. Autotransfusion of the shed blood is extremely valuable in theater as fresh whole blood or packed red blood cells may be limited. To perform autotransfusion, the blood collected from the chest tube is reinfused through a blood filter. In anticipation of autotransfusion in the field, the chest tube collection device should be spiked with

50–100 cc of citrate phosphorous dextrose (CPD) for every 500 cc of blood collected. Although the idea of autotransfusion of shed whole blood was thought to have coagulopathic properties, clinical studies have shown no clinically significant coagulopathy but significant safety and efficacy in the use of the casualties' own blood [66].

For damage control thoracotomies, patients are placed in the supine position on the operating room table with a shoulder bump sufficient to facilitate an anterior lateral thoracotomy. In the trauma setting, exposure obtained from a posterior lateral thoracotomy is usually too restrictive and does not allow access to the contra-lateral chest. In a Role 2 setting, patients are often operated on the stretcher that they came in on. Performing anterior lateral thoracotomy on a stretcher can be problematic as it is difficult to raise the left arm above the shoulder and keep it there when the casualty is still in the stretcher. In addition, the side rails of the stretcher are high in relation to the casualty as they sink down in the stretcher, and the rail is at approximate mid-axillary level. In order to get around this problem, a torso elevator can be easily made so that the torso is elevated when the stretcher with the casualty is placed on the device. This device is a rectangular box that is about 4 ft in length shorter than the width of the stretcher so that as the stretcher is placed on it, the side rails of the stretcher fall lower than the torso.

If thoracotomy is needed and the chest is entered, there is always a hematoma clot, and this is removed first and inspection is begun for the bleeding source. To facilitate exploration, the inferior pulmonary ligament should be mobilized. Tractotomies and nonanatomic wedge resections with GIA staplers can be quickly accomplished to address bleeding/significant air leaks and are favored to more formal, time-consuming anatomic resections. It will be assumed for this discussion that the thoracotomy was urgently or emergently needed, and thus a double lumen endotracheal tube is not available.

Second-order bronchus injuries can be treated with lobe resection. This is accomplished by dissecting freely the lobar vessels and ligating artery and vein with suture ligatures. The bronchus may be stapled with a TA device and then oversewn or handsewn in multiple layers.

More proximal injuries are highly lethal [60, 61]. Hilar clamping or twisting is associated with rapid increase in pulmonary vasculature resistance and rapid onset of right heart failure. Often this also results in a venous tourniquet and thus is not advised. If the hilar structures require control, then a standard angled clamp is the most effective. If there is no clamp or any sort that is available, then ties with large structures such as umbilical tape can be used, but again it must be tied down extremely tightly to occlude the bronchus and arterial blood supply or it will again be a venous tourniquet which can increase bleeding. While there are reported survivors, this technique should only be used as a quick bridge to identification of hemorrhage source and its control. Traumatic pneumonectomy is a procedure of last resort as its mortality approaches 42% even in the most robust US academic trauma centers [62]. Those undergoing traumatic pneumonectomy develop right heart failure and respiratory failure and may require extracorporeal lung support (ECLS). ECLS is available from the acute lung rescue team based at Landstuhl Regional Medical Center (LRMC) but is 8–10 h away in the best circumstances [63–65]. If pneumonectomy is required, fluid balance is of particular importance post-op as while resuscitation is required to recover from hypovolemia, hypervolemia can cause deadly right heart failure. Diuresis may be required in this particular scenario postoperatively starting on day two.

If great vessel injuries are noted on exploration, they are best handled by primary repair, though survival is very low even in the best circumstances.

3.13 Cardiac Injuries

If cardiac injury is suspected (either by injury pattern, ultrasound, or physiology), the heart is approached via a left anterior lateral thoracotomy or median sternotomy if a Lebsche knife is available as sternal saws are not available at the Role 2 level. The pericardium is opened along a line par-

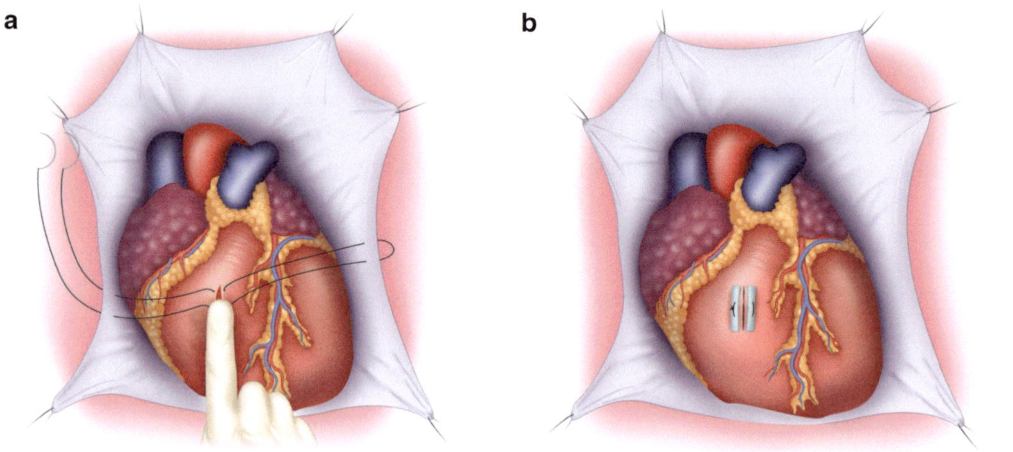

Fig. 3.1 Digital pressure providing hemostasis while pledgeted "U" stitch is being placed for formal hemorrhage control

allel to the floor and anterior to the left phrenic nerve if approached via anterolateral thoracotomy. The heart is delivered into the field and inspected for injuries. Most cardiac injuries are amenable to digital control until suture can be obtained. Cardiac lacerations should be closed with double armed 2–0 or 3–0 nonabsorbable "U" stitch suture sewing under the finger if possible. Pericardial pledget is an option but is generally not required, and pledget of any kind can hinder the source of hemorrhage. Care must be taken not to oversew coronary vessels. In fact, for lacerations adjacent to coronary vessels, the "U" stitch must traverse underneath the vessels (Fig. 3.1).

In patients with multiple life-threatening injuries, temporizing cardiac injuries may be necessary. This may be accomplished by placing a Foley balloon catheter into the laceration, inflating the balloon, and providing anterior traction—enough to prevent leakage around the balloon, but not too much traction that would tear the myocardium. In the left ventricle, the balloon often tears and enlarges the laceration while hinding preload. Digital control of hemorrhage is best preferred. Smaller injuries can be temporized with a sterile skin stapler until sutures are available.

Inspection of posterior cardiac injuries must be conducted slowly and in coordination with anesthesia as lifting the heart will "kink" the vena cava rendering the right side of the heart temporarily empty, potentially inciting cardiac arrest. Repairs are made as described above, but sutures are placed one throw at a time—allowing for time to place the heart back into normal anatomic position between suture throws. Grasping the posterior pericardium with two Allis clamps and pulling downward will often lift the heart and expose the laceration for repair.

3.14 Esophageal/Tracheal Injuries

Esophageal injuries should be approached with caution. Small lacerations may be repaired with primary closure, covered with intercostal muscle flap, and widely drained both internally and externally. Destructive injuries should be excluded with a stapling device and widely drained. To handle oral secretions, a sumping nasal tube should be sutured to the nose with the tip just proximal to the cephalad staple line. A gastric tube should be placed as well to allow for interval decompression and feeding. Cervical esophagostomy is an option to divert flow from the injury. Cervical or pharyngeal esophagus is different than thoracic or mediastinal esophagus, and they can easily be repaired simply and if a spit fistula later forms, it will most often close spontaneously if properly drained.

Similar to esophageal injuries, small tracheal injuries should undergo primary repair. If this is not feasible or if the injury is destructive, the endotracheal tube should be advanced beyond the injury to allow for continued lung ventilation. Alternatively, if this is not possible, an endotracheal tube can be placed through the wound to either be occlusive or to allow for ventilation.

3.14.1 Summary

Damage control surgery in the military takes much of the principles from civilian trauma but differs mainly due to the austere setting and limited resources. In the forward surgical capabilities, there are minimal hospital beds, physicians, supplies, and equipment. In the larger Role 3 hospitals, they have tremendous capability including a CT scan, surgical subspecialists, and ability to transport severely injured long distances to military bases out of theater. In this chapter we have focused on what might be needed in the Role 2 facilities which often only has two general or trauma surgeons with or without orthopedic surgeons. In this setting where critical care is not available and blood bank supplies are limited, abbreviation of surgery is often required due to lack of supply rather than due to exhaustion of physiologic reserves. The combat scenario dictates what should or could be done. In general, if the supply is adequate and the walking blood bank is available, providing fresh whole blood, and most importantly there are minimal limited number of casualties, then completion surgery is preferred. However, if needed due to high volume of patients and shortage of supply, then abbreviation of surgery after hemorrhage and contamination can be done. Shunts are very useful in the forward setting, but completion vascular repairs are possible if experience is available. Fasciotomies should be applied liberally and selective fasciotomies cannot be reliably applied. Future experience in military combat damage control surgery may find that the liberal use of REBOA may be quite useful.

References

1. Eastridge BJ, et al. Death on the battlefield (2001–2011): implications for the future of combat casualty care. J Trauma Acute Care Surg. 2012;73(6 Suppl 5):S431–7.
2. Garner J, et al. Mechanisms of injury by explosive devices. Anesthesiol Clin. 2007;25(1):147–60.
3. Belmont PJ Jr, et al. Incidence and epidemiology of combat injuries sustained during "the surge" portion of operation Iraqi Freedom by a US Army brigade combat team. J Trauma. 2010;68(1):204–10.
4. Mabry RL, et al. United States Army Rangers in Somalia: an analysis of combat casualties on an urban battlefield. J Trauma. 2000;49(3):515–28.
5. Chandler H, et al. Extremity injuries sustained by the UK military in the Iraq and Afghanistan conflicts: 2003–2014. Injury. 2017;48(7):1439–43.
6. Blackbourne LH, et al. Military medical revolution: prehospital combat casualty care. J Trauma Acute Care Surg. 2012;73(6):S372–7.
7. TCCC guidelines. https://www.jsomonline.org/TCCC/TCCC%20Guidelines%20for%20Medical%20Personnel%20170131%20Final.pdf. Accessed 6 Sept 2017.
8. Hodgetts TJ, et al. Putting role 1 first: the role 1 capability review. J R Army Med Corps. 2012;158(3):162–70.
9. Wheatley RJ. The role 1 capability review: mitigation and innovation for Op Herrick 18 and into contingency. J R Army Med Corps. 2014;160(3):211–2.
10. Chambers LW, et al. The experience of the US Marine Corps' Surgical Shock Trauma Platoon with 417 operative combat casualties during a 12 month period of operation Iraqi Freedom. J Trauma. 2006;60(6):1155–64.
11. Brisebois CR, et al. The role 3 multinational medical unit at Kandahar Airfield 2005-2010. Can J Surg. 2011;54(6):S124–9.
12. Beckett A, et al. Multidisciplinary trauma team care in Kandahar, Afghanistan: current injury patterns and care practices. Injury. 2012;43(12):2072–7.
13. Kotwal RS, et al. The effect of a Golden Hour policy on the morbidity and mortality of combat casualties. JAMA Surg. 2016;151(1):15–24.
14. Bennett BL, et al. Management of external hemorrhage in Tactical Combat Casualty Care: chitosan-based hemostatic gauze dressings—TCC guidelines- change 13-05. J Spec Oper Med. 2014;14(3):40–57.
15. Beekley AC, et al. Prehospital tourniquet use in Operation Iraqi Freedom: effect on hemorrhage control and outcomes. J Trauma. 2008;64(2 Suppl):S28–37.

16. Tactical Combat Casualty Care Guidelines for Medical Personnel, January 31, 2017. http://www.usaisr.amedd.army.mil/pdfs/TCCCGuidelinesforMedicalPersonnel170131Final.pdf. Accessed 30 April 2018.
17. King DR, et al. Tourniquet use at the Boston Marathon bombing: lost in translation. J Trauma Acute Care Surg. 2015;78(3):594–9.
18. Lakstein D, et al. Tourniquets for hemorrhage control on the battlefield: a 4-year accumulated experience. J Trauma. 2003;54(5 Suppl):S221–5.
19. Kragh JF, et al. Minor morbidity with emergency tourniquet use to stop bleeding in severe limb trauma: research, history, and reconciling advocates and abolitionists. Mil Med. 2007;176(7):817–3.
20. Kragh JF, et al. Junctional tourniquet training experience. J Spec Oper Med. 2015;15(3):20–30.
21. Klotz JK, et al. First case report of SAM(r) Junctional tourniquet use in Afghanistan to control inguinal hemorrhage on the battlefield. J Spec Oper Med. 2014;14(2):1–5.
22. Holcomb JB, et al. Damage control resuscitation. J Trauma. 2007;62(6 Suppl):S36–7.
23. Cotton BA, et al. Damage control resuscitation is associated with a reduction in resuscitation volumes and improvement in survival in 390 damage control laparotomy patients. Ann Surg. 2011;254(4):598–605.
24. Morrison JJ, et al. Military application of tranexamic acid in trauma emergency resuscitation (MATTERs) study. Arch Surg. 2012;147(2):113–9.
25. Joseph B, et al. Assessing the efficacy of prothrombin complex concentrate in multiply injured patients with high-energy pelvic and extremity fractures. J Orthop Trauma. 2016;30(12):653–8.
26. Spinella PC, et al. Resuscitation and transfusion principles for traumatic hemorrhagic shock. Blood Rev. 2011;23(6):231–40.
27. Damage control resuscitation. Joint trauma system clinical practice guideline. http://www.usaisr.amedd.army.mil/cpgs/DamageControlResuscitation_03Feb2017.pdf. Accessed 6 Oct 2017.
28. Fresh whole blood transfusion. Joint trauma system clinical practice guideline. http://www.usaisr.amedd.army.mil/cpgs/Fresh_Whole_Blood_Transfusion_24_Oct_12.pdf. Accessed 6 Oct 2017.
29. Parker PJ, et al. Casualty evacuation timelines: an evidence-based review. J R Army Med Corps. 2007;153(4):274–7.
30. Hypothermia prevention, monitoring, and management. Joint trauma system clinical practice guideline. http://www.usaisr.amedd.army.mil/cpgs/Hypothermia_Prevention_20_Sep_12.pdf. Accessed 6 Oct 2017.
31. Pain, anxiety, and delirium. Joint trauma system clinical practice guideline. http://www.usaisr.amedd.army.mil/cpgs/Pain_Anxiety_Delirium_13Mar2017.pdf. Accessed 6 Oct 2017.
32. Lubin D, et al. Modified Veress needle decompression of tension pneumothorax: a randomized crossover animal study. J Trauma Acute Care Surg. 2013;75(6):1071–5.
33. Martin M, et al. Does needle thoracostomy provide adequate and effective decompression of tension pneumothorax? J Trauma Acute Care Surg. 2012;73(6):1412–7.
34. Butler FK, et al. Management of open pneumothorax in tactical combat casualty care: TCCC guidelines change 13-02. J Spec Oper Med. 2013;13(3):81–6.
35. Kotwal RS, et al. The effect of a golden hour policy on the morbidity and mortality of combat casualties. JAMA Surg. 2016;151(1):15–24.
36. American College of Surgeons, Committee on Trauma, "Advanced Trauma Life Support, 9th edition". Chicago, Illinois, American College of Surgeons, 2013.
37. Hathaway E, et al. Exploratory laparotomy for proximal vascular control in combat-related injuries. Mil Med. 2016;181(5 Suppl):247–52.
38. Dismounted complex blast injury: report of the army dismounted complex blast injury task force. 2011. http://armymedicine.mil/Documents/DCBI-Task-Force-Report-Redacted-Final.pdf. Accessed 6 Oct 2017.
39. Andersen RC, et al. Dismounted complex blast injury. J Surg Orthop Adv. 2012;21(1):2–7.
40. Rodriguez CJ, et al. Risk factors associated with invasive fungal infections in combat trauma. Surg Infect. 2014;15(5):521–6.
41. Radowsky JS, et al. A surgeon's guide to obtaining hemorrhage control in combat-related dismounted lower extremity injury. Mil Med. 2016;181(10):1300–4.
42. Advanced Surgical Exposures in Trauma (ASSET). https://www.facs.org/quality-programs/trauma/education/asset. Accessed 6 Oct 2017.
43. Brenner M, et al. Basic endovascular skills for trauma course: bridging the gap between endovascular techniques and the acute care surgeon. J Trauma Acute Care Surg. 2014;77(2):286–91.
44. Reva VA, et al. Field and en route REBOA: a feasible military reality? J Trauma Acute Care Surg. 2017;83(1):S170–6.
45. Fisher AD, et al. The role 1 resuscitation team and resuscitative endovascular balloon occlusion of the aorta. J Spec Oper Med. 2017;17(2):65–73.
46. Demetriades D, et al. Penetrating injuries to the subclavian and axillary vessels. J Am Coll Surg. 1999;188(3):290–5.
47. Sciarretta JD, et al. Subclavian vessel injuries: difficult anatomy and difficult territory. Eur J Trauma Emerg Surg. 2011;37(5):439.
48. Owens BD, et al. Comparison of irrigation solutions and devices in a contaminated musculoskeletal wound survival model. J Bone Joint Surg Am. 2009;91(1):92–8.
49. Vascular injury. Joint trauma system clinical practice guideline. http://www.usaisr.amedd.army.mil/cpgs/Vascular_Injury_12_Aug_2016.pdf. Accessed 8 Sept 2017.
50. Acute extremity compartment syndrome (CS) and the role of fasciotomy in extremity war wounds. Joint trauma system clinical practice guideline. http://www.usaisr.amedd.army.mil/cpgs/Acute_Compartment_

Syndrome-Fasciotomy_25Jul2016.pdf. Accessed 8 Sept 2017.

51. Filiberto DM, et al. Preperitoneal pelvic packing: technique and outcomes. Int J Surg. 2016;33(Pt B):222–4.
52. Urologic trauma management. Joint trauma system clinical practice guidelines. http://www.usaisr.amedd.army.mil/cpgs/Urologic_Trauma_Management_2_Apr_12.pdf. Accessed 8 Sept 2017.
53. Eskridge SL, et al. Injuries from combat explosions in Iraq: injury type, location, and severity. Injury. 2012;43(10):1678–82.
54. Blunt abdominal trauma, splenectomy, and post-splenectomy vaccination. Joint trauma system clinical practice guideline. http://www.usaisr.amedd.army.mil/cpgs/Blunt_Abdominal_Splenectomy_Vacc_12_Aug_2016.pdf. Accessed 8 Sept 2017.
55. Burlew CC, et al. Sew it Up! A Western Trauma Association multi-institutional study of enteric injury management in the post-injury open abdomen. J Trauma. 2011;70(2):273–7.
56. Sullivan PS, et al. Outcome of ligation of the inferior vena cava in the modern era. Am J Surg. 2010;199(4):500–6.
57. Lauerman MH, et al. Delayed interventions and mortality in trauma damage control laparotomy. Surgery. 2016;160(6):1568–75.
58. Keneally R, et al. Thoracic trauma in Iraq and Afghanistan. J Trauma Acute Care Surg. 2013;74(5):1292–7.
59. Inaba K, et al. Does size matter? A prospective analysis of 28-32 versus 36-40 French chest tube size in trauma. J Trauma Acute Care Surg. 2012;72(2):422–7.
60. Alfici R, et al. Total pulmonectomy in trauma: a still unresolved problem- our experience and review of the literature. Am Surg. 2007;73(4):381–4.
61. Wilson A, et al. The pulmonary hilum twist as a thoracic damage control procedure. Am J Surg. 2003;186(1):49–52.
62. Halonen-Waras J, et al. Traumatic pneumonectomy: a viable option for patients in extremis. Am Surg. 2011;77(4):493–7.
63. Bien T, et al. Transportable extracorporeal lung support for rescue of severe respiratory failure in combat casualties. J Trauma Acute Care Surg. 2012;73(6):1450–6.
64. Allan PF, et al. The introduction of extracorporeal membrane oxygenation to aeromedical evacuation. Mil Med. 2011;176(8):932–7.
65. Fang R, et al. Closing the “care in the air” capability gap for severe lung injury: the Landstuhl Acute Lunge Rescue Team and extracorporeal lung support. J Trauma. 2011;71(1 Suppl):S91–7.
66. Rhee P, et al. Early autologous fresh whole blood transfusion leads to less allogeneic transfusions and is safe. J Trauma Acute Care Surg. 2015;78(4):729–34.

4 En Route Care

Joel Elterman, Daniel Cox, and Jay Johannigman

Abstract

The history of aeromedical evacuation parallels that of manned flight. The first fixed wing aeromedical evacuations occurred on limited basis during the First World War with a significantly increased experience occurring during the Second World War. The Korean War introduced the role of rotary-wing transport in decreasing transport time from the forward area of battle to medical care units. Vietnam expanded on this rotary-wing evacuation experience and introduced a limited set of medical interventions for the casualty during the transport process. The experience of aeromedical evacuation in the military during Vietnam was largely responsible for the subsequent proliferation of civilian aeromedical evacuation services in the trauma system of the United States during the latter part of the twentieth century.

J. Elterman, M.D., F.A.C.S.
University of Cincinnati College of Medicine, United States Air Force Center for Sustainment of Trauma and Readiness Skills (CSTARS), Cincinnati, OH, USA

D. Cox, M.D., F.A.C.S.
University of Cincinnati College of Medicine, Office of the Command Surgeon, Air Mobility Command, Cincinnati, OH, USA

J. Johannigman, M.D., F.A.C.S., F.C.C.M. (✉)
University of Cincinnati College of Medicine, Cincinnati, OH, USA
e-mail: jay.johannigman@uc.edu

The last 15 years of conflict as a result of the Global War on Terrorism has provided an extended experience in the art and medical science of aeromedical evacuation. The scope of this chapter will focus on current concepts of aeromedical evacuation as it evolves into a process of en route care. The evolution from safe transport via the air to a continuous process of medical care and continuous resuscitation marks the pivotal changes that have emerged over the last decades of care in the air. The evolution of terminology from aeromedical evacuation to en route care highlights the focus on principles of care rather than mode of transportation.

This chapter will focus on the challenges of the aeromedical environment, the composition of the advanced care teams (Critical Care Air Transport Teams), and the processes of provision of care in this uniquely challenging space. The current team composition and equipment sets will be discussed along with opportunities for new technologies to positively impact on the provision of en route care.

4.1 Introduction

The concept of transporting combat casualties by air parallels the history of military aviation. Many texts cite the aeromedical evacuation of casualties by balloon during the Franco-Prussian War

J. Duchesne et al. (eds.), *Damage Control in Trauma Care*,
https://doi.org/10.1007/978-3-319-72607-6_4

(1870) as the first successful instance of aeromedical evacuation. More recent publications have challenged and refuted this claim [1]. The true initiation of aeromedical evacuation awaited the successful development of the fixed-wing aircraft. During the First World War, British, French, German, and American forces all utilized fixed-wing evacuation on a very limited basis. These first aeromedical evacuations provided the opportunity for medics to overcome the "tyranny of distance" facing the medic and the casualty. The introduction of flight evacuation during the First World War offered the advantage of speed and time while avoiding the arduous task of ground evacuation via carriage or rudimentary gas-powered vehicles of the era.

During the Second World War, more than a million injured combatants would be evacuated by British, American, and German aircrafts. During this period, aeromedical evacuation was largely reserved for very stable or ambulatory casualties who had been managed at established rear hospital facilities (weeks to months following wounding) and were sufficiently recovered to sustain (and survive) the relatively difficult transport process in unpressurized aircraft.

The Korean conflict was the first to demonstrate the advantages of rotary-wing evacuation and its ability to clear casualties from the forward area of battle. The introduction of helicopter evacuation during the Korean War demonstrated the extension of aeromedical care into the far-forward area of prehospital care. The venerable OH-13 Sioux helicopter was utilized to evacuate casualties over the inhospitable and mountainous terrain of Korea. Combat casualties were delivered to nearby MASH units within minutes rather than hours or days. The role of rotary-wing evacuation became even more preeminent during the United States' combat role in Vietnam. The widely visible success of the US Army's MEDEVAC units (DUSTOFF) in clearing casualties and providing rapid delivery to definitive trauma care hospitals would be widely copied by the civilian trauma system then developing in the US (1970–1980). The Vietnam Dustoff era is also recognized as the first time when rudimentary medical care (hemorrhage control and IV fluids) was delivered by medical personnel while en route from the point of wounding to the first level of surgical care (Fig. 4.1).

The model of aeromedical evacuation (AE) developed since Korea through the First Gulf War comprised a dichotomous, two-step process. The first step consisted of forward (tactical) evacuation of casualties from the point of wounding and was

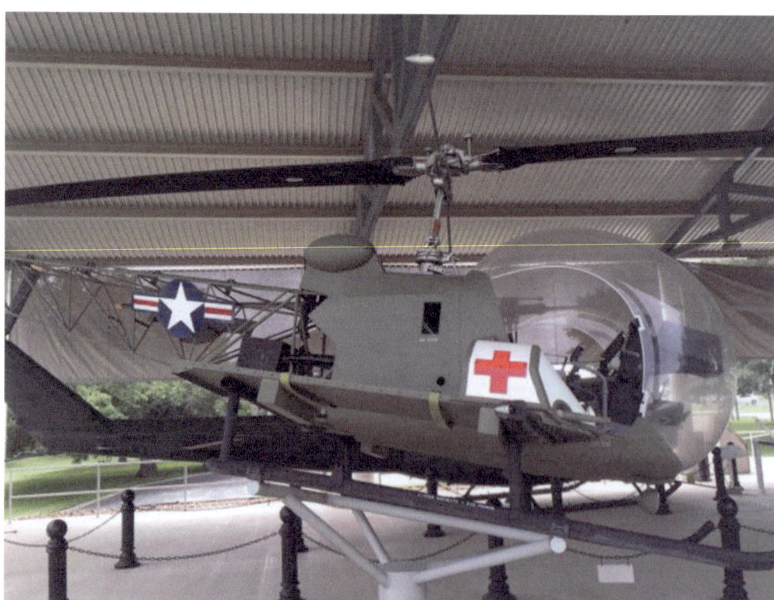

Fig. 4.1 The OH-13 "MASH" helicopter (authors picture)

accomplished via rotary-wing transport to an established surgical unit. The primary focus of this phase was the provision of rapid transport out of a hostile/combat environment. The opportunity to provide medical care during these transports was not a primary objective, and care en route was rudimentary at best. Once at a more established facility (mobile or theater surgical facility), the casualty would recover until sufficiently stable to tolerate the second phase of the process. This second phase (strategic aeromedical evacuation) consisted of transport of the casualty over much greater distances using fixed-wing aircraft.

The scope of this chapter will be to examine the continued evolution of the AE process during the last 15 years including the Global War on Terror and Operation Iraqi Freedom and Operation Enduring Freedom. This evolution has changed the scope of AE from a process which hoped to deliver casualties from the forward area of battle safely and without further harm to today's system which emphasizes the provision of sophisticated en route critical care ensuring rapid transport while providing for, and improving upon, the medical conditions of the patient. The ideal system state sought is a continuum of care which begins at the forward area and continues to provide movement capability in a timely and integrated process to deliver the casualty to progressively more sophisticated and capable facilities across the echelons of care. The challenge to be met is to ensure that the provision of medical care to the injured soldier remains continuous, capable, and as sophisticated/intense as the ground-based combat medical treatment facilities.

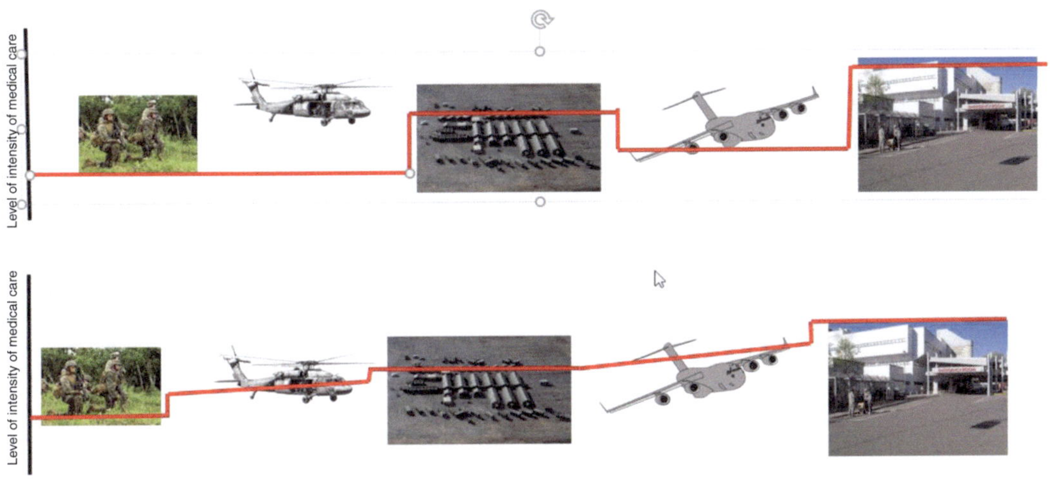

4.2 Development of Critical Care Air Transport Teams

Review of medical care delivery during the First Gulf War (1991) resulted in critical introspection of the capabilities (or lack thereof) of the military health service and its ability to provide medical support for combat operations. Medical doctrine was realigned to emphasize mobility and proximity of surgical support to an increasingly agile and mobile fighting force. Small, mobile surgical teams moved forward to provide surgical stabilization capability in far-forward and austere settings. The proximity and capabilities of these robust surgical support teams (US Army FST, US Navy FRSS, US Air Force MFST) proved themselves capable of salvaging critically injured soldiers with practices such as whole blood transfusion, permissive hypotension, and damage control surgery. The demonstrated lifesaving capabilities of these far-forward teams created a new class of patient, namely, the patient who had been surgically stabilized but was far from medically stable. This new class of patients were those who would have previously died at the point of injury (KIA) or succumbed while en route or at a far-forward battalion aid station. Supporting these critically ill, surgically stabilized patients necessitated either moving ICU resources and capabilities to every far-flung resuscitation team (not logistically or practically possible) or formulating a process capable of moving critically ill patients through time and space in a combat theater of operation. En route care and the US Air Force's Critical Care Air Transport Teams were that answer to this dilemma.

The need for realignment of the abilities of aeromedical evacuation into a more sophisticated and continuous process of en route care was further emphasized during the peacekeeping mission in Mogadishu ("Black Hawk Down"—October 1993). The patient care requirements for a requested long-range aeromedical evacuation of a critically injured soldier from the US Army medical facility in Mogadishu exceeded the capabilities of the assigned Air Force AE crew team. This capability shortfall was recognized on the tarmac of the airfield in Mogadishu and required the surgeon from the Army facility to accompany the patient during the evacuation to Germany. Shortly after this mission departed Mogadishu, the 75th Ranger Regiment became engaged in a firefight that resulted in 18 deaths and 73 wounded while one of the three surgeons assigned to the Army's Mogadishu FST team was en route to Germany. The review of this action drove two key elements of the foundation of modern en route care. The first was to ensure that medical capability of the en route care team could provide critical care support to a stabilized but not necessarily stable patient. The second requirement was that the en route care team had to be self-sustaining with respect to personnel and equipment in order not to strip critical elements of manpower or equipment from the far-forward surgical resuscitation teams.

The US Air Force set about the process of formulating a solution that would address the needs of the dynamically changing AE requirements. The US Air Force is doctrinally responsible for the strategic movement of wounded combatants of all branches. The Critical Care Air Transport (CCAT) Team would be developed as a solution to the perceived capability gaps developed by the changing nature of conflict in the twenty-first century. In past conflicts, AE movement was a process of providing transport with concomitant basic medical support for casualties. The new paradigm challenge facing the CCAT process was to prepare, and assume responsibility for, the provision of uninterrupted intensive care for critically ill soldiers from the furthest forward and austere location to the rearward area(s). The challenge was to ensure that the medical intensity of care never degraded or suffered because of the transport process or environment. It was no longer acceptable to simply ensure the safe transport of the casualty to the next point of care. The challenge was to match the intensity and capability of the far-forward resuscitation surgical teams and continue the process of stabilization and intensive medical care while simultaneously moving the patient across a distance small or great. ICU care was no longer the sole domain of ground-based theater facilities. Now CCAT teams were charged with ensuring the uninterrupted provision of critical care and patient optimization throughout the continuum from point of wounding to return to the Continental United States (CONUS).

The original concept and first CCAT teams were developed in the early 1990s at Wilford Hall Medical Center, San Antonio Texas. The original intent of the teams was to provide effective and capable means of transporting care-eligible active duty, dependent, and retirees from outside civilian ICUs throughout the United States back to Wilford Hall Medical Center. The opportunity to evolve these teams as a key element of the concomitant reengineering of combat medical care capability was recognized by Lt Gen PK Carlton Jr., (USAF/SG retired). Over the next decade, the CCAT process would grow from concept to accepted doctrine under the vigilant leadership of Lt Gen Carlton along with a handful of young AF Medical Service officers.

By November 9, 2001, the CCAT team was a recognized component of the larger AE movement process yet largely an untested concept. Combat operations following 9/11 would be the first large-scale test of the CCAT team(s) and their concept of operations. The initial years of combat casualty care (2001–2004) provided challenges to meet the extremely fluid, dispersed, and varied context of combat medical operations. Medical facilities in the combat zone were varied in size and shape as well as frequently relocating to remain relevant and near the soldiers they were supporting. Initially deployed CCAT teams were positioned at major air hubs such as Landstuhl Regional Medical Center or Al Udeid Air Base (Qatar). CCAT teams would fly "downrange" into theater onboard strategic cargo aircraft and assume responsibility for the stabilization and subsequent return transfer of patients from the forward-deployed facilities. New operational paradigms were developed as combat operations and casualties expanded and as theater medical facilities matured. CCAT teams were forward embedded at the location of major medical facilities in the theater of operations (Balad Air Base Iraq and Bagram Air Base Afghanistan) and subsequently other facilities such as the Navy's hospital in Kandahar Afghanistan. By 2005 a significant number of CCAT teams were deployed to these various facilities within the theater of operations. The forward positioning of CCAT teams provided the advantage of additional critical care personnel at the theater medical facilities as well as a knowledge base of how to prepare and position a critically ill patient in anticipation of a long-range CCAT.

The challenge for the CCAT teams was to ensure and sustain the intensity of medical care (that was being delivered in the forward facilities) throughout the transport process. In some cases, this meant the provision of critical care for a shorter (1–2 h) period during an intra-theater transport onboard a C-130 Hercules cargo plane. In most cases, it meant preparing for, and sustaining care throughout, strategic intercontinental flights from theater (Iraq or Afghanistan) to Landstuhl Regional Medical Center in Germany. The mission profile was flown onboard various cargo aircrafts such as the C-141 (now retired from inventory), the C-130, the C-17, or the KC-135 tanker. The missions were usually accomplished at night, and the duration of each mission often extended into the range of 8–12 h. Over the course of combat operations, the time window to CCAT movement would be increasingly shortened as trauma medical care and capabilities became increasingly practiced. By 2006 it was common for a wounded casualty to undergo one to two surgical stabilization procedures in theater and subsequently be transported to Germany within a 30–36 h period. A ten year review of CCATT team activity during OIF/OEF revealed that ninety three percent of all seriously wounded casualties arrived at the Role IV military treatment center in Landstuhl Germany within 72 hours. This is an even more remarkable statistic when one considers that this chain of care usually included one to three surgical procedures in theater (at Role II and Role III facilities) prior to a ten to twelve hour strategic, Critical Care evacuation flight to Germany. [2]

4.3 The CCAT Team

4.3.1 CCAT Team Composition

The current composition of a CCAT team includes a physician, a nurse, and a respiratory therapist. This three-person team may be tasked with caring for up to six critically ill patients including three critically ill patients requiring mechanical ventilation. Although members of the team come from a varied background, emphasis is placed on a collective understanding of all individual roles. This includes mastery of all equipment and a baseline fund of knowledge to ensure redundancy within the group. Each member of the team must have the ability and training to function independently if the physician is not immediately available or if immediate lifesaving interventions are required. This is due to operational realities that the team may have to split for periods of the transport when moving multiple patients. A well-constructed team includes a mix of skill, strong team dynamics, and a high level of situational awareness.

4.3.1.1 Physician

The physician functions as team leader and accepts responsibility for each patient being transported. The CCAT physician role requires critical care capability and is drawn from the specialties of emergency medicine, anesthesia, pulmonary critical care, cardiology, and general surgeons. Regardless of background training, clinical currency in the care of critically ill patients remains essential to provide the degree of support necessary to establish stabilization prior to transport and to perform critical interventions while en route (see training requirements below). In addition to the baseline medical knowledge required, the physician must also maintain operational and situational awareness to anticipate and reduce the occurrence of clinical incidents.

4.3.1.2 Critical Care Nurse

The CCAT nurse fills a vital role in the transport of the critically ill patients and is essential to the team. Most CCAT nurses have experience caring for critically ill patients on a daily basis in some form of ICU setting. This role has also been filled by advanced care nurse practitioners and certified registered nurse anesthetists. The RN must be current in advanced cardiac life support (ACLS); have worked in critical care or special care unit, emergency department, or postanesthesia care unit within 2 years of selection; and have a minimum of 1 year experience. Trauma Nursing Core Course (TNCC) is highly encouraged, but not required.

4.3.1.3 Cardiopulmonary/Respiratory Therapist

The CCAT respiratory therapist (RT) fills the final essential role on the team. This member must have 1 year of critical care experience, receive annual training in an intensive care unit, and must have worked with ventilated patients within the past year to be eligible for participation. The CCAT RT is held to the standard of being an expert with the transport ventilator, understanding all aspects of its functions and operations. In addition to the other roles, the respiratory therapist functions as the "medical mechanic" for the team. This role includes a thorough understanding of all the equipment in the allowance standard to be able to troubleshoot malfunctions smoothly during transport.

CCAT Training Requirements

CCAT training begins with the assumption: that the provider entering the training pipeline is clinically current and competent in the environment and delivery of critical care. The goal of the course is not to develop the existing critical care skill set of the individual but rather to teach the provider how to adapt the clinical skills that they already possess into the context of the en route care environment. The familiarization process begins with recognition that the en route environment is an austere environment where additional capabilities and resources are limited. The en route environment imposes limits upon many normally utilized clinical capabilities, and the impact of these limitations must be recognized, understood, and compensated for by the provider to ensure seamless care for the casualty (see environmental considerations below).

Members who have deployed as CCAT medics utilize the term "situational awareness" to describe the unique challenges posed by the provision of critical care in a remote and often austere environment that traverses many different platforms of care. The term situational awareness originates in the aviation community and refers to the ability of a pilot to maintain a comprehensive appreciation of where the aircraft is with respect to space, time, and energy. The term situational awareness in a medical sense implies the ability of the clinician to constantly assess the patient and their current status regardless of the environmental or situational distractors. A primary focus of the CCAT curricula is to teach the provider to recognize that traditional medical cues and signs utilized in daily bedside care (the tone of an oximeter, auscultation of breath or heart sounds, sufficient light to observe the patient, etc.) are compromised in the environment of care that occurs in the dark, with loud ambient noise and multiple situational distractors. Emphasis is placed on the provider maintaining patient "situational awareness" despite the challenges of a combat environment in the back of an aircraft executing a combat takeoff in a turbulent airspace.

One focus of the CCAT curricula is to develop an ingrained familiarity with the allowance standard (soft goods and medications) as well as patient movement items (equipment). Emphasis is placed upon patient preparation and the ability to anticipate and intervene in physiologic events that may occur because of the patient's preexisting condition or secondary to the rigors of the en route movement. The initial course is standardized across team members and regardless of background medical training. This helps to ensure that CCAT team members can move between teams as operational circumstances dictate. While maintaining the integrity of any single CCATT team is desirable, replacing a member of the team at any time when needed (illness, emergency) assures operational flexibility.

The initial stage of CCAT training consists of the selection process of team members from the various clinical specialties. Members selected are commissioned officers and enlisted personnel from Active Duty (AD), Air National Guard (ANG), or Air Force Reserve Command (AFRC) components of the US Air Force. All members must demonstrate regular participation in the care of critically ill patients. Once chosen, the member must successfully complete two separate courses before being qualified to fly operational CCAT missions.

The *CCAT Initial Course* is a 10-day curricula designed to introduce and prepare providers performing CCAT duties to meet the wartime and peacetime missions of caring for critically ill and injured patients in the aeromedical evacuation environment. The course takes place at the US Air Force School of Aerospace Medicine (USAFSAM) located at Wright-Patterson Air Force Base in Ohio. The focus of the initial course is to acquire an understanding of the aeromedical evacuation environment, as well as gain familiarization with aeromedical evacuation aircraft and the CCAT equipment set. The course also provides and extensive introduction to altitude physiology. Along with a detailed review of the CCAT mission, equipment, and organization, members receive hands-on training in altitude physiology including flights in a hypobaric chamber. Members also receive an introduction to the Joint Trauma System Clinical Practice Guidelines (CPGs) and receive training on how to adapt their baseline clinical skills to both the deployed and en route environment.

The second course is the CCAT Advanced Course which is held at the University of Cincinnati Medical Center in Cincinnati Ohio. The University of Cincinnati Medical Center is home to USAF Cincinnati CSTARS (Center for Sustainment of Trauma and Readiness Skills) and is one of five designated civilian strategic military collaborating hospitals that serve as military trauma training facilities within the United States. The advanced course builds on the concepts introduced at the CCAT Initial Course and further emphasizes core critical care principles routinely encountered in the deployed environment. Didactic portions of the course focus on delivering care in the deployed environment and understanding the treatment goals within the context of the CPGs. Effort is devoted to training to lessons learned from current real-world missions. Students and instructors join in on the weekly video teleconference call from the theater to maintain situational awareness of current operational challenges.

To ensure timely and relevant mission scenarios, the instructor cadre stationed at the University program routinely deploy into theater as part of a continuous deployment model. The CCAT Advanced Course is unique among military courses in terms of its flexibility and ability to rapidly adjust course content to real-world operations. As a clinically focused course, cadre have the discretion to adjust course material to ensure it is reflective of current operations with the aim of optimally preparing students for the deployed environment they are about to enter.

The hallmark of the CCAT Advanced Course is the employment of high-fidelity simulation to immerse teams in training in real-world patient care scenarios. High-fidelity mannequins reside in a training center designed to replicate the cabin of a C-130—complete with low light and aircraft noise. The simulator center and scenarios are intended to provide a realistic and life-like training environment where the provider team must effectively manage challenging clinical scenarios. Over the two-week period of the advanced course, CCAT student teams will spend over 10 h in simulated flights and medical scenarios that emphasize not

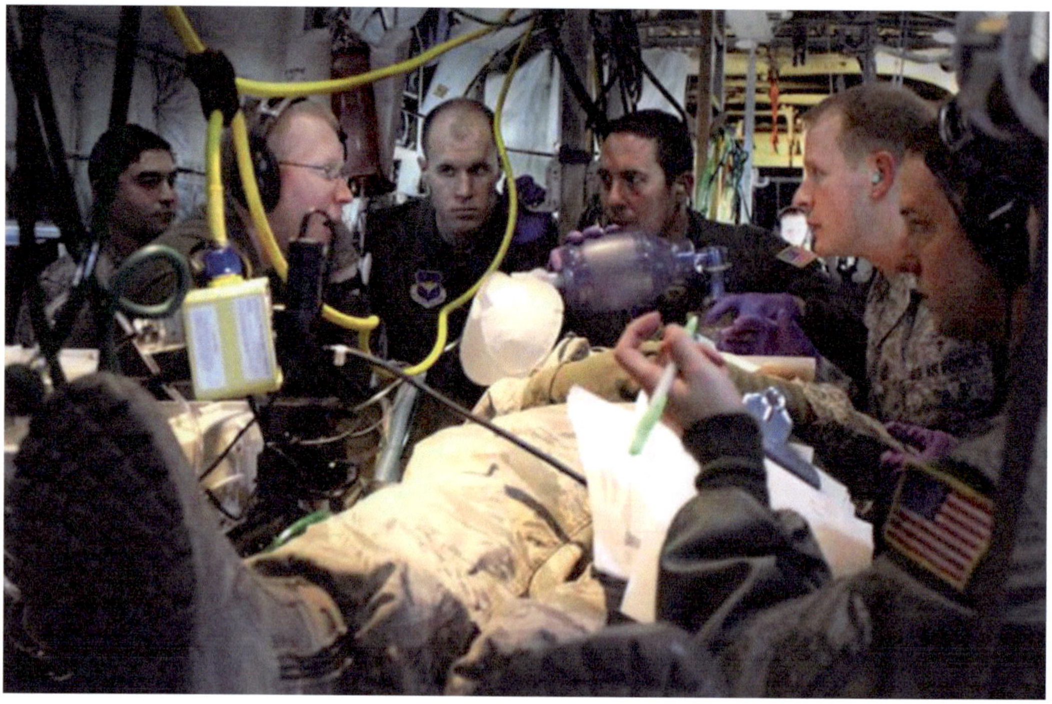

Fig. 4.2 CCAT students and their instructor discuss a patient scenario while in flight onboard a C-130

only medical management but also team building and crew resource management. During the second week, students and their instructors will participate in a full-day scenario that includes transportation of simulated patients by ambulance bus to a nearby airport. Once at the airport, the teams continue to monitor and prepare their patients for fixed-wing evacuation. A C-130 from the Kentucky Air Guard meets the teams at the airport and enplanes the teams and their instructors for a flight modeling a realistic mission profile (3 h) (Fig. 4.2).

The CCAT Advanced Course is categorized by USAFSAM as a validation course. The teams are evaluated in their ability to provide safe and efficient care during these high-fidelity simulated clinical scenarios. Providers who are unable to demonstrate the ability to effectively deliver care in the austere en route environment do not validate the course and are not eligible for deployment as a CCAT provider. The student is given recommendations on opportunities to further develop their skill set and offered the opportunity to participate in a future advanced course. Recurrent training is required to remain qualified for CCAT deployment, and each member is required to attend and validate the CCAT Advanced Course every 36 months.

4.4 CCAT Environmental Considerations

The environmental milieu of combat casualty aeromedical evacuation presents challenges to matching the intensity and precision of critical care in a more fixed facility. As previously asserted, the challenge of the CCAT mission is to ensure that the intensity and quality of critical care delivery remains sustained despite the movement of the patient through space and time onboard an aeromedical evacuation platform. The unique environmental stressors of the en route movement include hypobaria, temperature, noise, vibration, decreased humidity, acceleration forces, and fatigue. Each of these elements may have a significant impact on the mission as well as patient physiology and is described below.

4.4.1 Hypobaria and Hypoxia

One of the most prominent environmental factors influencing aeromedical evacuation remains changes in barometric pressure with increases in altitude and the resultant effect on oxygen delivery and gas expansion. The gas laws most applicable to changes in altitude include Boyle's Law, Henry's Law, and Dalton's Law.

4.4.1.1 Boyle's Law: P1/P2 = V2/V1

This equation relates how a volume of air within a closed space expands with decreases in atmospheric pressure. As an aircraft (or person) ascends in altitude, the experienced surrounding pressure decreases in an exponential fashion. At 18,000 feet, a volume of gas will be approximately doubled the volume as that at sea level. Trapped gasses can affect medical crew, patients, and equipment. The most common sites of trapped gas in healthy individuals are the sinuses, the middle ear, the gastrointestinal tract, and occasionally the teeth. Additional consideration is required for aeromedical evacuation of patients that are critically ill. Patients must be screened for evidence of a pneumothorax which may impact a physiologic response secondary to the expansion of gas at altitude. Air in the GI tract may be more problematic if the patient has an ileus or has had a recent abdominal surgery. Gastric decompression may be required for patients on mechanical ventilation or with evidence of intestinal ileus. Patients with a traumatic brain injury or an ocular injury must be screened for trapped air, as small increases in volume in these fixed compartments can have devastating effects. Gas expansion at altitude also affects medical equipment. For example, ventilators must have altitude compensation to provide accurate tidal volumes and maintain adequate minute ventilation. Additional equipments which require consideration include endotracheal tubes, Foley catheters, and IV solution bags.

4.4.1.2 Henry's Law: P1/P2 = A1/A2

This principle describes how gas dissolved in a solution varies with changes in pressure. For example, the amount of nitrogen dissolved in tissue will decrease and return to a gaseous form with decreases in atmospheric pressure. This most frequently manifests as altitude-induced decompression sickness. Symptoms can vary from mild joint pain and headaches to acute respiratory failure or neurologic dysfunction.

4.4.1.3 Dalton's Law: P = P1 + P2 + P3

This law relates that the total pressure of a gas is equal to the partial pressure of each gas within a mixture. This law explains how decreased atmospheric pressures at altitude contribute to a decrease in the availability of oxygen. For example, oxygen represents 21% of gas at sea level with an atmospheric pressure of 760 mmHg which makes the partial pressure of oxygen 159.6 mmHg. At 10,000 feet, the atmospheric pressure drops to 523 mmHg while the percentage of oxygen remains at 21%, and therefore the partial pressure of oxygen decreases proportionally to 109.8 mmHg. As the partial pressure of oxygen is reduced, diffusion across the alveolar-pulmonary capillary membrane is also reduced and contributes to hypoxia.

Cabin pressurization mitigates the effects of these gas laws to some extent. Most aircrafts pressurize the cabin by drawing in air from the outside, compressing it, and then delivering the compressed air to the cabin. The desired pressure is maintained in the cabin by controlling the flow of compressed air out of the cabin and into the environment. The pressure achieved represents a pressure equivalent to a certain altitude and thus is referred to as the cabin altitude pressure. Cabin altitude pressures fluctuate during the flight but averages range from 6000 to 8000 feet for most of the flight. The ability to further reduce the cabin altitude pressure exists; however, the aircraft must fly at lower altitudes with increased travel times and marked increases in fuel consumption.

The impact of hypobaria on human physiology is reasonably well qualified for certain organ systems such as the gastrointestinal tract, the inner ear, and alveolar oxygen exchange to name a few. Over the course of the last decade, the military has begun to focus medical and basic scientific research to discern if there are potential additional effects of hypobaria on the injured casualty. One of the most notable of these efforts has been studies examining the potential impact of aeromedical flight on the patient with traumatic brain injury. To date the conclusion of these efforts remains unclear but is sure to be a continued area of interest for the CCAT and aeromedical community [3].

4.4.2 Temperature and Humidity

Ambient temperature decreases by approximately 2 °C with each 1000 ft. increase in altitude. Because of this relationship, the temperature in the aircraft can vary widely between the ground and at altitude. Further, depending on the airframe, there may be a significant difference in the cabin temperature from the front (fore) of the aircraft to the back (aft). This can be particularly problematic for critically ill patients with depressed thermoregulatory function. Additionally, critical pieces of equipment (such as blood analysis equipment) often function at an optimal temperature. Extremes of temperature impose an additional environmental stressor that may lead to degradation of human as well as equipment performance or even equipment failure. CCAT teams must monitor temperature closely and protect both the patient and equipment as needed.

As altitude increases, the level of moisture (humidity) in the air decreases significantly. As described above, air for pressurization of the interior of the aircraft is drawn from the surrounding air space. As the aircraft ascends, the humidity of the entrained air for pressurization falls and creates a very low humidity cabin environment. Patients and providers may experience an increase in insensible fluid losses, and dehydration is exacerbated. Consideration should be given to utilization of humidified air for patients who require supplemental oxygen.

4.4.3 Noise, Light, and Vibration

Noise represents a substantial barrier to care of the critically ill patient. Current CCAT platforms are primarily cargo or refueling platforms, and these aircraft do not typically have engine or cabin noise abatement. The engine noise within the cabin of these aircraft often exceeds 80 dB. Hearing protection (earplugs or headsets) are mandatory for all crew members and patients. This level of ambient noise degrades communications both within the team and potentially between the patient and providers. Routine tasks such as auscultation of the lungs for breath sounds become impossible. Team members are taught that frequent visualization of the patient and a reliance on visual alarms are essential since auditory alarms will not be heard or recognized in most cases.

An equally important consideration are the lighting conditions encountered in many missions. During combat support operations, most CCAT movements will occur at night to minimize the potential targeting of the teams or patients. Limited light sources such as red or green head lamps may be used to support visualization of key components or the patient. Takeoff and landings in theater are invariably conducted under light discipline conditions which require a darkened (or dark) environment. The CCAT provider must once again recognize the limitations imposed by these environmental and operational constraints and how they may impact on recognition of standard events routinely noted in a normal ICU environment.

Vibration represents yet another unavoidable environmental condition that may impede patient care during aeromedical evacuation. Vibration may range from barely perceptible (transmitted engine vibration) to life-threatening (evasive maneuvering, turbulence, downdrafts, etc.). The presence of vibration in the cabin applies yet another additive stressor for both the providers and the patient. Vibration can have deleterious effects on the performance of some equipment such as noninvasive blood pressure cuffs and some monitors. Additionally, care must be taken to ensure all equipment is properly secured to avoid damage and potential safety hazards which occur as unsecured medical equipment is transformed into projectiles in the setting of severe maneuvering or turbulence.

4.4.4 Acceleration and Deceleration Forces

Gravitational forces acting on the aircraft during takeoff and landing have implications on critically ill patients that may be negligible for healthy individuals. Transiently, these forces lead to pooling of blood and can influence central hemodynamics. Fluctuations in intracranial pressure have been demonstrated during both takeoff and landing and must be recognized and managed in patients with severe TBI. Attention to these concerns can guide patient positioning and location on the aircraft (Fig. 4.3).

4.5 CCAT Equipment

The safe aeromedical evacuation of critically ill patients requires modern biological monitoring equipment which has been rigorously tested. Prior to being certified as "safe to fly," all CCAT equipment undergoes a rigorous set of testing to ensure that they meet the military standards established for the aeromedical environment. Testing of equipment includes altitude testing (10,000 feet), rapid decompressions, extremes of temperature, as well as exposure to humidity changes and vibration. In addition to the stressors of flight, equipment must be able to function safely in conjunction with radiofrequency transmitting equipment and must not produce electromagnetic interference which can hinder communication and navigation systems. Also, most airframes operate on 110 V of alternating current at 400 Hz in contrast to commercial power which provides 110 V at 60 Hz. Equipment must therefore have long battery life for transport or be capable of converting to the aircraft power source at 400 Hz. Providers must be educated on the power requirements of every device and monitor battery status and reserve during flight.

4.5.1 The Allowance Standard

The equipment utilized by CCAT teams is referred to as the allowance standard.

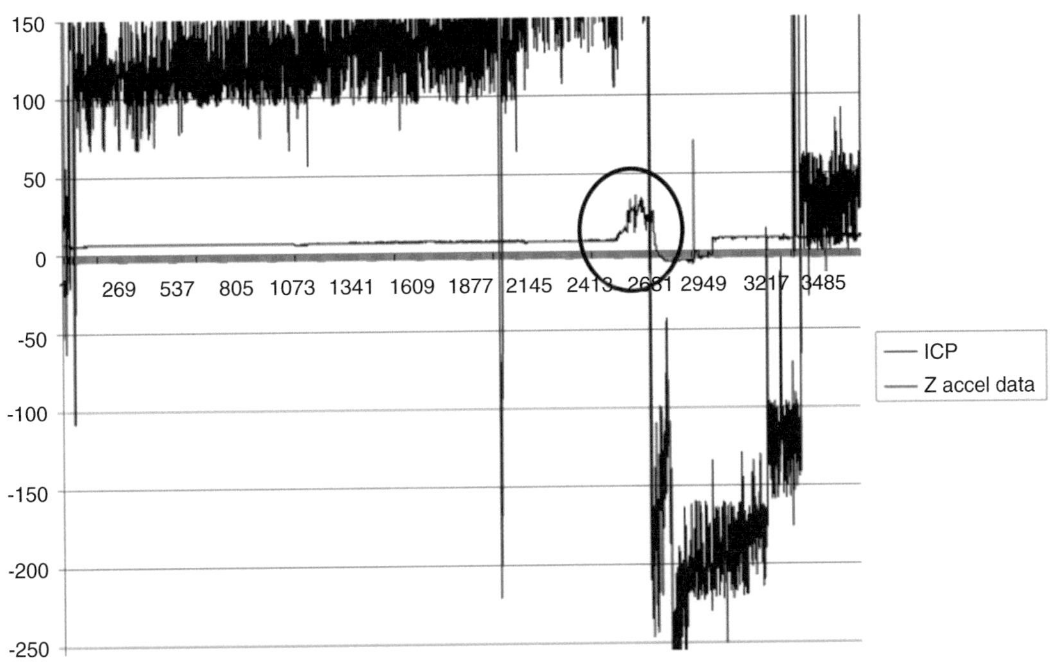

Fig. 4.3 G force (thick line) and ICP (thin line) encountered by traumatic brain injury patient during combat takeoff. The circle highlights a relative increase in intracranial pressure during takeoff

Standardization of equipment and bag sets is critical for CCAT teams to train and deploy effectively. It allows for bag sets to be exchanged between teams or between mission while maintaining confidence in knowing what the team has available and where it is located.

This allowance standard has been modified over time and is currently being deployed in its third version. The approximate weight is 650 lbs. The goal of the allowance standard is to have the capability to care for up to three high-acuity ventilated patients or six lower-acuity stabilized patients for up to 72 h. This includes several commonly used medications, supplies for common procedures (central lines, chest tubes), personal protective equipment, and communication equipment.

4.5.1.1 Patient Movement Items (PMI)

The patient movement items are stored in the gear bag. There are three identical gear bags that contain all the necessary equipment for the transport of a single ventilated patient. While a detailed description of the inventory in each bag is beyond the scope of this chapter, the main pieces of equipment located in the gear bag are described below.

4.6 Propaq MD

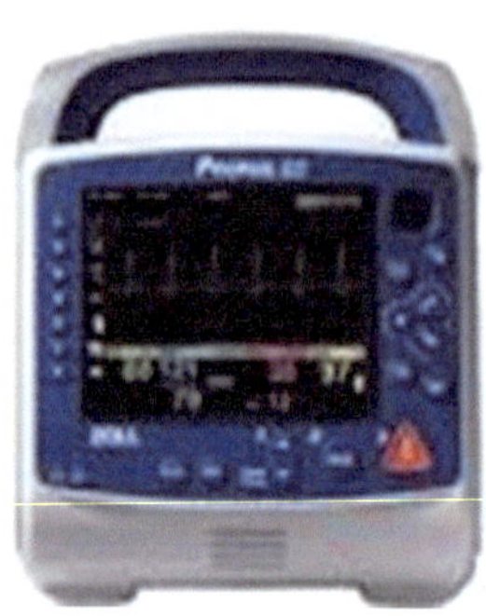

The Zoll Propaq MD combines the Propaq monitor with the Zoll defibrillator and noninvasive pacing technologies. This includes temperature, noninvasive blood pressure monitoring, heart rate, oxygen saturation, and ECG tracing. There are three ports for invasive monitors such as arterial pressure, central venous pressure, and intracranial pressure.

The operating time on battery power is 6 h and the battery requires 4 h to charge to full capacity.

4.7 Impact 731 Ventilator

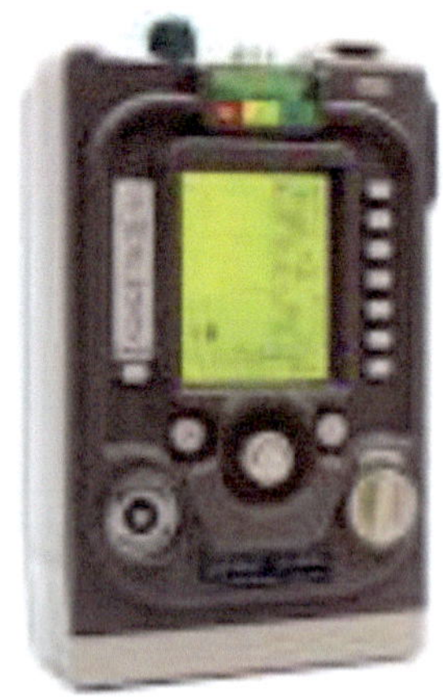

The Impact 731 ventilator by Zoll is the current ventilator utilized for most patient transports. It weighs 9.7 lbs and is capable of multiple modes of ventilation including AC modes (volume control or pressure control), SIMV, and pressure support. It is reported to have a 10 h battery run-time and recharges in 2 h. The 731 ventilator has been utilized in the development of a novel autonomous control of inspired oxygen study that has been funded by the DoD [4]. The FDA has recently (2016) approved an investigative new device exemption study to further evaluate the potential of closed loop control of this device in a deployed setting.

4.7.1 IVAC MedSystem III

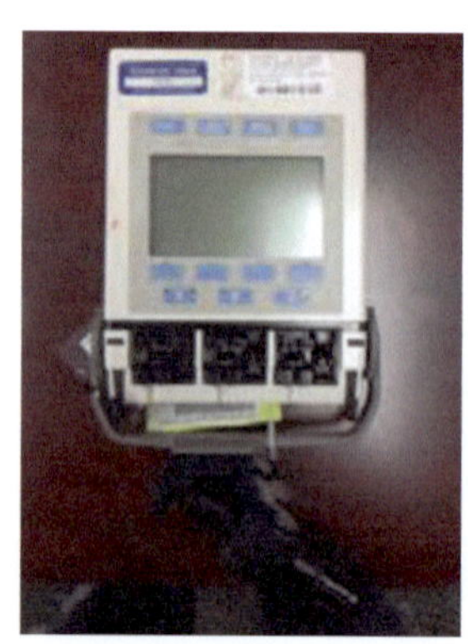

The infusion device currently employed in the allowance standard is the IVAC MedSystem III. It has the capacity for three independent infusion channels. It operates for 6 h on battery power with all three channels running.

4.7.2 Zoll Model 326: Suction Device

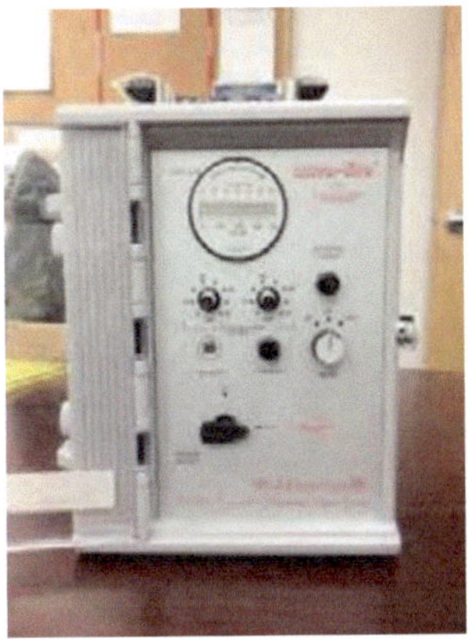

The multifunction aspirator can be used for oropharyngeal and tracheal suctioning as well as provide necessary suction for chest tubes and temporary abdominal closures.

4.8 CCAT Mission Profile

In an effort to understand the primary mission profile of CCAT teams in patient movement during recent conflicts in Iraq (OIF) and Afghanistan (OEF), we must first describe how patients transitioned through five defined "roles" of care at the military treatment facility (MTF). They are listed as:

- Role I—Self-aid and buddy care
- Role II—Battalion aid station or forward surgical team
- Role III—Combat support hospital
- Role IV—Established MTF outside of the theater of operations
- Role V—Military treatment facility in the United States

As described, CCAT teams were designed to care for the "stabilized" (but not necessarily stable) patient. Patients were "stabilized" at the Role II and Role III facilities as defined by four specific criteria. First, the casualty must have a stable or definitively established airway. The term "stabilized" also assumes that all fractures have been immobilized, active hemorrhage controlled, and resuscitation initiated. CCAT teams were deployed to the Role III hospitals within the theater of operations so that they could be quickly activated if patients required movement through the aeromedical evacuation system. With the robust trauma system present in OEF/OIF, CCAT teams could utilize the resources of the Role III hospital before prolonged inter-theater transport to include obtaining further medications from the pharmacy as well as blood products to further increase the capabilities of the base allowance standard. Standard missions of CCAT teams included (Figs. 4.4 and 4.5):

- Intra-theater Role II to Role III missions, primarily on C-130s by teams based at the deployed Role III
- Inter-theater Role III to Role IV missions, primarily on C-17s by teams either based at the deployed Role III or teams located at the Role IV
- Inter-theater Role IV to Role V missions, primarily on C-17s by teams based at the Role IV hospital

4.9 Tactical Critical Care Evacuation Team

With the success of safe patient movement by CCAT teams during OEF and OIF, efforts were made to utilize the skills of critical care providers in a further forward environment of patient movement. The concept of joint en route care was designed by the Army and Air Force to have a greater ability to provide critical care to the patient in this far-forward environment. The Air Force developed the Tactical Critical Care Evacuation Team (TCCET) in response to this

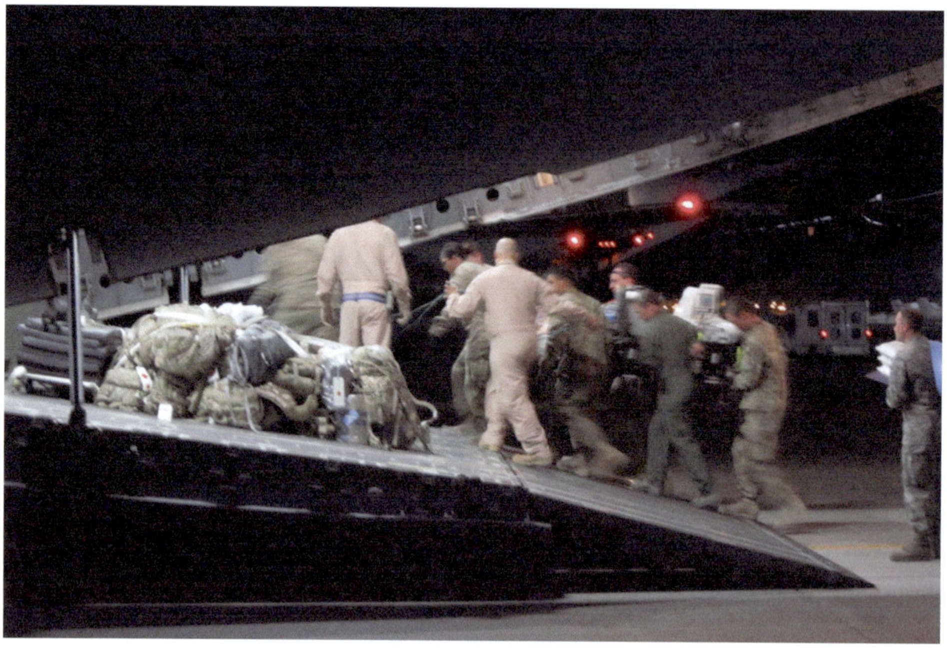

Fig. 4.4 Onloading of CCAT patient to C-17 Globemaster during night operations

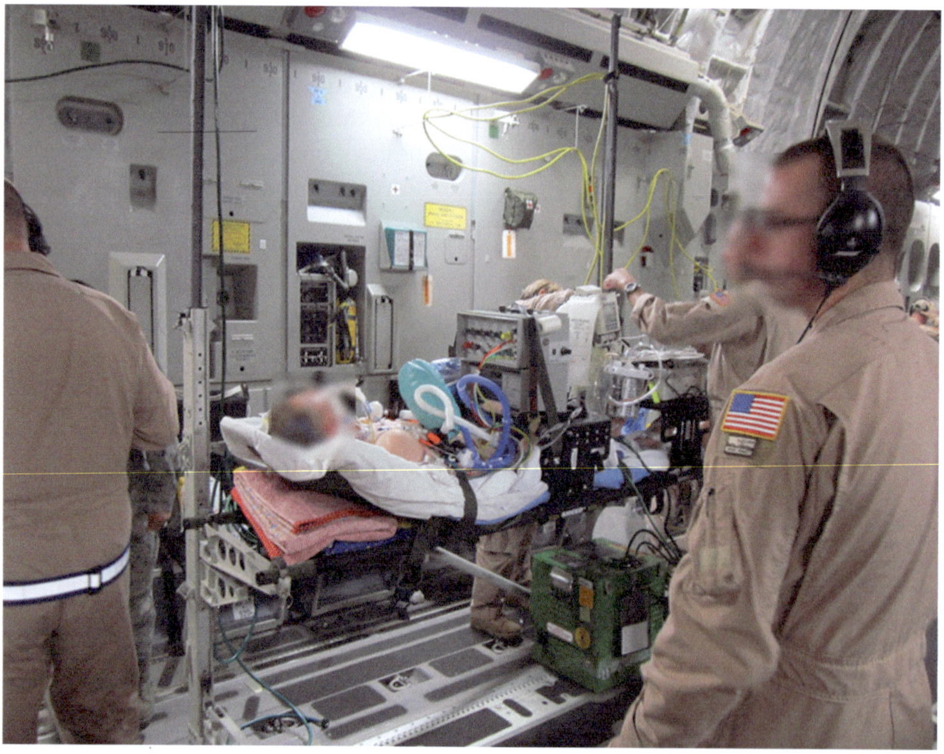

Fig. 4.5 CCAT patient in patient care stanchion prior to takeoff

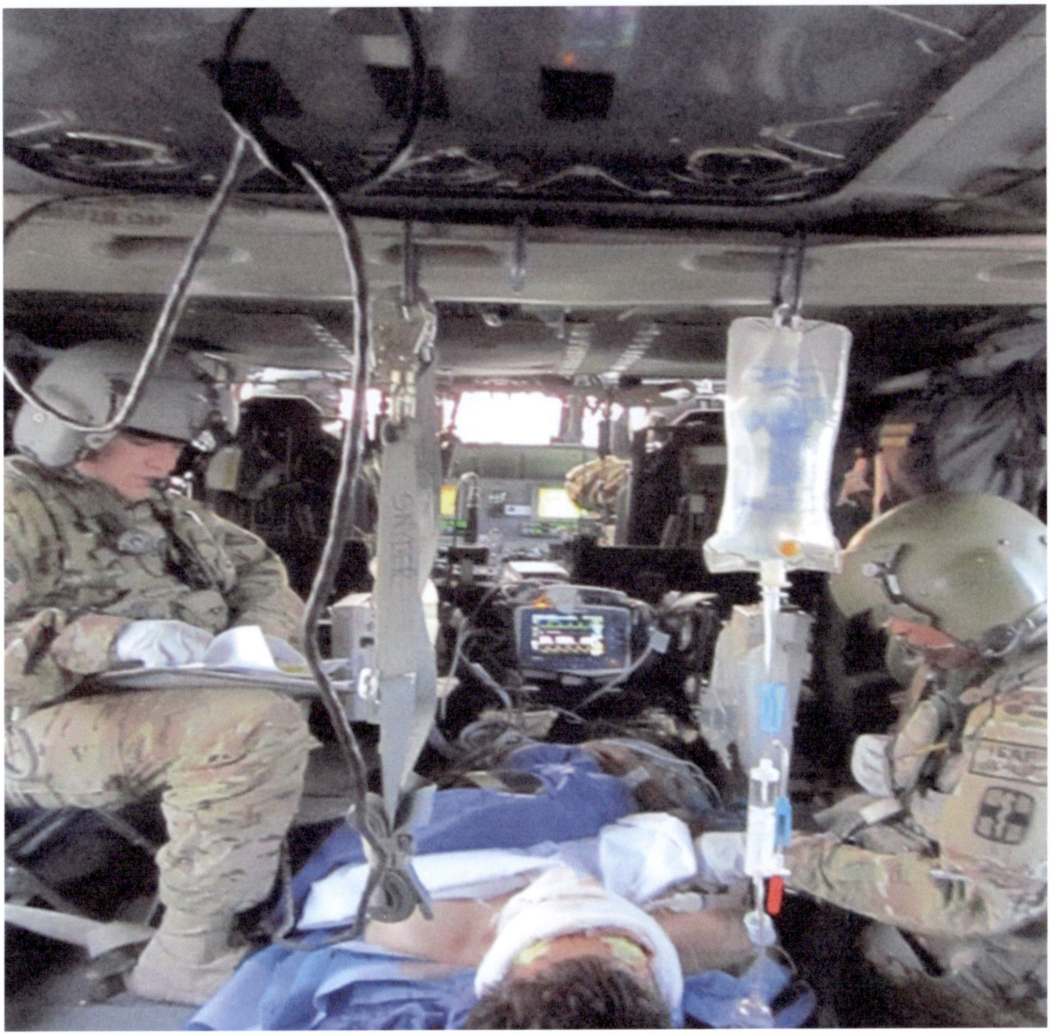

Fig. 4.6 Typical configuration in rotary-wing cabin for TCCET transport (authors picture)

need. The TCCET consist of an ER or critical care physician, a certified registered nurse anesthetists (CRNA), and an ER or critical care nurse. The allowance standard is reduced to three bags, and the aircraft used are usually rotary-wing airframes or C-130s. The focus of their mission is to treat immediately life-threatening conditions, control compressible hemorrhage, and initiate the resuscitation during transportation at or very near the point of injury. These teams increased critical care capability in the POI to Role II and Role II to Role III phases of patient movement (Fig. 4.6).

4.10 Future Considerations

The CCATT community faces two major challenges when considering future operational environments. The first is supporting small, remote surgical/medical teams outside of a robust trauma system when no combat support hospital exists to prepare the patient for long-distance evacuation. The joint trauma system present during OEF/OIF and the relatively large medical footprint in those theaters of operation allowed for practice patterns to develop within CCAT that may not be possible in future operations. The advanced capabilities and holding capacity of Role III hospitals in Iraq and Afghanistan permitted for greater discretion in determining if a patient was ideally stabilized for inter-theater transport. The expected attention to pre-mission stabilization and optimization of the patient physiology for en route care that the Role III hospitals provided may not be present in future conflicts. Due to limits in capability (i.e., dialysis, neurosurgical capability, etc.) or resources (size of holding capacity), CCAT teams must prepare for managing less "stabilized" patients as the medical footprint decreases in size and more austere surgical teams are positioned throughout the globe. While CCAT teams have certainly moved less stabilized patients from Role II to Role III facilities, these have typically been short-duration intra-theater missions. As more austere surgical teams without a supporting Role III facility become the norm, these less stabilized patients will occur more frequently and require longer mission times to a higher level of medical capability. This environment will further test the resuscitative capabilities of CCAT teams.

An emerging consideration is for CCAT teams to be prepared to respond to situations where there is no medical capability at the destination site. CCAT teams are doctrinally beginning to prepare for the potential of caring for critically wounded casualties that have had limited pre-transport surgical stabilization. The potential for prolonged evacuation distances with limited on-ground surgical capability has led to the development of en route surgical teams which are embedded with, or blended into, an extended CCAT mission team. As this surgical capability continues to evolve, the support of critical care to the en route surgical team by CCAT is critical to ensuring ICU-level capability.

The transition from the height of operations during OEF/OIF to decreased medical ground resources is already taking place and the CCATT community is actively adapting to this new state. Ultrasound has recently been added to the diagnostic tools available to CCAT teams to help enhance the ability to care for the less stabilized patient. The CCAT Advanced Course continuously adjusts clinical tabletop discussions to real-world mission-based clinical scenarios, thus giving students exposure to the "new-normal" mission. These prolonged Role II transports have also been added to high-fidelity simulation scenarios. The CCAT allowance standard is also regularly reviewed and updated, ensuring the bag-set meets the needs of deployed teams as the CCAT mission continues to evolve.

Conclusion

Throughout the first 10 years of conflict from September 11, 2001 through 2010, 2899 patients were transported by CCAT teams as part of Operation Iraqi Freedom and Operation Enduring Freedom. This experience was recently reviewed and demonstrated the following:

One of the most noteworthy findings of this inquiry is that 93% of all CCAT patients (representing the most grievously injured combat casualties of this conflict) arrived at LRMC within 72 hours of wounding. Equally remarkable is the finding that 98.5% of all critically wounded soldiers were at LRMC by the 96-hour mark. The documented success and attendant minimal mortality of movement of CCAT patients within hours of surgery represent a paradigm shift for trauma surgeons and trauma surgery doctrine. The overall 30-day mortality for all patients transported by CCATs is 2.1%, and the transport mortality en route is well less than 1% despite the transport of significantly injured combat casualties (mean ISS, 23.7). This historically low mortality rate is a tribute to and reflection of the dedication of the entire chain of survival established by the military and its medical corps. The chain of survival begins with the medic providing care under fire and continues until the casualty is returned to home station, family, and community.

This low mortality rate speaks to the success of the AE "system" that enters a patient into the movement system, determines when a patient is safe to fly, and links an available aircraft/mission to an AE crew and CCAT team. This system involves multiple checks involving the current medical providers, local and theater flight surgeons, receiving providers, and transporting teams all aimed at ensuring patient safety. As successful as this aeromedical evacuation system has been, new expectations and standards now exist. Through constant evolution in training and equipment, the CCAT community remains ready to meet the challenge of moving our most critically injured warriors anywhere in the world, anytime.

Disclaimer We are pleased to participate in the publication of this important work by contributing this chapter regarding Enroute Care. The authors have been asked to contribute similar contributions to many other publications over the past twelve months. In preparation for this chapter the authors began from their text of a similar contribution to Eastridge et al (citation). This chapter has been edited in its entirety, and, as appropriate, updated.

References

1. Lam DM. To pop a balloon: aeromedical evacuation in the 1870 siege of Paris. Aviat Space Environ Med. 1988;59:988–91.
2. Ingalls N, Zonies D, Bailey J, Martin K, Iddins B, Carlton PK, Hanseman D, Branson R, Dorlac W, Johannigman J. A review of the first 10 years of critical care aeromedical transport during Operation Iraqi Freedom and Operation Enduring Freedom: the importance of evacuation timing. JAMA Surg. 2014;149(8):807–13.
3. Goodman MD, Makley AT, Lentsch AB, Barnes SL, Dorlac GR, Dorlac WC, Johannigman JA, Pritts TA. Traumatic brain injury and aeromedical evacuation: when is the brain fit to fly? J Surg Res. 2010;164:286–93.
4. Johannigman JA, Branson R, Lecroy D, Beck G. Autonomous control of inspired oxygen concentration during mechanical ventilation of the critically injured trauma patient. J Trauma. 2009;66(2):386–92.

Adaptation of Military Damage Control in Civilian Settings

5

Kelly A. Fair and Martin A. Schreiber

Abstract

Damage control techniques originated during battlefield experience millennia ago. In the early twentieth century, damage control was utilized to limit hemorrhage from liver injuries. Since then damage control has evolved to include damage control surgery and damage control resuscitation in the military setting, which has been translated and integrated into civilian trauma and emergency general surgery practice. Application of damage control techniques in the military and civilian settings has been studied extensively. Damage control resuscitation in particular has made rapid and marked progress in the past 20 years. Hemostatic resuscitation became common practice in the military during modern Iraq and Afghanistan conflict. This led to application and study in the civilian setting. Differences between military and civilian settings include austere military environments, limited resources, and complex evacuation requirements. Future application of damage control in the civilian setting requires integration and collaboration between the military and civilian sectors.

Abbreviations

DC	Damage control
DCR	Damage control resuscitation
DCS	Damage control surgery
OEF/OIF	Operation Iraqi Freedom/Operation Enduring Freedom
PROMMTT	Prospective, Observational, Multicenter, Major Trauma Transfusion
PROPPR	Pragmatic Randomized Optimal Platelet and Plasma Ratios

5.1 Introduction

5.1.1 Defining Damage Control Techniques

The principle of damage control originated from a navy term used to describe the "capacity of a ship to absorb damage and maintain mission integrity" [1]. The term "damage control" as it applies to surgical and trauma patients was coined by Rotondo in 1993 in a population of patients with penetrating abdominal trauma. This series described initial control of hemorrhage and

K.A. Fair, M.D. (✉)
Division of Trauma, Critical Care, and Acute Care Surgery, Oregon Health and Science University, Portland, OR, USA
e-mail: fair@ohsu.edu

M.A. Schreiber, M.D. (✉)
Division of Trauma, Critical Care and Acute Care Surgery, School of Medicine, Oregon Health and Science University, Portland, OR, USA
e-mail: schreibm@ohsu.edu

J. Duchesne et al. (eds.), *Damage Control in Trauma Care*,
https://doi.org/10.1007/978-3-319-72607-6_5

contamination and application of damage control resuscitation, with a markedly improved survival of 77% compared to 11% in patients undergoing definitive laparotomy [2]. Since then, damage control neurosurgery, orthopedic surgery, thoracic, and vascular techniques have been described [3–5].

In practice, damage control is a strategy for management of patients with critical injuries and physiologic derangements which aims to:

- Rapidly address life threatening hemorrhage and gastrointestinal soilage following injury.
- Prevent and treat the lethal triad of hypothermia, acidosis, and coagulopathy via resuscitation, blood product transfusion, and rewarming.
- Return to the operating room for definitive treatment when the patient is stable [6–9].

Damage control resuscitation (DCR) is a multifaceted approach which includes limiting hemorrhage in the field with the use of tourniquets and hemostatic dressings [10, 11]. Avoidance of high volume crystalloid resuscitation aims to limit dilutional coagulopathy, exacerbation of acidosis by avoiding solutions containing high chloride concentrations, and secondary abdominal compartment syndrome [12, 13]. Hemostatic resuscitation is a DCR strategy which provides 1:1:1 transfusion ratios of red blood cells (RBC) to plasma to platelets that is associated with reduced mortality in trauma patients [14–16].

5.2 History of Damage Control

Damage control techniques in their current state have evolved through decades of military experience and application to civilian circumstances. The first damage control techniques originated on the battlefield. As early as 400 B.C., Hippocrates described soldiers exsanguinating from extremity wounds who underwent lifesaving amputation [17, 18]. In 1908, Pringle described measures to treat traumatic liver injuries, including use of packs to control hemorrhage [19]. In the 1980s, Stone et al. described the success of initial laparotomy, packing for hemorrhage control and arrest of the planned procedure, correction of coagulopathy, and return to the operating room for completion of the planned surgical procedure [20–22].

Historically, innovations in the care of trauma patients have been born from wartime experiences. Limited resources, unpredictable conditions, and prolonged evacuation times characteristic of the battlefield have promoted ingenuity in the development of new techniques, and many of these techniques are then applied to the civilian setting. Advancements in trauma care borne from military experience have been well recognized in the trauma literature [11, 23–25]. The past decade has seen the longest period of military conflict in American history, and this period in particular has led to important battlefield innovations including modern damage control techniques [11]. Advances in care of military patients have been promoted by military investment of trauma research through the development of the Department of Defense Joint Trauma System and trauma registry [11, 24].

As treatment of war-related injuries has evolved, mortality rates have improved. Though modern combat is associated with more destructive and complex injuries, the lethality associated with injuries sustained in the war in Iraq is the lowest in history at just 9.1% [26, 27]. In contrast, the rate of mortality in the Revolutionary War exceeded 40%. Death rates decreased to 24% by the Vietnam era, though most deaths occurred before the injured were able to be treated in a field hospital [28].

A study of deaths in patients treated in military forward combat hospitals in Iraq and Afghanistan using the Joint Theater Trauma Registry (JTTR) compared outcomes prior to implementation of damage control resuscitation (DCR) and after implementation of DCR in 2006. Patients treated with DCR were found to receive significantly less crystalloid, as well as more fresh frozen plasma. The ratio of PRBC to FFP shifted from 2.6:1 pre-DCR to 1.4:1 post-DCR. This was associated with a decrease in deaths among potentially salvageable patients [29].

5.3 Translation to Civilian Settings

5.3.1 Unique Challenges in Military and Combat Damage Control

The evolution of military damage control has led to advancements in the care of civilians, and damage control is currently considered the standard of civilian trauma care. While both military and civilian damage control measures are aimed at rapid assessment and control of injury to facilitate stabilization prior to definitive surgical intervention, there are critical differences. Combat damage control poses several unique challenges related to austere conditions, lack of resources, and unique injury patterns. Injured patients may require transport across thousands of miles to reach definitive care.

5.3.2 Character of Injuries

Most injuries during modern military conflict, including Operation Iraqi Freedom/Operation Enduring Freedom (OEF/OIF), are related to high-powered explosive devices, rockets, and mortars (55%) or automatic rifles [27, 30]. Injuries may be characterized by blunt, penetrating, and burn mechanisms simultaneously [28]. The majority of combat-related deaths are not survivable. Deaths in this setting result primarily from truncal hemorrhage (67%) and junctional hemorrhage (19%) [26]. Conversely, civilians are more likely to sustain blunt mechanisms of injury or penetrating injuries from handguns or knife wounds [30]. Improvised explosive devices have led to extensive shrapnel injuries and an unprecedented burden of mangled limbs with severe soft tissue, neurovascular, and bony injuries requiring extensive and complex soft tissue debridement, amputation, and wound care [28].

Schreiber et al. compared patients treated at a combat support hospital in Iraq from 2004 to 2005 with those treated at a level I trauma center in the United States. Patients treated at the CSH were more likely to be injured by high-powered penetrating mechanisms (62% explosions), while civilians were more likely to be injured by blunt mechanisms (33% motor vehicle collision, 24% falls, and 19% motorcycle/bicycle collision). Patients treated at the CSH were also more likely to require soft tissue procedures compared to those in the civilian setting. Despite these differences, mortality was similar among both civilian (6.1%) and combat (6.9%) patients [31].

Sambasivan et al. investigated outcomes of damage control procedures in a combat setting and at a US level I trauma center. In their series, military patients experienced mostly high-powered explosion-related penetrating trauma (96%), similar to other literature [27, 30–32]. Patients in the civilian setting experienced blunt trauma more frequently (83%). Patients treated in the military setting required more thoracic operations, skin and soft tissue operations, and more serial wound debridements. While patients in both settings had similar transfusion requirements, patients in the combat setting received whole blood, while those in the civilian setting did not. Regarding outcomes, there was no difference in the rate of abdominal closure after damage control 7 days after injury in both groups nor any difference in mortality [32].

5.3.3 Resources and Transport

Perhaps one of the most notable differences between military and civilian damage control is the austere environment in which military damage control is performed. Civilian environments are replete with skilled personnel, ancillary staff, radiology, and laboratory services. Modern civilian trauma systems such as the United States are composed of a network of hospitals and transfer systems. Much care of complex traumatic injuries occurs at well-equipped level I trauma centers, with most or all care occurring within a single facility. Required resources and transfer criteria are defined by the American College of Surgeons [32, 33].

Conversely, initial damage control in the modern military setting is accomplished by forward surgical teams (FST) equipped to follow troops as a mobile functioning hospital. Forward surgical teams were first utilized by the military in the 1990 Panama conflict with the goal of providing damage control to a small number of patients closer to the point of initial injury [23]. While an FST is able to provide rapid care and damage control of patients on the battlefield, resources are limited, as an FST does not include radiography, angiography, or means for long-term patient support [28]. Forward surgical teams serve to accomplish the same initial goals of damage control: limiting hemorrhage and contamination, rapid closure, and avoidance of the lethal triad of hypothermia, acidosis, and coagulopathy while in a remote environment [2, 6, 7, 34].

Combat damage control is a more prolonged and complex endeavor, requiring multiple stages. Patients sustaining injuries on the battlefield are initially cared for by the FST. Damage control begins with initial resuscitation and abbreviated operation to control bleeding and gastrointestinal soilage. FSTs (military level II) have limited resources for ongoing resuscitation. Most units have 20–50 units of packed red blood cells, and some carry fresh frozen plasma. Minimal acceptable resuscitation goals aim to divide the limited number of units available among the maximum number of patients. Combat damage control patients require evacuation to combat support hospitals (CSH), which are considered military level III. CSHs have additional resources such as X-ray, fluoroscopy, and computed tomography. Damage control patients undergo additional resuscitation and second look operations at the CSH. When stable, patients are then evacuated to a level IV center such as Landstuhl Regional Medical Center in Germany (American College of Surgeons level II trauma center). Those requiring long-term care and rehabilitation are transported to a military level V center in the United States [28, 33].

5.3.4 The Development of Damage Control Resuscitation and Its Application to Civilians

Recent military conflict in Iraq and Afghanistan has led to a profound paradigm shift in the resuscitation of injured patients. As transfusion practice shifted away from whole blood transfusion and toward component therapy, recognition of the risks of transfusion and excessive use of crystalloid led to development of hemostatic resuscitation [6, 35, 36]. Hemostatic resuscitation was studied extensively in combat settings during the Iraq and Afghanistan wars.

Borgman demonstrated improved survival and decreased death from hemorrhage in 246 patients receiving a massive transfusion with a high ratio of plasma to RBCs treated at a US Army combat support hospital [14]. Similarly, Spinella studied patients with combat-related injuries receiving at least one unit of product transfusion. Each unit of FFP was independently associated with improved survival, while each unit of RBC was associated with decreased survival [16].

Military surgeons soon adopted DCR practice in the civilian setting. Demonstration of improved survival in military patients receiving hemostatic resuscitation led to study in civilians. Campion et al. implemented a military DCR strategy in 2007 at a civilian trauma center. The authors found that patients received more plasma and platelets and less crystalloid after implementation of the DCR strategy. Furthermore, this was associated with less acute hypoxia in trauma patients undergo operative intervention and receiving a massive transfusion (greater than 10 units PRBC) [37].

The Prospective, Observational, Multicenter, Major Trauma Transfusion (PROMMTT) study examined outcomes and transfusion practices in ten level I trauma centers. Patients in this study did not receive constant ratios of plasma:RBC nor platelet:RBC in the first 24 h of their resuscitation. However, increased ratios of plasma:RBC were independently associated with decreased 6-h mortality, when death was more likely due to hemorrhage [38, 39].

The Pragmatic, Randomized Optimal Platelet and Plasma Ratios (PROPPR) trial sought to examine the outcomes associated with 1:1:1 vs. 1:1:2 ratios of plasma, platelets, and red blood cells. No significant differences in 24-h or 30-day mortality were observed. However, patients receiving a hemostatic 1:1:1 achieved earlier hemostasis and fewer experienced death due to exsanguination at 24 h [40].

To determine the extent to which civilian trauma systems have adopted damage control techniques, Haider et al. surveyed trauma medical directors at level I–III trauma centers in the United States. A large majority (82%) of trauma medical directors stated that military data supporting damage control resuscitation (DCR) has led to changes in civilian practice at their institutions. Of those surveyed, 68% stated they were most likely to use a 1:1:1 ratio of packed red blood cells to fresh frozen plasma to platelet transfusion and had a written massive transfusion protocol in place.

Extensive combat experience has led to damage control resuscitation practices highlighting hemostatic 1:1:1 transfusion goals. Hemostatic resuscitation has been extensively studied after its implementation in OEF/OIF, and its favorable outcomes led to application and study in the civilian setting. PROPPR was a prospective, randomized phase 3 trial of hemostatic resuscitation in civilians, which confirmed both safety of increased use of plasma and platelets and also increased hemostasis and decreased death from hemorrhage in patients receiving 1:1:1 resuscitation.

5.3.5 Damage Control Surgery in the Civilian Setting

Much of damage control surgery, like damage control resuscitation, has originated from wartime experience. Indications for damage control surgery in civilians are similar to those for military patients. Indications for damage control surgery in civilians include inability to control bleeding by conventional methods; use of large volume resuscitation or inability to close the abdomen due to visceral edema or signs of abdominal compartment syndrome, ongoing hypothermia, acidosis, or coagulopathy; and complex injury patterns such as hepatobiliary or pancreatic injuries [20, 41, 42]. Use of damage control resuscitation practices in civilians results in improved survival in patients undergoing DCR [43].

5.3.6 Special Circumstances in Civilian Populations

5.3.6.1 Remote Damage Control Resuscitation

Application of military damage control to urban civilian settings has been widespread. However, several civilian circumstances may approximate military environments more accurately due to remote environments. Austere civilian environments are situations in which the use of damage control may be particularly useful. Examples of austere civilian environments include both rural and maritime settings.

The demonstrated survival benefit and greater likelihood of achieving hemostasis in PROPPR highlight the need to address prehospital product transfusion, as well as alternative options such as whole blood and lyophilized plasma [44]. In civilian maritime environments, severe hemorrhage can be a major event. Ships may be greater than 24 h from a port, and operative intervention is usually not an option. This has led to the development of a whole blood transfusion program. Though this is not accepted by the FDA, many ships proceed with this practice in international waters when treating patient in extremis [45].

5.3.6.2 Damage Control in Emergency General Surgery

As the acute care surgery model has developed, the use of damage control surgery and resuscitation in civilian patients has expanded. The acute care surgery model often includes care of trauma and non-trauma general surgeries and surgical critical care patients by a trauma/critical care surgeon [46]. This has led to application of trauma damage control techniques to non-trauma emergency general surgery patients. A series of emergency general surgery patients with gastrointestinal sepsis, intra-abdominal hemorrhage, and necrotizing pancreatitis demonstrated benefit from application of damage control measures to this population, including a trend toward a lower mortality rate. Similar to other literature, there was a high rate of abdominal infectious complications including fistula (44%) and abscess (33%) [47, 48].

5.4 Future Directions

A major barrier to implementation of damage control practices in civilian settings includes lack of research regarding its outcomes. Haider stressed that civilian surgeons were more likely to adopt damage control resuscitation owing to its extensive study in both military and civilian populations but were less likely to adopt other interventions such as tourniquet use or use of hemostatic agents [11].

This highlights the need for collaboration between military and civilian surgeons. Cancio emphasized the important link between civilian and military combat research and spread of information regarding damage control resuscitation via attendance at scientific meetings [49]. Multiple authors have advocated for integration of military and civilian training programs to facilitate maintenance of military surgeon skills and education during peacetime [50–53].

Finally, the Health and Medicine Division of the National Academy of Sciences described the great advancements in military and civilian trauma care during the wars in Iraq and Afghanistan, as well as the need for future collaboration and research:

> *Trauma care advances were driven by an urgency to save lives that precluded reliance on slow and costly clinical trials to inform improvements in trauma care practices and drove the Military Health System and its emerging Joint Trauma System to embrace a more agile approach to advancing both combat casualty care and a culture of continuous performance improvement. This learning approach aligns remarkably with the attributes of a learning health system, in which data from each care experience are captured and care practices evolve incrementally and pragmatically based on the best available evidence.*
> *However, sustaining needed expertise and capacity in the military trauma care system is simply impossible absent integration with civilian trauma care systems, given the essential role of the civilian sector in facilitating combat-relevant research and providing training opportunities for the military trauma care workforce.* [54]

Acknowledgments The authors would like to thank the staff of the Trauma Research Laboratory at Oregon Health & Science University.

References

1. Defense Do. U.S. Navy Surface ship survivability. Washington, D.C.; 1996. P. 3–20.
2. Rotondo MF, Schwab CW, McGonigal MD, Phillips GR, Fruchterman TM, Kauder DR, et al. 'Damage control': an approach for improved survival in exsanguinating penetrating abdominal injury. J Trauma. 1993;35(3):375–82. discussion 82-3
3. Rosenfeld JV. Damage control neurosurgery. Injury. 2004;35(7):655–60.
4. Wall MJ, Villavicencio RT, Miller CC, Aucar JA, Granchi TA, Liscum KR, et al. Pulmonary tractotomy as an abbreviated thoracotomy technique. J Trauma. 1998;45(6):1015–23.
5. Hildebrand F, Giannoudis P, Kretteck C, Pape HC. Damage control: extremities. Injury. 2004;35(7):678–89.
6. Schreiber MA. The beginning of the end for damage control surgery. Br J Surg. 2012;99(Suppl 1):10–1.
7. Moore EE. Thomas G. Orr Memorial Lecture. Staged laparotomy for the hypothermia, acidosis, and coagulopathy syndrome. Am J Surg. 1996;172(5):405–10.
8. Cosgriff N, Moore EE, Sauaia A, Kenny-Moynihan M, Burch JM, Galloway B. Predicting life-threatening coagulopathy in the massively transfused trauma patient: hypothermia and acidoses revisited. J Trauma. 1997;42(5):857–61. discussion 61-2
9. Kashuk JL, Moore EE, Millikan JS, Moore JB. Major abdominal vascular trauma--a unified approach. J Trauma. 1982;22(8):672–9.
10. Galante JM, Smith CA, Sena MJ, Scherer LA, Tharratt RS. Identification of barriers to adaptation of battlefield technologies into civilian trauma in California. Mil Med. 2013;178(11):1227–30.
11. Haider AH, Piper LC, Zogg CK, Schneider EB, Orman JA, Butler FK, et al. Military-to-civilian translation of battlefield innovations in operative trauma care. Surgery. 2015;158(6):1686–95.
12. Bickell WH, Wall MJ, Pepe PE, Martin RR, Ginger VF, Allen MK, et al. Immediate versus delayed fluid resuscitation for hypotensive patients with penetrating torso injuries. N Engl J Med. 1994;331(17):1105–9.
13. Balogh Z, McKinley BA, Cocanour CS, Kozar RA, Valdivia A, Sailors RM, et al. Supranormal trauma resuscitation causes more cases of abdominal compartment syndrome. Arch Surg. 2003;138(6):637–42. discussion 42-3
14. Borgman MA, Spinella PC, Perkins JG, Grathwohl KW, Repine T, Beekley AC, et al. The ratio of blood products transfused affects mortality in patients receiving massive transfusions at a combat support hospital. J Trauma. 2007;63(4):805–13.
15. Holcomb JB, Wade CE, Michalek JE, Chisholm GB, Zarzabal LA, Schreiber MA, et al. Increased plasma and platelet to red blood cell ratios improves outcome in 466 massively transfused civilian trauma patients. Ann Surg. 2008;248(3):447–58.

16. Spinella PC, Perkins JG, Grathwohl KW, Beekley AC, Niles SE, McLaughlin DF, et al. Effect of plasma and red blood cell transfusions on survival in patients with combat related traumatic injuries. J Trauma. 2008;64(2 Suppl):S69–77. discussion S-8
17. Stansbury LG, Branstetter JG, Lalliss SJ. Amputation in military trauma surgery. J Trauma. 2007;63(4):940–4.
18. Kinch KJ, Clasper JC. A brief history of war amputation. J R Army Med Corps. 2011;157(4):374–80.
19. Pringle JHV. Notes on the arrest of hepatic hemorrhage due to trauma. Ann Surg. 1908;48(4):541–9.
20. Stone HH, Strom PR, Mullins RJ. Management of the major coagulopathy with onset during laparotomy. Ann Surg. 1983;197(5):532–5.
21. Waibel BH, Rotondo MM. Damage control surgery: it's evolution over the last 20 years. Rev Col Bras Cir. 2012;39(4):314–21.
22. Roberts DJ, Ball CG, Feliciano DV, Moore EE, Ivatury RR, Lucas CE, et al. History of the innovation of damage control for management of trauma patients: 1902-2016. Ann Surg. 2017;265(5):1034–44.
23. Glassberg E, Nadler R, Erlich T, Klien Y, Kreiss Y, Kluger Y. A decade of advances in military trauma care. Scand J Surg. 2014;103(2):126–31.
24. Thorson CM, Dubose JJ, Rhee P, Knuth TE, Dorlac WC, Bailey JA, et al. Military trauma training at civilian centers: a decade of advancements. J Trauma Acute Care Surg. 2012;73(6 Suppl 5):S483–9.
25. Hooper TJ, Nadler R, Badloe J, Butler FK, Glassberg E. Implementation and execution of military forward resuscitation programs. Shock. 2014;41(Suppl 1):90–7.
26. Eastridge BJ, Mabry RL, Seguin P, Cantrell J, Tops T, Uribe P, et al. Death on the battlefield (2001-2011): implications for the future of combat casualty care. J Trauma Acute Care Surg. 2012;73(6 Suppl 5):S431–7.
27. Holcomb JB, McMullin NR, Pearse L, Caruso J, Wade CE, Oetjen-Gerdes L, et al. Causes of death in U.S. Special Operations Forces in the global war on terrorism: 2001-2004. Ann Surg. 2007;245(6):986–91.
28. Gawande A. Casualties of war--military care for the wounded from Iraq and Afghanistan. N Engl J Med. 2004;351(24):2471–5.
29. Langan NR, Eckert M, Martin MJ. Changing patterns of in-hospital deaths following implementation of damage control resuscitation practices in US forward military treatment facilities. JAMA Surg. 2014;149(9):904–12.
30. Champion HR, Bellamy RF, Roberts CP, Leppaniemi AA. Profile of combat injury. J Trauma. 2003;54(5 Suppl):S13–9.
31. Schreiber MA, Zink K, Underwood S, Sullenberger L, Kelly M, Holcomb JB. A comparison between patients treated at a combat support hospital in Iraq and a level I trauma center in the United States. J Trauma. 2008;64(2 Suppl):S118–21. discussion S21-2
32. Sambasivan CN, Underwood SJ, Cho SD, Kiraly LN, Hamilton GJ, Kofoed JT, et al. Comparison of abdominal damage control surgery in combat versus civilian trauma. J Trauma. 2010;69(Suppl 1):S168–74.
33. Blackbourne LH. Combat damage control surgery. Crit Care Med. 2008;36(7 Suppl):S304–10.
34. Blackbourne LH, McMullin N, Eastridge B, Baskin T, Holcomb J. Aggressive proactive combat damage control surgery. US Army Med Dep J. 2007:3–6.
35. Pfeffermann R, Rozin RR, Durst AL, Marin G. Modern war surgery: operations in an evacuation hospital during the October 1973 Arab-Israeli war. J Trauma. 1976;16(9):694–703.
36. Silliman CC, Moore EE, Johnson JL, Gonzalez RJ, Biffl WL. Transfusion of the injured patient: proceed with caution. Shock. 2004;21(4):291–9.
37. Campion EM, Pritts TA, Dorlac WC, Nguyen AQ, Fraley SM, Hanseman D, et al. Implementation of a military-derived damage-control resuscitation strategy in a civilian trauma center decreases acute hypoxia in massively transfused patients. J Trauma Acute Care Surg. 2013;75(2 Suppl 2):S221–7.
38. Holcomb JB, Fox EE, Wade CE, Group PS. The prospective observational multicenter major trauma transfusion (PROMMTT) study. J Trauma Acute Care Surg. 2013;75(1 Suppl 1):S1–2.
39. Holcomb JB, del Junco DJ, Fox EE, Wade CE, Cohen MJ, Schreiber MA, et al. The prospective, observational, multicenter, major trauma transfusion (PROMMTT) study: comparative effectiveness of a time-varying treatment with competing risks. JAMA Surg. 2013;148(2):127–36.
40. Holcomb JB, Tilley BC, Baraniuk S, Fox EE, Wade CE, Podbielski JM, et al. Transfusion of plasma, platelets, and red blood cells in a 1:1:1 vs a 1:1:2 ratio and mortality in patients with severe trauma: the PROPPR randomized clinical trial. JAMA. 2015;313(5):471–82.
41. Roberts DJ, Bobrovitz N, Zygun DA, Ball CG, Kirkpatrick AW, Faris PD, et al. Indications for use of thoracic, abdominal, pelvic, and vascular damage control interventions in trauma patients: a content analysis and expert appropriateness rating study. J Trauma Acute Care Surg. 2015;79(4):568–79.
42. Roberts DJ, Bobrovitz N, Zygun DA, Ball CG, Kirkpatrick AW, Faris PD, et al. Indications for use of damage control surgery in civilian trauma patients: a content analysis and expert appropriateness rating study. Ann Surg. 2016;263(5):1018–27.
43. Cotton BA, Reddy N, Hatch QM, LeFebvre E, Wade CE, Kozar RA, et al. Damage control resuscitation is associated with a reduction in resuscitation volumes and improvement in survival in 390 damage control laparotomy patients. Ann Surg. 2011;254(4):598–605.
44. Yonge JD, Schreiber MA. The pragmatic randomized optimal platelet and plasma ratios trial: what does it mean for remote damage control resuscitation? Transfusion. 2016;56(Suppl 2):S149–56.
45. Jenkins D, Stubbs J, Williams S, Berns K, Zielinski M, Strandenes G, et al. Implementation and execution of civilian remote damage control resuscitation programs. Shock. 2014;41(Suppl 1):84–9.

46. Austin MT, Diaz JJ, Feurer ID, Miller RS, May AK, Guillamondegui OD, et al. Creating an emergency general surgery service enhances the productivity of trauma surgeons, general surgeons and the hospital. J Trauma. 2005;58(5):906–10.
47. Stawicki SP, Brooks A, Bilski T, Scaff D, Gupta R, Schwab CW, et al. The concept of damage control: extending the paradigm to emergency general surgery. Injury. 2008;39(1):93–101.
48. Waibel BH, Rotondo MF. Damage control for intra-abdominal sepsis. Surg Clin North Am. 2012;92(2):243–57. viii
49. Cancio LC, Rasmussen TE, Cannon JW, Dubick MA. The vital civilian-military link in combat casualty care research: impact of attendance at scientific conferences. J Trauma Acute Care Surg. 2015;79(4 Suppl 2):S221–6.
50. Dubose J, Rodriguez C, Martin M, Nunez T, Dorlac W, King D, et al. Preparing the surgeon for war: present practices of US, UK, and Canadian militaries and future directions for the US military. J Trauma Acute Care Surg. 2012;73(6 Suppl 5):S423–30.
51. Hight RA, Salcedo ES, Martin SP, Cocanour CS, Utter G, Galante JM. Level I academic trauma center integration as a model for sustaining combat surgical skills: the right surgeon in the right place for the right time. J Trauma Acute Care Surg. 2015;78(6):1176–81.
52. Knuth TE. The peacetime trauma experience of U.S. Army surgeons: another call for collaborative training in civilian trauma centers. Mil Med. 1996;161(3):137–42.
53. Schreiber MA, Holcomb JB, Conaway CW, Campbell KD, Wall M, Mattox KL. Military trauma training performed in a civilian trauma center. J Surg Res. 2002;104(1):8–14.
54. Academies N. A national trauma care system: integrating military and civilian trauma systems to achieve zero preventable deaths after injury. 2016. http://nationalacademies.org/hmd/~/media/Files/Report%20Files/2016/Trauma-Care/Trauma-Care-Recs.pdf.

Prehospital Damage Control Resuscitation

6

Timothy E. Scott and Lance Stuke

The fate of the wounded rests in the hands of the one who applies the first dressing.
—Col. Nicholas Senn (1844–1908)
Founder, Association of Military Surgeons of the United States

Abstract

Prehospital trauma medicine is both one of the most demanding and rewarding fields of medicine available to health-care providers. The challenge of delivering fast and effective medical interventions in a chaotic, potentially dangerous, or environmentally uncomfortable circumstances will suit only a small proportion of the medical fraternity. To succeed, information must be gathered quickly and shared with the medical team and a plan generated. Quick and decisive decision-making is of paramount importance as is the communication of information within the team and with relevant outside agencies. Effective team working is essential. The predominate aims of the team are to limit further blood loss, to protect the airway and to provide adequate analgesia. In a mass casualty event, triage and medical organization assume priority as effective command and control becomes vital.

Well-trained and resourced clinicians can deliver high-quality medical care in any environment that results in reduction in mortality, effective pain control, and a well-organized transfer to hospital that will result in a myriad of unmeasurable but nonetheless important effects for the victims of trauma, their families, and other first responders alike.

6.1 Introduction

Severely injured patients must receive the highest quality of prehospital care in the earliest moments following injury to ensure the best chance of survival. Systems of prehospital care vary among different countries and between civilian and military emergency medical services (EMS); however many of the principles remain the same. The prehospital provider must work in an environment completely different from the safety and security of a hospital. Poor lighting, severe weather conditions, dangerous scene situations, and lack of support staff all contribute to the challenges encountered in the prehospital world. EMS members often work alone in the tight confines of an ambulance or helicopter with limited equipment and none of the conveniences found in the trauma bay.

As in the civilian sector, military prehospital medicine is one of the most challenging and rewarding areas of medicine in which to practice. It is a unique environment that offers EMS personnel a significant risk of personal injury or loss of life in environmentally difficult circum-

T.E. Scott, M.R.C.P., F.R.C.A., E.D.I.C. (✉)
Academic Department of Military Anaesthesia and Critical Care, Royal Centre for Defence Medicine, ICT Centre, Birmingham, UK
e-mail: timscott4@me.com

L. Stuke, M.D., M.P.H., F.A.C.S.
LSU Department of Surgery, New Orleans, LA, USA

J. Duchesne et al. (eds.), *Damage Control in Trauma Care*,
https://doi.org/10.1007/978-3-319-72607-6_6

stances with limited resources. In return, this environment, more than any other, allows medics to utilize their skill sets in a manner that demonstrates immediate benefits in young fit adults who are exceptionally grateful for their help. Not only does military prehospital medicine deliver significant clinical improvements, it also delivers an important nonclinical effect that is difficult to measure. For deployed troops in combat, the knowledge that there is a skilled medical team in close support is a powerful message that improves confidence and moral.

6.2 History of the Emergency Medical Services

Advancements in civilian EMS often follow times of military conflict and arise from lessons learned in the combat setting. Jean Larrey, one of Napoleons chief surgeons, was one of the first physicians to recognize the benefits of bringing care to the wounded on the battlefield. He formed the *ambulance volante* ("flying ambulance") with the goal of providing initial trauma care as close to the battlefield as possible. Larrey is credited with developing the first triage and prehospital transport system.

In the United States, the Rucker ambulance, designed by Brigadier General Daniel Rucker, was inspired by the poorly executed evacuation of injured troops following the Battle of Bull Run in Manassas, Virginia. Soldiers could either sit or be placed on stretchers. It also had the capacity to carry supplies and water.

Following the American Civil War, the earliest civilian EMS services were initially hospital based and staffed by intern physicians in training. Charity Hospital in New Orleans, Grady Hospital in Atlanta, Bellevue Hospital in New York City, and Cincinnati General Hospital all developed the initial horse-drawn ambulances.

Progress in civilian prehospital care during the first half of the twentieth century remained relatively stagnant, despite advances made in trauma resuscitation during the two World Wars and the Korean War. Many ambulances were actually based out of funeral homes as the stretchers could fit in the back of a hearse. There was no formal training; communication between police, fire, and EMS was nonexistent; and rescue techniques were rudimentary. In the early 1960s, J.D. "Deke" Farrington began promoting the idea of translating lessons learned on the battlefield into civilian practice. He, along with Sam Banks, developed the first course for ambulance personnel in 1962 with the Chicago Fire Academy. Farrington is now recognized as the father of modern EMS [1].

In the United States, the landmark white paper *Accidental Death and Disability: The Neglected Disease of Modern Society* was published in 1966 by the National Academy of Sciences/National Research Council. It specified weakness in prehospital care and suggested guidelines for the training of EMS personnel, development of an EMS system, and advances in ambulances and equipment [2]. Congress passed the National Highway Safety Act that same year, which established the Department of Transportation (DOT). States were required to develop EMS systems under the threat of losing federal highway funds. The DOT funded development of the Emergency Medical Technician-Ambulance (EMT-A) curriculum, first published in 1969. The Emergency Medical Services System Act, passed by Congress in 1973, funded development of region-wide EMS systems during the period of 1974–1981. The legislation outlined 15 components which were needed in order to have an integrated EMS system. One of those components was education, which led to the development of the EMT-basic, EMT-intermediate, and EMT-paramedic levels of certifications.

Subsequently, the National Registry of Emergency Medical Technicians (NREMT, or "Registry") was established as a national standard for testing and credentialing for all levels of EMTs.

Prehospital emergency medicine (PHEM) is now recognized in many parts of the world as a discrete medically specialty for which board certification (or equivalent) is available and which is increasingly required by the physicians that lead these services. Physician-lead EMS is the model adopted by civilian agencies in Europe and Australia as well as by the UK military. Such services reduce mortality in the severely injured casualty when injury occurs at a location remote from a major trauma center.

6.3 EMS Systems

EMS care can be provided by any number of agencies, including the fire department, police department, hospital, private agency, or a "third service." A third service is an independently funded government agency with the sole responsibility of providing prehospital care, separate from police and fire. Regardless of the type of agency which provides EMS coverage, prehospital care is divided into basic life support (BLS), advanced life support (ALS), and a tiered response.

A BLS service is able to provide noninvasive care delivered at the EMR and EMT level. BLS provides advanced first aid, basic airway management, CPR, oxygen administration, spine immobilization, and childbirth. Some BLS systems are able to utilize automatic external defibrillators (AED) for patients in cardiac arrest. While a BLS service is easier to establish and less expensive to maintain than an ALS service, it is also limited in capability.

An ALS system provides care at a higher level than BLS. ALS providers are certified at the AEMT or paramedic level and possess a higher skill set. ALS systems are able to provide advanced airway management, including endotracheal intubation. They are able to establish intravenous (IV) access, administer a multitude of cardiac medications, interpret 12-lead EKGs, and undertake chest needle decompression. ALS systems are able to provide advanced care on the scene, prior to arrival at an emergency department. ALS care has shown excellent results for prehospital cardiac arrest but is more controversial for care of the trauma patient, in which expeditious transport is more important than on-scene interventions.

A tiered-response system combines elements of both the BLS and ALS systems. The basic goal of a tiered-response system is to match the level of EMS response with the needs of the patient. Non-emergent calls can be handled by a BLS ambulance, leaving the ALS response for critically ill patients. In many tiered-response systems, the initial response is often BLS, with an ALS ambulance being dispatched only if deemed necessary. This allows ALS ambulances to be utilized only for those patients who are seriously ill or severely injured.

6.4 Principles of Civilian Prehospital Damage Control Resuscitation

Damage control for civilian EMS follows many of the same principles taught in the military. Discussion will focus on scene time, control of catastrophic hemorrhage (including resuscitative thoracotomy), fluid and blood product resuscitation, airway management, chest decompression, tourniquet use, tranexamic acid administration, and spine immobilization.

6.5 Scene Time

There is controversy as to whether total prehospital time is a risk factor for mortality. While common sense dictates that scene time should be as short as possible, several studies do not support the theory [3, 4]. Analyses of subgroups of trauma patients, such as those with traumatic brain injury or shock, had variable conclusions [5]. One subgroup which seemed to benefit from a shorter prehospital time was shock patients who required early critical resources [6]. Additional data from Philadelphia support short prehospital scene times for the trauma patient with penetrating trauma who arrives to the trauma center in extremis [11]. They compared patients who were transported by police (with no interventions) to those who arrived via EMS having had procedures en route such as endotracheal intubation, IV access, and medication administration. Patients brought directly from the scene by the police had a higher survival than those brought by EMS. Their data suggests that in an urban environment time to the trauma center is more important than any prehospital intervention. The PHTLS course teaches the non-physician prehospital provider to have a goal of maintaining a scene time of less than 10 min, unless hampered by external factors such as prolonged vehicle extrication, multiple patients, or a delay in accessing the patient due to a violent scene, geography, or building design [7]. EMS team composition and transfer times are also important considerations when determining how much time should be spent on scene. Where possible, any prehospital interventions should be undertaken in a sheltered area (i.e., an ambulance) and every effort made to maintain normothermia.

6.6 Control of Catastrophic Hemorrhage

Most avoidable trauma deaths in civilian practice occur due to hemorrhage, and it is here that EMS personnel have most to gain through rapid and effective intervention [8]. The tools available to EMS providers to achieve this include hemostatic dressings, pressure bandages, tourniquets, pelvic binders, and in extremis resuscitative thoracotomy (personnel and training dependent).

Tourniquet use in the civilian setting is becoming standard of care, largely due to the experience of the military in the recent Iraq and Afghanistan wars. While civilian studies are underway to assess the role of tourniquets in the civilian setting, common sense suggests they are beneficial and should be utilized by civilian EMS. Tourniquets are inexpensive, simple to apply, and easy to manage and, other than pain, have no significant side effects if applied correctly. Tourniquets are most effective when applied early (prior to the onset of shock). If tourniquet application is held until the patient is already in shock, then survival is only 10% [9]. A summary of key points regarding tourniquet use is listed in Table 6.1.

Similarly, application of pelvic binders is increasingly commonplace. Pelvic binders are safe and effective when applied correctly to patients at risk of significant pelvic injury (Table 6.2). There is no longer a role for "springing" the pelvis in the prehospital setting, and the decision to apply a binder is based entirely on the mechanism of injury or obvious deformity. They should be applied directly to skin across the greater trochanters. Tying the feet together can augment pelvic stability in these circumstances. Lower limb traction devices that apply pressure to the ischial tuberosity can still be used in combination with a pelvic binder.

When hemorrhage occurs at an anatomic junctional area (groin or axilla), then conventional tourniquets cannot be used. In this circumstance a hemostatic dressing should be applied in accordance with the manufacturer's instructions. These dressings consist of a ribbon, gauze, or pellets coated with a hemostatic agent (chitosan

Table 6.1 Use of tourniquets

– Prehospital tourniquets are indicated if direct pressure fails to control hemorrhage
– The tourniquet is tightened until hemorrhage ceases (medullary ooze may persist). A second tourniquet should be used if required
– Tourniquets should be placed prior to extrication and transport. There is a clear survival advantage if placement occurs prior to the onset of shock
– The time of tourniquet application should be documented and relayed to the trauma team upon arrival at the hospital
– Care must be taken adequately; tighten the tourniquet on application to prevent occlusion of venous outflow but not arterial inflow to a limb
– As blood pressure increases following resuscitation, ongoing adequacy of the tourniquet needs reassessing
– An in-hospital "staged release" of tourniquets that have been in place for several hours should be undertaken to mitigate against the risk of myocardial reperfusion injury and hyperkalemia

Table 6.2 Mechanisms of injury that may cause significant pelvic injury. Such an injury requires a blunt high-energy transfer injury

– Fall from height greater than 15 ft (5 m)
– Motor vehicle collision (MVC)
– Motorcycle accident
– Struck pedestrian
– Less likely in children than adults due to more flexible pelvis

or kaolin) which is packed into the wound with direct pressure applied. Such dressings are not used in inter-cavity bleeding. Novel devices for use in junctional trauma are discussed below.

6.7 Blood Product and Fluid Resuscitation

Prehospital resuscitation follows the tenants of the low volume, hypotensive resuscitation commonly practiced in trauma centers around the world. A goal systolic blood pressure of 80–90 mmHg (or a MAP of 50 mmHg) is adequate, unless a head injury is suspected, in which case the goal systolic pressure should be 100–110 mmHg. Alternative targets are to resuscitate to achieve a radial pulse or, in the event of penetrating thoracic injury, a femoral pulse. Ideally, warmed blood products and crystalloid fluid in 250 mL boluses are used to achieve this. Patients allowed to remain hypotensive prior to surgical control of hemorrhage have a survival advantage [10]. Increasingly, both civilian and military EMS providers are equipped with group O negative blood, group AB plasma, lyophilized plasma substitute (e.g., LyoPlas), or in some cases even fresh whole blood. Optimal management would be to obtain a blood sample from the casualty prior to administration of blood products though the scene situation may not facilitate this.

Prehospital IV access should be considered a luxury and not a necessity, particularly in an urban setting with short transport times. Intraosseous access is faster and may be the route of choice in children, intravenous drug users, etc. A review of over 700,000 patients from the National Trauma Data Bank (NTDB) noted patients receiving prehospital IV fluid had a higher mortality than those who had no IV placed [11]. Reasons cited for the higher mortality associated with prehospital IV placement include the increased scene time often associated with the placement of the IV and "popping the clot" due to the raised systolic blood pressure and dilution from the IV fluid. Casualties in receipt of blood products prehospitally should also receive tranexamic acid (TXA, 15 mg kg^{-1}) and 10% calcium chloride solution (0.2 mL s kg^{-1}).

Tranexamic acid (TXA) is an antifibrinolytic that inhibits the activation of plasminogen to plasmin. It has been used for decades during tooth extractions in hemophilia patients as well as for intraoperative bleeding in gynecologic, orthopedic, and cardiac procedures. The CRASH-2 trial, while controversial, showed a mortality improvement when administered to trauma patients [12]. The MATTERs trial reviewed TXA administration in severely injured soldiers and noted a survival benefit in those requiring transfusion, although a slight increase in thromboembolic events was seen [13]. A subgroup analysis of CRASH-2 data examined the timing of administration and noted a significant reduction in mortality if TXA was administered within 1 h of injury [14]. The benefit was still significant, although less, if given between 1–3 h of injury. TXA was shown to be harmful if given after 3 h of injury. The drug is an excellent option for the prehospital setting, as it is easy to administer and inexpensive and has few side effects. A recent position statement by the American College of Surgeons Committee on Trauma (ACS-COT), the American College of Emergency Physicians (ACEP), and the National Association of EMS Physicians (NAEMSP) note TXA has an adjunct to the hemorrhaging trauma patient [15]. In their statement, they recognize the significance of trauma system integration of TXA use, the importance of trauma center transport, and development of a quality improvement initiative to monitor TXA use. Civilian studies are currently underway to assess the benefit of TXA in the prehospital setting.

6.8 Resuscitative Thoracotomy

In the event of significant deterioration or traumatic cardiac arrest, an appropriately trained EMS team, distant from a major trauma center, may consider undertaking a resuscitative thoracotomy. The indication for this procedure is outlined in Table 6.3. Survival rates following prehospital thoracotomy vary between 40 and 60% for penetrating trauma and 2 and 10% for blunt injury [16]. The injury most amenable to reversal following this intervention is pericardial

Table 6.3 Indications for resuscitative thoracotomy

– Traumatic cardiac arrest with organized electrical activity on the EKG
– In an agonal state within 15 min of respiratory effort following penetrating trauma
– Persisting critical hypotension despite adequate resuscitation

Table 6.4 Resuscitative thoracostomy

– Undertake finger thoracostomies in the fourth intercostal space at the mid-axillary line bilaterally
– Identify and mark out the fourth intercostal across the midline
– Use a scalpel to incise through the skin and fat layer
– Use trauma scissors to cut through the muscle layer and sternum (this may require a Gigli saw in larger males)
– Retract chest wall up and manually compress descending aorta. Extend incision to posterior axillary line if access restricted
– Apply suction and then identify bleeding point and/or exclude tamponade – If coarse ventricular fibrillation is present, close chest and defibrillate as usual
– If fine ventricular fibrillation is present, commence internal cardiac massage and blood product resuscitation. Administer calcium chloride
– Cover chest with cling film prior to transfer. Remain alert for rebleeding in the event of return of spontaneous circulation (i.e., the internal mammary arteries)

tamponade resulting from knife injury, but it has also a good track record for non-compressible hemorrhage below the diaphragm. The procedure is briefly described in Table 6.4. In the event that such a patient is pregnant with a gestation greater than 24 weeks, perimortem cesarian section undertaken within 5 min of the onset of CPR has a small but growing evidence base in favor of both maternal and fetal survival [17]. Delivering a viable fetus from a dying mother clearly gives that fetus a chance of survival, but mothers realize an increase in venous return following the procedure that increases their chance of a return of spontaneous circulation.

Restoration of the circulating volume remains the priority should traumatic cardiac arrest becomes established, and there is no role for CPR or adrenaline unless a medical event precipitated the traumatic incident or ultrasound examination demonstrates an adequately filled but poorly contractile left ventricle.

6.9 Airway Management

Airway management in the prehospital setting can be divided into BLS and ALS interventions. In many cases, BLS management with an oral airway and bag-valve mask may be all that is necessary. If a fully conscious casualty has bleeding into a traumatized airway, attempts can be made to manage them in a sitting-up and forward position. Taking time to orally intubate a hemorrhaging trauma patient is counterproductive and likely not beneficial. The preferred BLS airway maneuver is the jaw thrust, especially in patients with a possible cervical spine injury [18]. The jaw thrust had significantly less cervical displacement when compared to the head tilt-chin lift. In patients requiring an advanced airway, consideration should be given to placing an extraglottic airway device (EGD), such as a laryngeal mask airway (LMA), esophageal-tracheal combitube, or a King laryngeal tube. Placement of an EGD can be done faster than endotracheal intubation, with less risk of dislodgement or esophageal intubation. No difference in survival has been noted in blunt trauma patients managed with an EGD compared to traditional endotracheal intubation [19]. A subset of trauma patients will require rapid sequence intubation (RSI), such as those about to be transported for a prolonged distance or via helicopter. Prehospital success rates with RSI are comparable to in-hospital RSI [20]. Older data suggest no benefit to prehospital RSI. However, a recent multicenter study from Australia does note a survival benefit to those patients with a traumatic brain injury who receive prehospital RSI [21].

Apneic oxygenation prior to and during RSI (in addition to BVM preoxygenation) with high-flow oxygen through nasal cannula will mitigate against hypoxia, and the procedure may require ongoing airway suctioning throughout. The choice of drugs and the implementation of cricoid pressure are determined at the discretion and experience of the intubator. For hemodynamically shocked casualties, induction with ketamine (0.5–1 mg kg^{-1}) and rocuronium (1 mg kg^{-1}) is optimal [22]. In more stable patients, propofol and fentanyl can be used. Anesthesia can be maintained in a variety of ways. Profoundly shocked individuals will only require occasional bolus top-ups of the induction agent. As physiology improves, a combined infusion of ketamine and midazolam is effective (200 mg ketamine mixed with 5 mg midazolam in a 50 mL syringe and run at 0.5mL kg^{-1} h^{-1}), and in hemodynamically stable patients, the standard propofol and fentanyl infusions can be used (other than in very small children). Anesthetizing severely injured casualties for "humanitarian" reasons, that is, to ease suffering, to facilitate aggressive medical intervention, and to manage tourniquet pain, is now a normal practice. This also enables rapid transfer to both CT and the operating room on arrival at the MTF. In this environment, provision of anesthesia is always suboptimal, and small doses of midazolam may mitigate against inadvertent awareness. All members of the prehospital team should be trained in sighting emergency surgical airway devices. Establishing a "kit dump" on-scene in a predetermined fashion combined with the use of challenge-response pre and post RSI checklists can make a difficult procedure more manageable and safer. End-tidal carbon dioxide monitoring ($ETCO_2$) in ventilated patients is essential. The airway of the traumatized military casualty can be managed in the same manner as in the civilian sector. Anatomically difficult airways are unusual because of the age and health of the population at risk, and we can expect to reach casualties before trauma- or burn-induced edema occurs.

6.10 Breathing and Chest Decompression

All casualties with compromised physiology should receive supplemental oxygen when possible. Other causes of respiratory compromise such as primary blast lung injury or inhalation of toxic substances may need to be considered, especially if multiple casualties start to present with similar symptoms. Spontaneously breathing patients should have open chest wounds covered with an occlusive dressing or a one-way chest seal. Ventilated patients will need a chest seal to manage such wounds. Chest decompression, either via a needle thoracostomy or finger thoracostomy, is becoming a commonly used prehospital procedure for patients with suspected tension pneumothorax. Additionally, many prehospital protocols for traumatic cardiac arrest or peri-arrest include mandatory bilateral chest decompression to rule out tamponade as a cause of the arrest. Success rates are low for needle decompression, most commonly due to using a needle too short for the chest wall thickness. One study noted a significant increase in success rates after switching from a 5 cm catheter to an 8 cm catheter [23]. In UK practice, finger thoracostomies have now replaced needle thoracostomy (other than in children) due to greater initial success and a reduced incidence of occlusion and subsequent re-accumulation of air.

There is no definitive answer regarding the management of a massive hemothorax with ongoing blood loss in these circumstances; the treating clinician will need to manage the casualty according to the particular circumstances and their personal experience. Some EMS providers consider this to be an indication for a thoracostomy.

6.11 Spine Immobilization

Spine immobilization is becoming a controversial topic in prehospital trauma care. For decades, the dogma of spine immobilization was prevalent in EMT and paramedic courses around the world. Little data actually supports the use of routine spine immobilization. However, cervical collar placement and spine immobilization are not benign procedures. While treating a hemorrhaging trauma patient, in which seconds count, taking the time to immobilize a patient can be catastrophic. In one study, the time required for

Table 6.5 PHTLS guidelines for spinal immobilization in penetrating trauma (2011)

– There are no data to support routine spine immobilization in patients with penetrating trauma to the neck or torso
– Spinal immobilization may be performed after penetrating injury when a focal neurological deficit is noted on physical examination although there is little evidence of benefit even in these cases
– There are no data to support routine spine immobilization in patients with isolated penetrating trauma to the cranium
– Spine immobilization should never be done at the expense of accurate physical examination or identification and correction of life-threatening conditions in patients with penetrating trauma

experienced emergency medical technicians to properly immobilize a cervical spine was 5.64 min (±1.49 min) [24]. Cervical collars make examination of the neck difficult. This can be particularly important in the patient with penetrating trauma, where examination for an expanding hematoma, tracheal deviation, or airway compromise is critical. Endotracheal intubation is more difficult in those patients with a cervical collar in place, and more attempts are required for a successful intubation [25, 26]. The theoretical benefit of spine immobilization, to prevent propagation of a spinal injury, is simply not proven, has a very high number needed to treat, and is difficult to fit in this context and not required [27]. Immobilization with blocks and tape is adequate. This is particularly in penetrating trauma, where the damage is instantaneous and permanent. The PHTLS recommendations for spinal immobilization in patients with penetrating trauma are detailed in Table 6.5 [28].

6.12 Principles of Military Prehospital Damage Control Resuscitation

The population at risk in the military context falls into four broad categories. Coalition military personnel, entitled personnel (civilian contractors, civilian law enforcement agencies, and aid agency staff), enemy combatants (or captured personnel—CPERS), and injured local nationals (LNs). Combatant military personnel are normally extremely fit with significant physiological reserve whom can survive a significant injury burden of injury. Entitled civilian personnel are not normally medically screened to any extent and may share the same physiology and disease burden as our domestic populations. Enemy combatants are also not medically screened but are normally "fighting aged males." Local national casualties can take any form from newborns to elderly and include heavily pregnant females.

Independent of the type of casualty, it is imperative that they are "sanitized" before transfer. All casualties (including women and children) must be thoroughly searched for weapons or explosive materials which are left with the "ground call sign" to manage. Personal weapons of allied personnel can be carried at the discretion of your team once they have been made safe. Where possible, noncritically ill enemy combatants should be accompanied by a military escort. Children and, in some cultures in particular, females of childbearing age should be accompanied by an adult family member when circumstances allow.

The environment at the point of injury will be either permissive (no enemy or other threat) or nonpermissive (viable enemy threat or threat from fire, flood, or poisonous substances). Doctrine will vary between services and nationalities, but it serves no purpose for medical staff to expose themselves to unnecessary risk. This may serve only to increase the number of casualties and deny your population at risk of your services. Generally, we should let our combatant colleagues "win the firefight" first and hand their casualties over in a secured area. In a nonpermissive environment, a casualty's personal protective equipment (helmet, body armor, etc.) should be left in situ unless it is interfering with immediate lifesaving interventions. When evacuating a casualty by helicopter, eye and ear protection should be offered when appropriate. It is likely that the ground call sign delivering the casualty to you will have used a significant proportion of their medical supplies (including their stretcher) in caring for them prior to your arrival. Consideration should be given to replacing core components of this equipment at handover with a prepacked supply as well as providing bottles of water in hotter climates.

6.13 Personnel, Equipment, and Training

Team composition will depend on the size of the vehicle being used for casualty transfer and the degree of enemy threat at the casualty location. In general, the most senior medical team available should be offered to the casualty, and ideally this will include the decision-making capability and skill set of an anesthetic or emergency medicine physician [29]. Prehospital medicine should be part of the teams' normal practice in their civilian or domestic medical occupation. The degree of enemy threat will determine whether "medics with some military skills" or "combatants with some medical skills" retrieve the casualty. When military medics are used, they should have sufficient military training to facilitate determined self-defense, escape, and evasion if required. When larger aircraft such as the CH-47 Chinook and the V22 Osprey or larger combat support boats (CSBs) are utilized, there may be space for extra personnel such as a force protection element or firefighters to assist with vehicle extraction (Fig. 6.1.). Such personnel can provide enthusiastic and effective help when a permissive environment is reached. In the MERT (medical emergency response team) model adopted by the UK during the Afghan conflict, such extra personnel helped with log-rolling patients, syringing blood through intraosseous devices, and obviously escorting CPERS.

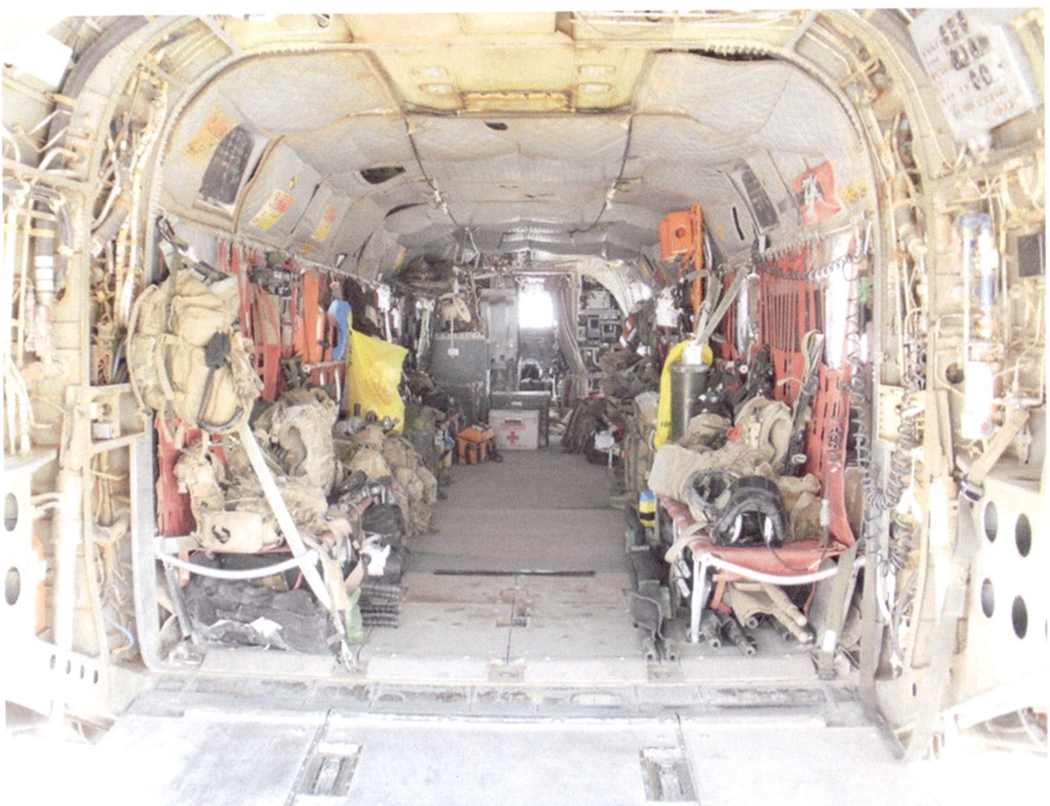

Fig. 6.1 A CH-47 Chinook helicopter being used for prehospital casualty retrieval. The floor space allows all-round access to litter patients, and the aircraft is large enough to accommodate a four-person medical team as well as a military escort consisting of four to six soldiers

The MERT model of military prehospital care consisted of a consultant anesthetic or emergency physician, an emergency medicine nurse, and two paramedics. Additionally, four to six soldiers provide force protection, and the MERT Chinook aircraft was escorted to the scene by an Apache attack helicopter. Aircraft such as the Osprey or Chinook are ideal for this role as they offer enough floor space for all-round access to a single casualty, thus facilitating "horizontal" resuscitation, and can accommodate multiple litter-borne casualties or a large number of walking wounded. They also allow easier access for litter cases and are powerful enough to facilitate armoring and have a good range in the absence of refueling.

6.14 Communication

As with all prehospital activity, communication is the weakest link in the care pathway. This is particularly so in the military context when communications need to be secure, are being interrupted by enemy activity, or are not possible at all. It is highly likely that the circumstances at the point of injury will have changed in the time it has taken to call for medical aid and your arrival. Flexibility is key, and when lines of communication are fragile, this should be clear and brief, bearing in mind that nonmedical intermediaries often staff military lines of communication so that medical language should be simplified in order to avoid error.

Within the North Atlantic Treaty Organization (NATO), the "9-Liner" signal is the standard signal format for requesting medical help and will be the basis on which medical facilities are alerted and dispatched. In addition to location and medical information, this signal will inform prehospital medical teams as to the nature of any enemy threat present (including chemical, biological, radiological, or nuclear threats), the need for specialist equipment, and how the landing site will be identified (e.g., colored smoke, cylumes, or infrared devices).

The use of "operation" brevity codes is a useful mechanism for simplifying medical communication in the military prehospital environment. Printed cards displaying the codes can be easily shown to radio operators in low-light, noisy, or otherwise challenging situations to convey pertinent information to receiving medical treatment facilities. Examples of brevity codes used by coalition forces in the recent conflict in Afghanistan are given in Table 6.6.

Table 6.6 Operational brevity codes

Brevity code	Meaning	Actions required
Op Vampire	Blood products administered	MTF to instigate massive hemorrhage protocol and organize replacing prehospital shock packs
Op Tube	Patient is intubated and ventilated	MTF to provide anesthetic care practitioner to receive casualty
Op Hero	Casualty is deceased	Receiving trauma team to stand down, blood products and drugs returned

6.15 Catastrophic Hemorrhage

Most military deaths result from non-survivable head injuries [30]. Most avoidable military deaths result from catastrophic hemorrhage [31, 32], and it is here that the military prehospital medical team must concentrate their efforts and where damage control resuscitation starts. Catastrophic hemorrhage must be controlled rapidly, and this is the immediate priority for first responders who have available to them tourniquets, hemostatic dressings, and pelvic binders to help them achieve this. Without such intervention, deploying advanced medical teams forward would be futile.

Once in the care of the prehospital team, the aim is to confirm that bleeding is controlled as well as possible and aggressively restore near normal physiology with the rapid hemostatic resuscitation with warmed blood products and hypothermia mitigation [33]. The position and effectiveness of tourniquets and pelvic binders should be checked and reapplied if necessary. Traumatic lower limb amputations should be managed with two tourniquets per limb and a pelvic binder. In penetrating injury, the patient needs to be log rolled to confirm control of hemorrhage only; there is no role for vertebral or rectal examination in this environment in a patient who will shortly be having a CT traumagram.

While large-bore intravenous access remains optimal, this is often unrealistic in severely injured casualties, particularly when being cared for in a tactically flying helicopter, in a CSB, or in the dark. Under these circumstances the initial choice for achieving vascular access should be either humeral head or sternal intraosseous access. Sternal devices can be inserted quickly and reliably and have the added benefit of not being knocked out accidentally during movement around the casualty or on rolling. Anterior humeral head devices facilitate faster transfusion of blood products which will require pressure support to flow.

Bleeding soft tissue wounds should be packed with hemostatic dressings and occlusive pressure bandages applied. Occasionally, unnecessary tourniquets are applied by first responders, and it is reasonable to reassess their need. When journey times to the nearest MTF are prolonged, this will involve the careful loosening and subsequent removal of tourniquets deemed not to be required.

Traumatic cardiac arrest due to hypovolemia is treated in the same manner as in civilian practice with the immediate focus being control of hemorrhage and restoration of circulating blood volume and not on chest compressions which will be futile. When appropriate, a resuscitative thoracotomy via a clamshell incision (described above) should be undertaken to achieve proximal control of bleeding and allow internal cardiac massage.

6.16 Novel Interventions

Managing non-compressible hemorrhage, either within a cavity or from an anatomic junctional zone, is a significant challenge prehospitally.

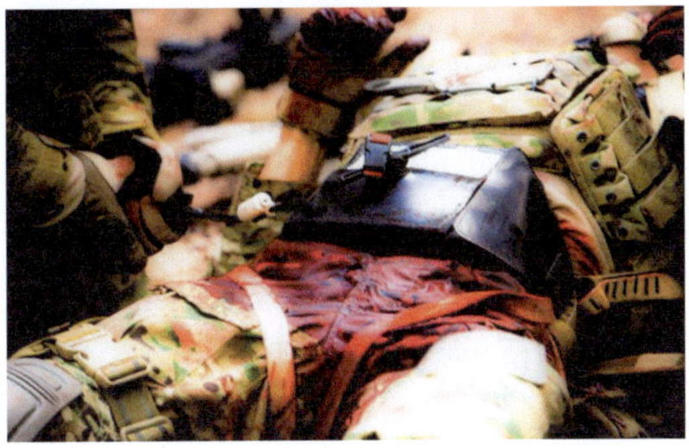

Fig. 6.2 The Abdominal Aortic and Junctional Tourniquet™ in use

Emerging and less invasive alternatives to thoracotomy are becoming available which aim to occlude or partially occlude the aorta through either extra-luminal pressure or intraluminal interruption of blood flow. Such approaches include the possible use of an Abdominal Aortic Junctional Tourniquet (AAJT) [34] (example shown in Fig. 6.2.) or the Resuscitative Endovascular Balloon Occlusion of the Aorta (REBOA) device [35, 36]. The REBOA device is an intraluminal catheter and balloon inserted via the femoral artery for the management of bleeding within the abdomen or pelvis in casualties with intact vasculature above the diaphragm. Its use either within the hospital or prehospital is in its infancy, but the concept is good. The AAJT can be applied to axillary and femoral bleeding as well as to the mid-abdomen to manage pelvic bleeding (assuming the subject is not pregnant or known to have a pre-existing abdominal aortic aneurysm). It is noninvasive and requires minimal training to apply and can be left in situ for up to 4 hours. Again, it is a technology in its infancy but may represent a significant tool for the prehospital management of hemorrhage.

6.17 Futility

Futility is important to recognize for several reasons. Most importantly, it allows EMS personnel to concentrate on the comfort and dignity of the patient rather than unpleasant and painful interventions as well as attending to the psychological well-being of other first responders or witnesses via some form of "hot debriefing" process. It also prevents unnecessary utilization of prehospital and in-hospital resources. Definitions of non-survivability will change with time, and each case must be considered individually, but the absence of electrical and mechanical myocardial activity after a period of effective resuscitation should prompt a discussion around futility [37].

6.18 Summary

Many of the principles taught in civilian EMS course can trace their roots to lessons learned by the military. Damage control in civilian EMS should follow the tenants of providing good BLS care, minimizing scene time and maintenance of normothermia while performing as many procedures as possible en route to the trauma center. Use of crystalloid should be minimized and shocked casualties resuscitated with blood when available. Tourniquet use is becoming standard of care in the civilian sector, and every agency should have tourniquets available to their medics. The use of TXA may prove to be beneficial in the prehospital setting. Spine immobilization should only be done when absolutely necessary and is not likely to be beneficial in the cases of penetrating trauma.

Prehospital damage control resuscitation in any arena will be the most challenging and rewarding practice medicine health-care providers will encounter. With appropriate training and excellent team working skills, a good outcome can be achieved for everyone involved but in particular for the casualty who fights on our behalf in the knowledge that they have the close support of their medical services.

References

1. Rockwood CA, Mann CM, Farrington DM, et al. History of emergency medical services in the United States. J Trauma. 1976;16:299.
2. National Academy of Sciences/National Research Council. Accidental death and disability: the neglected disease of modern society. Rockville: U.S. Department of Health, Education, and Welfare; 1966.
3. Harmsen AK, Giannakopoulos GF, Moerbeek PR, et al. The influence of prehospital time on trauma patients outcome: a systematic review. Injury. 2015;46:602–9.
4. Newgard CD, Schmicker RH, Hedges JR, et al. Emergency medical services intervals and survival in trauma: assessment of the "golden hour" in a north American prospective cohort. Ann Emerg Med. 2010;55:235–46.
5. Dinh MM, Bein K, Roncal S, et al. Redefining the golden hour for severe head injury in an urban setting: the effect of prehospital times on patient outcomes. Injury. 2013;44:606–10.
6. Newgard CD, Meier EN, Bulger EM, et al. Revisiting the "golden hour": an evaluation of out-of-hospital time in shock and traumatic brain injury. Ann Emerg Med. 2015;66:30–41.
7. PHTLS: Prehospital Trauma Life Support. 8th ed. Burlington: Jones and Bartlett; 2014.
8. Kauvar DS, Wade CE. The epidemiology and modern management of traumatic hemorrhage: US and international perspectives. Crit Care. 2005;9:S1–9.
9. Kragh JF, Walters TJ, Baer DG, et al. Survival with emergency tourniquet use to stop bleeding in major limb trauma. Ann Surg. 2009;249:1–7.
10. Bickell WH, Wall MJ, Pepe PE, et al. Immediate versus delayed fluid resuscitation for hypotensive patients with penetrating torso injuries. N Engl J Med. 1994;331:1105–9.
11. Haut ER, Kalish BT, Cotton BA, et al. Prehospital intravenous fluid administration is associated with higher mortality in trauma patients: a national trauma data bank analysis. Ann Surg. 2011;253:371–7.
12. Crash-2 Trial Collaborators, Skakur H, Roberts I, et al. Effects of tranexamic acid on death, vascular occlusive events, and blood transfusion in trauma patients with significant haemorrhage (CRASH-2): a randomized, placebo-controlled trial. Lancet. 2010;376(9734):23–32.
13. Morrison JJ, Dubose JJ, Rasmussen TE, Midwinter MJ. Military application of tranexamic acid in trauma emergency resuscitation (MATTERs) study. Arch Surg. 2012;147(2):113–9.
14. Crash-2 Trial Collaborators, Roberts I, Shakur H, et al. The importance of early treatment with tranexamic acid in bleeding trauma patients: an exploratory analysis of the CRASH-2 randomised controlled trial. Lancet. 2011;377(9771):1096–101.
15. Fischer PE, Bulger EM, Perina DG, et al. Guidance document for the prehospital use of tranexamic acid in injured patients. Prehosp Emerg Care. 2016; 17:1–3.
16. Forrest M, Lax P, Van der Velde J. Anaesthesia, trauma and critical care course manual. 2014.
17. Katz V, Balderston K, Defreest M. Perimortem cesarean delivery: were our assumptions correct? Am J Obstet Gynecol. 2005;192(6):1916–20.

18. Prasarn ML, Horodyski MB, Scott NE, et al. Motion generated in the unstable upper cervical spine during head tilt-chin lift and jaw thrust maneuvers. Spine J. 2014;14:609–14.
19. Kempema J, Trust MD, Ali S, et al. Prehospital endotracheal intubation vs extraglottic airway device in blunt trauma. Am J Emerg Med. 2015;33(8):1080–3.
20. Sloane C, Vilke GM, Chan TC, et al. Rapid sequence intubation in the field versus hospital in trauma patients. J Emerg Med. 2000;19(3):259–64.
21. Bernard SA, Nguyen V, Cameron P, et al. Prehospital rapid sequence intubation improves functional outcome for patients with severe traumatic brain injury. Ann Surg. 2010;252:959–65.
22. Jabre P, Combes X, Lapostolle F, et al. Etomidate versus ketamine for rapid sequence intubation in acutely ill patients: a multicentre randomised controlled trial. Lancet. 2009;374:293–300.
23. Aho JM, Thiels CA, El Khatib MM, et al. Needle thoracostomy: clinical effectiveness is improved using a longer angiocatheter. J Trauma Acute Care Surg. 2016;80(2):272–7.
24. Arishita GI, Vayer JS, Bellamy RF. Cervical spine immobilization of penetrating neck wounds in a hostile environment. J Trauma. 1989;29:1453–4.
25. Kennedy FR, Gonzalez P, Beitler A, et al. Incidence of cervical spine injury in patients with gunshot wounds to the head. South Med J. 1994;87:621–3.
26. Kaups KL, Davis JW. Patients with gunshot wounds to the head do not require cervical spine immobilization and evaluation. J Trauma. 1998;44:865–77.
27. Scott TE, Coates PJB, Davies SR, Gay DAT. Clearing the spine in the unconscious trauma patient: an update. J Intensive Care Society. 2012;13(3):227–31.
28. Stuke LE, Pons PT, Guy JS, Chapleau WP, Butler FK, McSwain NE. Prehospital spine immobilization for penetrating trauma: review and recommendations from the prehospital trauma life support (PHTLS) executive committee. J Trauma. 2011;71:763–9.
29. Davis PR, Rickards AC, Ollerton JE. Determining the composition and benefit of the pre-hospital medical response team in the conflict setting. J R Army Med Corps. 2007;153(4):269–73.
30. Keene DD, Penn-Barwell JG, Wood PR, et al. Died of wounds: a mortality review. J R Army Med Corps. 2016;162:355–60.
31. Eastridge BJ, Hardin M, Cantrell J, et al. Died of wounds on the battlefield: causation and implications for improving combat casualty care. J Trauma. 2011;71:S4–8.
32. Champion HR, Bellamy RF, Roberts P, Leppaniemi AA. Profile of combat injury. J Trauma. 2003;54:S13–9.
33. Midwinter MJ. Damage control surgery in the era of damage control resuscitation. J R Army Med Corps. 2009;155:323–6.
34. Croushorn J. Abdominal aortic and junctional tourniquet controls hemorrhage from a gunshot wound of the left groin. J Spec Oper Med. 2014;14(2):6–8.
35. Morrison JJ, Ross JD, Rasmussen TE, Midwinter MJ, Jansen JO. Resuscitative endovascular balloon compression of the aorta: a gap analysis of severely injured UK combat casualties. Shock. 2014;41(5):388–93.
36. Davidson AJ, Russo RM, DuBose JJ, Roberts J, Jurkovich GJ, Galante JM. Potential benefit of early operative utilization of low profile, partial resuscitative endovascular balloon occlusion of the aorta (P-REBOA) in major traumatic hemorrhage. Trauma Surg Acute Care Open. 2016;1:1–3.
37. Tarmey NT, Park CL, Bartels OJ, Konig TC, Mahoney PF, Mellor AJ. Outcomes following military traumatic cardiorespiratory arrest: a prospective observational study. Resuscitation. 2011;82:1194–7.

Damage Control Surgery

7

Elizabeth Benjamin, Kenji Inaba,
and Demetrios Demetriades

Abstract

Damage control is a combination of surgical techniques and damage control resuscitation. It can be performed in injuries involving the abdomen, chest, neck, vessels, bones, and soft tissues. It should be considered in patients with persistent bleeding and limited physiological reserve, in austere environments with limited resources, and in bleeding from anatomically difficult areas. It is a three-stage approach and involves temporary control of bleeding by packing, vascular shunting, or ligation and control of intestinal spillage in the operating room (first stage), physiological stabilization in the intensive care unit (second stage), and semi-elective definitive repair of all injuries in the operating room (third stage).

Damage control should be considered early, before major physiological decompensation. The timing of damage control should be determined by several factors including the type, anatomical site, and severity of injuries; the physiological condition, age and co-morbidities of the patient; the experience of the surgeon; and the available resources. Angio-embolization in the appropriate cases may be a useful adjunct to damage control procedures. This chapter reviews the indications, techniques, controversies, complications, and outcomes for damage control procedures in trauma.

E. Benjamin, M.D., Ph.D., F.A.C.S. (✉)
K. Inaba, M.D., F.A.C.S.
D. Demetriades, M.D., Ph.D., F.A.C.S.
Department of Surgery, LAC+USC Medical Center,
Los Angeles, CA, USA
e-mail: Elizabeth.Benjamin@med.usc.edu

7.1 Background

Damage control surgery for trauma utilizes techniques that rapidly temporize injuries, stop bleeding, and stabilize patients in extremis. This philosophy focuses on streamlining early interventions with definitive management delayed until the patient is physiologically stable. The rapid and targeted operative phase allows early transfer of the patient to the intensive care unit (ICU), where resuscitation, rewarming, and reversal of coagulopathy can occur. The patient may then return to the operating room in a semi-elective fashion for definitive management. Temporizing techniques have been described in various forms throughout the past century, and in more recent decades, damage control surgery and the philosophy of delayed definitive management have gained popularity in the military setting, and lessons learned from the battlefield have been applied and adapted to civilian trauma.

Historically, operative trauma has been managed with hemorrhage control and definitive management of the traumatic injuries at the index operation. These techniques can be highly effective in the setting of physiologic stability

J. Duchesne et al. (eds.), *Damage Control in Trauma Care*,
https://doi.org/10.1007/978-3-319-72607-6_7

and specific injury patterns. In cases of complex, destructive, or major arterial injury with instability, hypothermia, or coagulopathy, however, definitive management may contribute to ongoing physiologic demise. Reports of damage control techniques in the early 1900s progressed to small series publications in the latter half of the century that began to describe positive results using temporizing measures with a planned "second-look" operation [1, 2]. In the early 1980s, Stone et al. [3] published a series of 31 patients undergoing laparotomy for trauma in which the final 17 patients were managed with a staged method, rapid temporizing of the injuries, intra-abdominal packing, and delayed return to the operating room for definitive management. Patients treated with these damage control techniques had significantly lower transfusion requirements and improved mortality when compared to patients with standard management. By 1993, the stages of damage control were clearly defined [4] as first, hemorrhage and contamination control with temporary abdominal closure; second, ICU resuscitation; and third, re-exploration with definitive surgical management. The modern concept of damage control surgery includes not only the temporizing operative techniques but also the concepts of damage control resuscitation with clear transfusion, physiologic, and hemodynamic goals.

Although clear indication criteria for damage control surgery continue to evolve, as many as

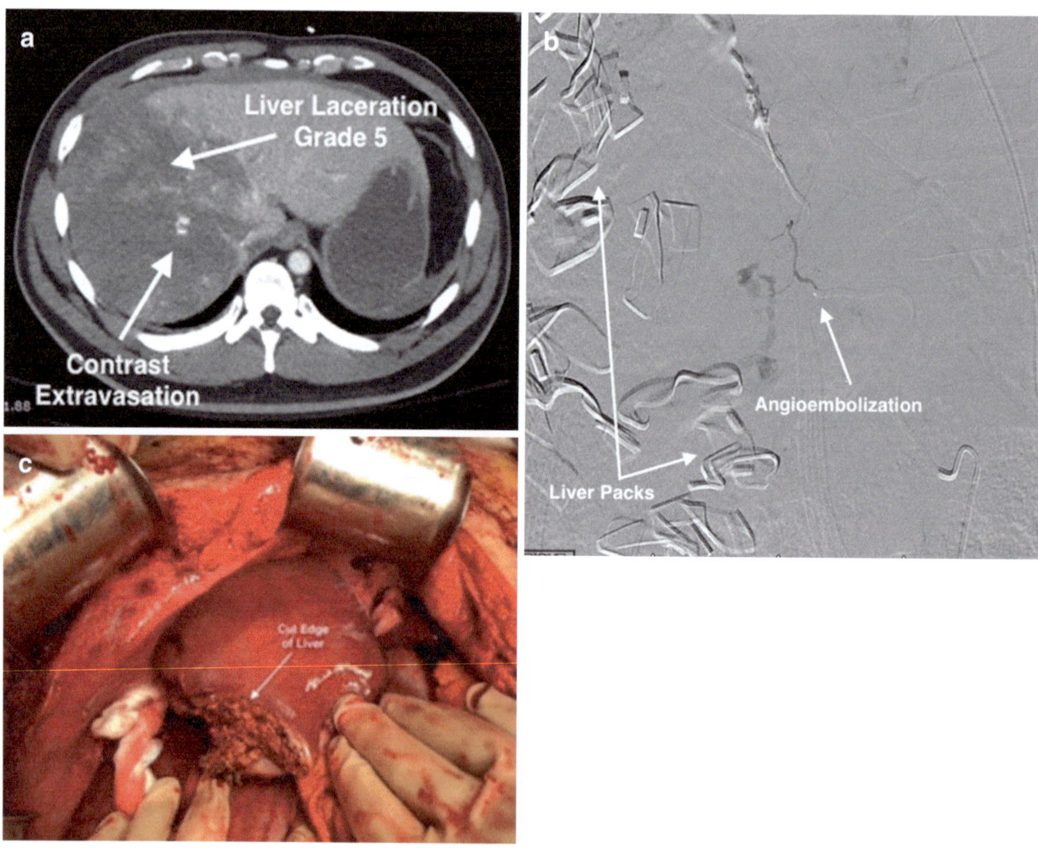

Fig. 7.1 Damage control operation in a young male who developed hypotension after being admitted with a grade 5 liver injury after blunt abdominal trauma. CT scan imaging obtained on arrival shows a grade 5 liver injury with active contrast extravasation (**a**). The patient underwent damage control laparotomy during which the liver hemorrhage was contained with multiple packs, and the patient was taken to the hybrid operating room for angioembolization (**b**). The patient was then resuscitated and stabilized in the ICU and returned to the operating room 24 h later for a liver resection and pack removal (**c**)

10% of trauma patients undergoing operation may benefit from these techniques, and a clear mortality advantage has been shown with this staged approach, especially when coupled with the principles of damage control resuscitation (Fig. 7.1) [4–7].

7.2 Indications for Damage Control

Damage control techniques are most commonly applied during massive exsanguination or in patients in poor physiological condition; however, they may also be applied in austere environments or in the treatment of complex injuries where further exploration or definitive management is outside the clinical expertise of the operating surgeon.

Damage control should be considered in patients in extremis, with severe metabolic or physiologic derangements. These physiologic abnormalities contribute to an overall shock state in which patients remain coagulopathic with ongoing hemorrhage despite maximal operative intervention. Ongoing hypotension, shock, tissue hypoperfusion, and acute coagulopathy after trauma have all been shown to significantly worsen outcomes [8–10]. It is in these patients that damage control procedures are most commonly recommended [6].

The classic premorbid parameters described after severe trauma include the "lethal triad" of hypothermia, coagulopathy, and acidosis. Hemodilution and consumptive coagulopathy combined with metabolic acidosis and increased fibrinolysis in the setting of hypothermia have all been clearly shown to contribute to ongoing bleeding and a patients' inability to tolerate prolonged operative interventions [11–14].

Hypothermia is a common problem in the trauma population that can exacerbate the effects of acidosis and worsen ongoing coagulopathy. Prehospital environmental causes are propagated by difficulties in rewarming during operative intervention, cool resuscitative fluids, and ongoing heat loss due to open cavities and wounds. Hypothermia alone is not an indication for damage control; however, hypothermia can exacerbate coagulopathy causing altered platelet function and abnormalities in the coagulation cascade [12, 15, 16], and it is associated with increased mortality after trauma [17]. In the hypothermic trauma patient, cold and wet clothing should be removed and skin covered with warm blankets. Intravenous fluid warmers and warm air convection devices are commonly used [18, 19]. Despite early reports supporting the correlation between ambient operating room and patient core temperature [20], modern analyses have failed to reproduce these benefits [21]. In the setting of persistent hypothermia during operative intervention, the most effective maneuver to rewarm the patient is with copious warm saline cavity irrigation. Establishing normothermia is a key component of coagulopathy reversal during damage control resuscitation.

Complex injuries such as severe liver injuries, bleeding from pelvic fractures, pancreaticoduodenal injuries, and many vascular injuries may benefit from damage control procedures. In an acute setting, these complex injuries can be difficult to expose, coagulopathy can exacerbate blood loss, and definitive management can be futile, increasing the risk of intraoperative mortality. Even the most experienced surgeon may choose to proceed with temporary control of the injury using packing or shunts with the definitive treatment delayed until the patient may physiologically tolerate the procedure. Additionally, suboptimal environments such as those with limited resources, inadequate blood product resources, austere environments, or lack availability of surgeons experienced in the needed procedure can all be indications for damage control interventions.

7.3 Stages of Damage Control

7.3.1 Stage 1

The first stage of damage control involves temporary control of bleeding and contamination. An initial surveillance assessment of the injuries should be performed with temporizing measures such as packing to allow a rapid cataloging of injuries. This is immediately followed by bleeding control with ligation, simple repairs, and solid organ removal, using tight packing as an adjunct when standard surgical techniques are insufficient. After these initial steps, the surgeon, in consultation with the anesthesia team, has sufficient information and control to determine if a damage control operation is necessary or if definitive management can safely progress. Consideration to temperature, acidosis, coagulopathy, injury burden, underlying medical conditions, and surgeon experience as described above will factor into this decision. A common mistake is to delay the decision to proceed with damage control until the patient has further deteriorated. This can be a fatal mistake. Damage control should be considered early and not be reserved as a procedure of last resort. If the surgeon decides to proceed with damage control, a rapid but thorough exploration of the abdomen should be performed prior to temporary abdominal closure. Injuries are commonly missed in the setting of significant trauma, and delayed management of ongoing bleeding or contamination can increase morbidity and mortality.

Hollow viscus injuries should be addressed with contamination control. Small or minimally destructive injuries can be primarily repaired, while extensive or devascularizing injuries should be resected. Although bowel ligation and discontinuity are described in the damage control setting, there is concern that this practice will increase bowel ischemia and ultimately worsen outcome [22]. In a multicenter study including 167 patients with damage control operations for hollow viscus injury, those managed with discontinuity were significantly more likely to have ischemia on repeat operation. For hollow viscus injury in damage control operations, injury identification, contamination containment, and restoration of continuity are the key elements to minimize morbidity and mortality [22, 23].

Vascular injuries need to be addressed at the index operation with definitive hemorrhage control. In the setting of complex injuries or physiologic derangements, a variety of temporary techniques have been described that can safely be used to delay definitive injury management. In the right setting, primary vessel repair is the first-line management option; however, in damage control settings, ligation, balloon occlusion, packing, and temporary shunts are all acceptable means to address vascular injuries. Nearly all complex venous injuries including the infrarenal IVC and iliac veins can be ligated with minimal long-term effect, and ligation should be considered as a damage control strategy if the vessel cannot be repaired without a complex reconstruction or significant stenosis. The exception to this rule is the superior vena cava, which should never be ligated. Ligation of the suprarenal vena cava carries significant morbidity with renal failure, and although not universally fatal, ligation of the portal vein and superior mesenteric vein should be avoided whenever possible due to the significant risk of bowel edema and necrosis that results. Intravascular shunts are most commonly used in extremity arterial trauma either during damage control operations or as part of a staged repair with orthopedics in treating a mangled extremity (Fig. 7.2); however, they may also be used in damage control operations on the carotid artery and/or abdominal arterial injury [24]. The

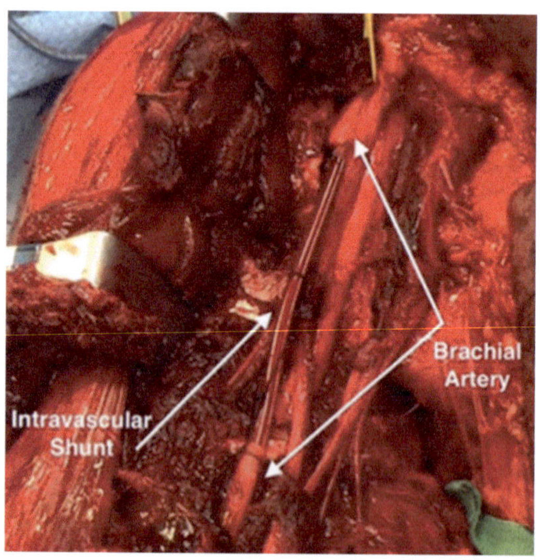

Fig. 7.2 Intravascular shunt placement in the right brachial artery of a mangled extremity during a damage control procedure. The patient returned to the operating room 24 h later and underwent graft placement and tissue coverage

use of intravascular shunts is well tolerated and has likely improved outcomes and limb salvage after damage control operation [24–27]. Definitive repair of arterial injuries treated with intravascular shunts should be prioritized, as the ideal dwell time remains uncertain.

In the stable patient with pelvic fracture-associated hemorrhage, angio-embolization is an ideal management algorithm. Pelvic hemorrhage in the setting of hemodynamic instability, however, can provide a more complex challenge. In this scenario, pre-peritoneal packing and, more recently, inflation of a REBOA catheter are damage control treatment options that can transiently stabilize a patient and potentially facilitate transfer to an angiography or hybrid suite [28–32]. Angiography may be used to address the pelvic bleeding; however, over 15% of all patients with pelvic fracture and almost one third of patients with severe pelvic fractures have associated intra-abdominal injuries [33]. For this reason, in patients with severe pelvic fractures, especially those with associated hemodynamic instability, open exploration should be strongly considered. During exploration, bilateral internal iliac artery ligation is a well-described damage control technique to address retroperitoneal pelvic bleeding [34]. This maneuver addresses distal pelvic fracture-associated arterial bleeding, decreases the arterial pressure head in the pelvis for venous bleeding, can be performed concurrently with an open abdominal exploration, and is generally well tolerated.

Topical hemostatic agents have gained in popularity and are useful adjuncts during this first stage of damage control. Hemostatic agents currently available include scaffold materials with impregnated matrices and topical clotting factors and materials that stimulate the coagulation cascade. These are available as powders, gels, foams, granules, impregnated sponges, or combined with expandable foams. In the civilian setting, these agents are not a substitute for surgical control of bleeding, but they have been used effectively as adjuncts, especially in the setting of trauma-induced coagulopathy.

Once the intra-abdominal bleeding has been controlled and injuries temporized, temporary abdominal closure is performed using either a sterilized plastic sheet or one of the many commercially available temporary closure devices. The skin should never be closed after a damage control operation due to the high risk of abdominal compartment syndrome during the resuscitative phase. The patient is then transitioned to the intensive care unit, a hybrid operating room, or to the angiography suite depending on the injury profile. Despite efforts to minimize the time spent in the operating room during this first stage of damage control, the patient must not leave the operating room with ongoing exsanguination. If the patient has transitioned to the ICU and persistent bleeding is identified, the patient must be returned immediately to the operating room for hemorrhage control.

7.3.2 Stage 2

The second stage of damage control is the resuscitative phase and most frequently occurs in the ICU. The overall goal of this phase is to physiologically normalize the patient through rewarming, product administration, fluid resuscitation, and reversal of metabolic derangements. This stage typically lasts 24–48 h and is designed to reverse the progression of coagulopathy by addressing the "lethal triad" through patient rewarming, correction of acidosis, clearance of lactate, correction of base deficit, and blood product administration. Although "damage control resuscitation" begins in the operating room, stabilization of the patient in the ICU requires a keen understanding of both the patient's resuscitative needs and the physiologic response to damage control interventions.

Contemporary resuscitation strategies focus on early blood product transfusion including component therapy in lieu of the traditional large volume crystalloid resuscitation that was previously recommended. The dilutional effects of crystalloid resuscitation with the resultant coagulopathy and acidosis have been largely replaced with aggressive and early implementation of balanced blood product administration [35–38]. Early administration of plasma in addition to

PRBC transfusion in a ratio approximating 1:1 has been shown to improve outcomes after trauma [39–43].

In the setting of severe liver injury or complex pelvic fractures, this second stage may require continued resuscitation in the radiology suite with postoperative angio-embolization for additional hemorrhage control. During this resuscitative phase, patients often remain critically unstable, and any interventions undertaken outside of the ICU setting require close monitoring and observation. In these cases, the ICU team and equipment including physicians and nurses must be transferred with the patient to the radiology suite to facilitate ongoing monitoring and resuscitation despite the need for off-site intervention.

7.3.3 Stage 3

The third stage of damage control involves the semi-elective return to the operating room for pack removal and definitive management of the identified injuries. Although adequate resuscitation is paramount prior to reoperation, packing material should be removed expeditiously to minimize infection risk. Once intra-abdominal injuries have been definitively addressed and packing material removed, abdominal fascia closure is a top priority. Delayed fascial closure can incur significant morbidity and mortality with increased risk of infection, fistula formation, anastomotic dehiscence, and hernia formation [44, 45].

Conclusions

Damage control surgery is a three-stage intervention strategy that focuses on rapid treatment of surgical injuries and high prioritization of patient resuscitation, followed by semi-elective definitive operative interventions. During the initial operation, hemorrhage and contamination control are achieved followed by transition to the ICU or angiography suite. Once resuscitated, the patient can return to the operating room for definitive injury management including pack removal or vascular reconstruction. These techniques are designed to perform only necessary operative interventions when the patient is most physiologically vulnerable and integrate damage control resuscitation strategies into the operative planning. The decision to proceed with damage control surgery should be made expeditiously and not be delayed until the patient has deteriorated significantly. Appropriate application of this staged approach has demonstrated improved outcome and survival.

References

1. Feliciano DV, Mattox KL, Jordan GL Jr. Intra-abdominal packing for control of hepatic hemorrhage: a reappraisal. J Trauma. 1981;21(4):285–90.
2. Lucas CE, Ledgerwood AM. Prospective evaluation of hemostatic techniques for liver injuries. J Trauma. 1976;16(6):442–51.
3. Stone HH, Strom PR, Mullins RJ. Management of the major coagulopathy with onset during laparotomy. Ann Surg. 1983;197(5):532–5.
4. Rotondo MF, Schwab CW, McGonigal MD, Phillips GR 3rd, Fruchterman TM, Kauder DR, et al. 'Damage control': an approach for improved survival in exsanguinating penetrating abdominal injury. J Trauma. 1993;35(3):375–82; discussion 82–3.
5. Teixeira PG, Salim A, Inaba K, Brown C, Browder T, Margulies D, et al. A prospective look at the current state of open abdomens. Am Surg. 2008;74(10):891–7.
6. Roberts DJ, Bobrovitz N, Zygun DA, Ball CG, Kirkpatrick AW, Faris PD, et al. Indications for use of thoracic, abdominal, pelvic, and vascular damage control interventions in trauma patients: a content analysis and expert appropriateness rating study. J Trauma Acute Care Surg. 2015;79(4):568–79.
7. Johnson JW, Gracias VH, Schwab CW, Reilly PM, Kauder DR, Shapiro MB, et al. Evolution in damage control for exsanguinating penetrating abdominal injury. J Trauma. 2001;51(2):261–9; discussion 9–71.
8. Brohi K, Singh J, Heron M, Coats T. Acute traumatic coagulopathy. J Trauma. 2003;54(6):1127–30.
9. Siegel JH, Rivkind AI, Dalal S, Goodarzi S. Early physiologic predictors of injury severity and death in blunt multiple trauma. Arch Surg. 1990;125(4):498–508.
10. Shafi S, Elliott AC, Gentilello L. Is hypothermia simply a marker of shock and injury severity or an independent risk factor for mortality in trauma patients? Analysis of a large national trauma registry. J Trauma. 2005;59(5):1081–5.
11. Brohi K, Cohen MJ, Davenport RA. Acute coagulopathy of trauma: mechanism, identification and effect. Curr Opin Crit Care. 2007;13(6):680–5.
12. Hess JR, Brohi K, Dutton RP, Hauser CJ, Holcomb JB, Kluger Y, et al. The coagulopathy of trauma:

a review of mechanisms. J Trauma. 2008;65(4): 748–54.
13. Simmons JW, Powell MF. Acute traumatic coagulopathy: pathophysiology and resuscitation. Br J Anaesth. 2016;117(suppl 3):iii31–43.
14. Engstrom M, Schott U, Romner B, Reinstrup P. Acidosis impairs the coagulation: a thromboelastographic study. J Trauma. 2006;61(3):624–8.
15. Rohrer MJ, Natale AM. Effect of hypothermia on the coagulation cascade. Crit Care Med. 1992;20(10):1402–5.
16. Valeri CR, Feingold H, Melaragno AJ, Vecchione JJ. Cryopreservation of dog platelets with dimethyl sulfoxide: therapeutic effectiveness of cryopreserved platelets in the treatment of thrombocytopenic dogs, and the effect of platelet storage at −80 degrees C. Cryobiology. 1986;23(5):387–94.
17. Jurkovich GJ, Greiser WB, Luterman A, Curreri PW. Hypothermia in trauma victims: an ominous predictor of survival. J Trauma. 1987;27(9):1019–24.
18. Perlman R, Callum J, Laflamme C, Tien H, Nascimento B, Beckett A, et al. A recommended early goal-directed management guideline for the prevention of hypothermia-related transfusion, morbidity, and mortality in severely injured trauma patients. Crit Care. 2016;20(1):107.
19. Tsuei BJ, Kearney PA. Hypothermia in the trauma patient. Injury. 2004;35(1):7–15.
20. Morris RH. Operating room temperature and the anesthetized, paralyzed patient. Arch Surg. 1971;102(2): 95–7.
21. Inaba K, Berg R, Barmparas G, Rhee P, Jurkovich GJ, Recinos G, et al. Prospective evaluation of ambient operating room temperature on the core temperature of injured patients undergoing emergent surgery. J Trauma Acute Care Surg. 2012;73(6):1478–83.
22. Talving P, Chouliaras K, Eastman A, Lauerman M, Teixeira PG, DuBose J, et al. Discontinuity of the bowel following damage control operation revisited: a multi-institutional study. World J Surg. 2017;41(1):146–51.
23. Harris BT, Franklin GA, Harbrecht BG, Richardson JD. Impact of hollow viscus injuries on outcome of abdominal gunshot wounds. Am Surg. 2009;75(5):378–84.
24. Inaba K, Aksoy H, Seamon MJ, Marks JA, Duchesne J, Schroll R, et al. Multicenter evaluation of temporary intravascular shunt use in vascular trauma. J Trauma Acute Care Surg. 2016;80(3):359–64; discussion 64–5.
25. Ball CG, Feliciano DV. Damage control techniques for common and external iliac artery injuries: have temporary intravascular shunts replaced the need for ligation? J Trauma. 2010;68(5):1117–20.
26. Hornez E, Boddaert G, Ngabou UD, Aguir S, Baudoin Y, Mocellin N, et al. Temporary vascular shunt for damage control of extremity vascular injury: a toolbox for trauma surgeons. J Visc Surg. 2015;152(6): 363–8.
27. Ball CG. Damage control surgery. Curr Opin Crit Care. 2015;21(6):538–43.
28. Morrison JJ, Percival TJ, Markov NP, Villamaria C, Scott DJ, Saches KA, et al. Aortic balloon occlusion is effective in controlling pelvic hemorrhage. J Surg Res. 2012;177(2):341–7.
29. Tesoriero RB, Bruns BR, Narayan M, Dubose J, Guliani SS, Brenner ML, et al. Angiographic embolization for hemorrhage following pelvic fracture: is it "time" for a paradigm shift? J Trauma Acute Care Surg. 2017;82(1):18–26.
30. Burlew CC, Moore EE, Smith WR, Johnson JL, Biffl WL, Barnett CC, et al. Preperitoneal pelvic packing/external fixation with secondary angioembolization: optimal care for life-threatening hemorrhage from unstable pelvic fractures. J Am Coll Surg. 2011;212(4):628–35; discussion 35–7.
31. Cullinane DC, Schiller HJ, Zielinski MD, Bilaniuk JW, Collier BR, Como J, et al. Eastern Association for the Surgery of trauma practice management guidelines for hemorrhage in pelvic fracture--update and systematic review. J Trauma. 2011;71(6):1850–68.
32. Saito N, Matsumoto H, Yagi T, Hara Y, Hayashida K, Motomura T, et al. Evaluation of the safety and feasibility of resuscitative endovascular balloon occlusion of the aorta. J Trauma Acute Care Surg. 2015;78(5):897–903; discussion 4.
33. Demetriades D, Karaiskakis M, Toutouzas K, Alo K, Velmahos G, Chan L. Pelvic fractures: epidemiology and predictors of associated abdominal injuries and outcomes. J Am Coll Surg. 2002;195(1):1–10.
34. DuBose J, Inaba K, Barmparas G, Teixeira PG, Schnuriger B, Talving P, et al. Bilateral internal iliac artery ligation as a damage control approach in massive retroperitoneal bleeding after pelvic fracture. J Trauma. 2010;69(6):1507–14.
35. Hirshberg A, Dugas M, Banez EI, Scott BG, Wall MJ Jr, Mattox KL. Minimizing dilutional coagulopathy in exsanguinating hemorrhage: a computer simulation. J Trauma. 2003;54(3):454–63.
36. Hewson JR, Neame PB, Kumar N, Ayrton A, Gregor P, Davis C, et al. Coagulopathy related to dilution and hypotension during massive transfusion. Crit Care Med. 1985;13(5):387–91.
37. Duchesne JC, McSwain NE Jr, Cotton BA, Hunt JP, Dellavolpe J, Lafaro K, et al. Damage control resuscitation: the new face of damage control. J Trauma. 2010;69(4):976–90.
38. Tieu BH, Holcomb JB, Schreiber MA. Coagulopathy: its pathophysiology and treatment in the injured patient. World J Surg. 2007;31(5):1055–64.
39. Holcomb JB, Tilley BC, Baraniuk S, Fox EE, Wade CE, Podbielski JM, et al. Transfusion of plasma, platelets, and red blood cells in a 1:1:1 vs a 1:1:2 ratio and mortality in patients with severe trauma: the PROPPR randomized clinical trial. JAMA. 2015;313(5):471–82.
40. Holcomb JB, Fox EE, Wade CE, Group PS. The PRospective observational multicenter major trauma

transfusion (PROMMTT) study. J Trauma Acute Care Surg. 2013;75(1 Suppl 1):S1–2.

41. Holcomb JB, del Junco DJ, Fox EE, Wade CE, Cohen MJ, Schreiber MA, et al. The prospective, observational, multicenter, major trauma transfusion (PROMMTT) study: comparative effectiveness of a time-varying treatment with competing risks. JAMA Surg. 2013;148(2):127–36.
42. Brown LM, Aro SO, Cohen MJ, Trauma Outcomes G, Holcomb JB, Wade CE, et al. A high fresh frozen plasma: packed red blood cell transfusion ratio decreases mortality in all massively transfused trauma patients regardless of admission international normalized ratio. J Trauma. 2011;71(2 Suppl 3):S358–63.
43. del Junco DJ, Holcomb JB, Fox EE, Brasel KJ, Phelan HA, Bulger EM, et al. Resuscitate early with plasma and platelets or balance blood products gradually: findings from the PROMMTT study. J Trauma Acute Care Surg. 2013;75(1 Suppl 1): S24–30.
44. Chiara O, Cimbanassi S, Biffl W, Leppaniemi A, Henry S, Scalea TM, et al. International consensus conference on open abdomen in trauma. J Trauma Acute Care Surg. 2016;80(1):173–83.
45. Miller RS, Morris JA Jr, Diaz JJ Jr, Herring MB, May AK. Complications after 344 damage-control open celiotomies. J Trauma. 2005;59(6):1365–71; discussion 71–4.

8 Role of a Hybrid Room in Damage Control Surgery

Dushyant Iyer, Chad G. Ball, and Scott K. D'Amours

Abstract

Time to hemorrhage control is the key performance indicator of a trauma system. Open and percutaneous techniques represent complementary therapeutic modalities that may both be necessary in achieving expedient hemorrhage control. In most trauma facilities, the operating theater and angiography suite are separate rooms, not infrequently located on different floors or buildings. Transfer between these locations increases time to hemorrhage control and the chances of a patient succumbing to physiological exhaustion. By unifying an operating theater and angiography suite, hybrid rooms offer the potential to minimize time to hemorrhage control through nullifying the dilemma of deciding the optimal location to best manage a patient's ongoing bleeding.

D. Iyer, B.Med., M.D.
Department of Trauma Surgery, Liverpool Hospital, The University of New South Wales, Sydney, Australia

C.G. Ball, M.D., M.Sc., F.R.C.S.C.
Department of Hepatobiliary and Pancreatic Surgery, University of Calgary, Calgary, Canada

Department of Trauma and Acute Care Surgery, University of Calgary, Calgary, Canada

S.K. D'Amours, M.D., C.M., F.R.C.S.C. (✉)
Department of Trauma Surgery and General Surgery, Liverpool Hospital, University of New South Wales, Sydney, Australia
e-mail: Scott.Damours@sswahs.nsw.gov.au

8.1 Time to Hemorrhage Control

Exsanguination is the primary cause of death on the battlefield and the second leading cause of death in civilian trauma [1, 2]. On autopsy, it has been found that many of these patients have technically repairable injuries and may have survived if hemorrhage control was obtained before the onset of irreversible shock [3, 4]. Thus, the emphasis on actively resuscitating and arresting bleeding in the "golden hour" has formed the basis for modern trauma care. Indeed, in recent decades, trauma systems around the world have streamlined prehospital care services to expedite transport to specialized trauma centers by bypassing other hospitals and improved the layout of their units to allow easy access to CT scanners, operating theaters, interventional radiology suites, and intensive care units from their emergency departments.

Recent literature has indicated the importance of time to hemorrhage control as a key performance indicator in the management of trauma patients. One retrospective analysis of hemodynamically unstable patients with severe abdominal injuries found that every 3-minute delay in laparotomy commencement was associated with an approximately 1% increase in mortality. Furthermore, a retrospective study investigating hemodynamically unstable trauma patients that required early therapeutic interventional radiological (IR) procedures found that a delay to

J. Duchesne et al. (eds.), *Damage Control in Trauma Care*,
https://doi.org/10.1007/978-3-319-72607-6_8

radiographic vascular occlusion was independently associated with more than a twofold risk of mortality and that for every hour delay, the risk of mortality increased by 47% [5].

Concurrent damage control resuscitation is imperative in extending the window for definitive hemorrhage control. Indeed, the acute coagulopathy of traumatic shock is a well-documented phenomenon that is independently associated with up to a fourfold increase in mortality [6, 7]. Successful damage control resuscitation involving the early administration of tranexamic acid and warmed blood products and the sparing use of crystalloids, potentially guided by viscoelastic tests (thromboelastography (TEG) and rotational thromboelastometry (ROTEM)), may prevent and reverse the lethal triad of hypothermia, acidosis, and coagulopathy.

8.2 Hemorrhage Control

Hemorrhage control may be achieved in an operating theater with open surgical techniques, such as the ligation of bleeding vessels or the application of direct pressure through packing. However, certain anatomical locations of bleeding such as the pelvis, retroperitoneum, and solid organs (e.g., the spleen) may be more expediently controlled through the application of endoluminal techniques in an angiography suite. Indeed, interventional radiology (IR) and the use of catheter-directed angiography, intravascular balloon occlusion, embolization of bleeding vessels, and the deployment of stents to repair damaged vessels have become an imperative component of modern trauma care [8–10].

This is highlighted by the evolution in the management of hemodynamically unstable patients with pelvic fractures. Historically, this cohort of patients has a significant reported mortality that ranges from 10% to 42% [11–13]. Indeed, the surgical exploration and ligation of bleeding pelvic arteries are technically challenging, time consuming, and potentially comorbid. The invasion of the retroperitoneal space and disruption of formed clots have the propensity to exacerbate bleeding. While elegant surgical techniques such as preperitoneal pelvic packing have been developed and used successfully in some centers [14, 15], pelvic angiography and transcatheter arterial embolization (TAE) have been shown to be effective, acute interventions for arterial hemorrhage control [16]. A systematic review of the literature found that the efficacy of rate of emergency TAE in controlling retroperitoneal arterial hemorrhage associated with unstable pelvic fractures found an efficacy rate of 81–100% with a very low rate of associated complications [8].

Given the complementary nature of open and percutaneous techniques, it is often difficult to choose where to transport a bleeding patient for hemorrhage control. Consider, for instance, a prehospital retrieval team en route to your emergency department with a young male involved in a motorcycle collision. The retrieval team informs you that the patient is hemodynamically unstable, has an unstable pelvis on clinical examination, and has a positive FAST scan indicating intraperitoneal free fluid. Such a patient will demand time-critical decisions in regard to diagnoses, resuscitative strategies, and use of techniques to arrest bleeding. Indeed, it is difficult to establish what the most active site of extravasation is and whether the operating theater or the angiography suite is the most optimal location to transport the patient. In most trauma facilities, these destinations are separate geographic rooms, not infrequently located on different floors or buildings. Unfortunately, if the hypothesis defining the most compelling site of extravasation is incorrect and patients require further transportation to an alternate location, the time to hemorrhage control and the chances of a patient dying because of physiologic exhaustion secondary to the lethal triad increase.

This scenario is not uncommon; a retrospective review of persistently hypotensive patients arriving to a Canadian level I trauma center in a 17-year period found that 35 (7%) of these patients required both angiography and an operative interventions for ongoing hemodynamic instability [17]. Interestingly, there was a 90% rate of mortality (<24 h) in patients transferred to the angiography suite after the operating theater.

The authors stated that death in these patients was almost entirely due to ongoing hemorrhage and physiological exhaustion and that transport from one site to another was clearly a significant factor contributing to this poor end result.

8.3 Hybrid Suites

A trauma hybrid operating theater represents a dedicated location where open operative and percutaneous procedures can be performed concurrently with the added benefit of offering rotational computerized imaging and ample space to resuscitate the patient. The term hybrid room is synonymous with a RAPTOR unit (resuscitation with angiography, percutaneous techniques, and operative repair). By uniting an operating theater and an angiography suite, hybrid rooms offer the potential to minimize time to hemorrhage control through nullifying the dilemma of deciding the optimal location to best manage a patient's ongoing bleeding. Additionally, time lost in transit between two locations can be saved when one technique cannot completely control bleeding.

Like many other hospitals with hybrid rooms, the construction of a RAPTOR suite at Liverpool Hospital has been the centerpiece of a broader initiative to improve the delivery of quality trauma care. In preparation for the suite's construction, the center developed a "hot floor" that was connected to the helipad and emergency department by a high-speed elevator system. This floor was designed with broad corridors and configured to contain operating theaters, diagnostic and interventional radiology suites, and the intensive care unit in close proximity to each other. The RAPTOR suite was constructed close to the entrance of the operating theater complex, minimizing its distance to the elevator and intensive care unit.

The RAPTOR suite is essentially a large operating theater configured around a floating radiolucent table that allows for a mobile C-arm to preform rotational angiography. All components apart from the table, including a high-resolution flat screen monitor, are mounted on frames attached to the ceiling. These frames are built for flexible positioning, including the important ability to be stowed away (Fig. 8.1). The components are controlled from a large glass-paneled room adjacent to the suite. Three sets of doors around the suite allow for large numbers of personnel to enter and exit and bring additional equipment such as ultrasound and near-infrared spectroscopy machines without interfering with ongoing procedures.

Recent updates to the suite include an automated positioning program that minimizes human error when moving the robotic C-arm.

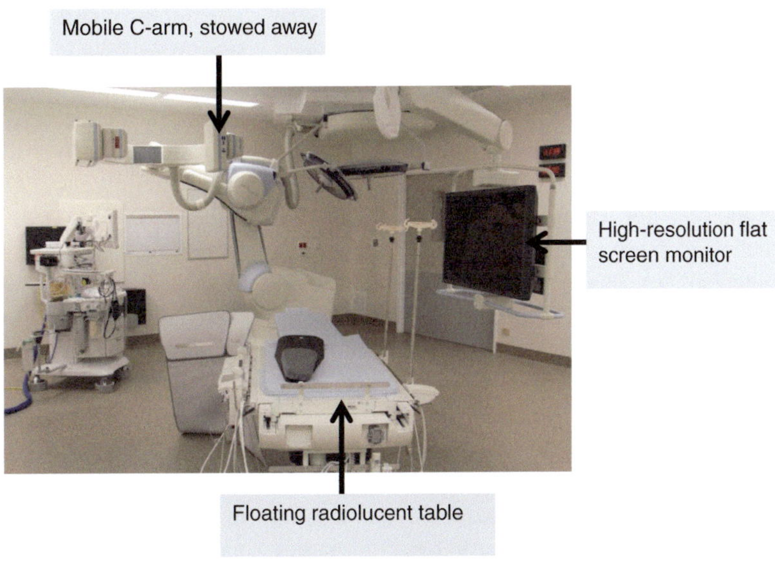

Fig. 8.1 RAPTOR suite at Liverpool Hospital

Wireless ultrasound transducers that connect to monitors via Bluetooth are useful in reducing congestion of valuable floor space and in reducing the potential for personnel to trip. Finally, while the rotational computerized imaging offered by the C-arm is not the same quality as that provided by a formal CT scanner, newer software enables the 3-D fusion of the static images obtained from a CT scanner with the real-time images obtained from rotational computerized imaging.

8.4 Overcoming Challenges Associated with Hybrid Suites

Traditionally, the early management of severely injured trauma patient has been compartmentalized into separate domains: the prehospital phase, the emergency department, the CT scanner, the operating theater, the angiography suite, and the intensive care unit. Each of these domains represents a distinct environment with unique objectives, equipment, and personnel with specific skills sets and team structures. Hybrid suites integrate these compartments and the personnel involved. Needless to say, it is a logistical challenge for the large numbers of clinicians required to effectively operate these suites to balance priorities, make collaborative decisions, and work in close proximity to each other. Furthermore, the team must respond effectively to dynamic information that may arise from real-time radiological and operative findings in the suite.

When conceptualizing their hybrid suite, the Calgary group recognized that with the increased propensity for complex decision-making and technical interventions, there was a greater potential for conflict and miscommunication [18]. Thus, before embarking on construction, the group assembled a multidisciplinary group consisting of architects, builders, clinicians, and allied health staff from emergency medicine, surgery, and anesthesia to optimize the final design of the suite. A plywood mockup of the preliminary model was constructed, and a committee of over 30 persons participated in a series of complex simulation scenarios under direct observation by several video cameras setup around the suite. The video footage, and specifically the movement of personnel, was analyzed to demonstrate high-traffic areas and "bump" points. This analysis led to a number of recommendations that translated in to changes in the suite's design [18].

One difficult issue experienced at Liverpool that is not unique to our hospital remains the high turnover of staff. With trainees regularly rotating through the emergency, surgical, radiology, anesthetic, and intensive care units, it is challenging to maintain a high level of competency with clinicians who may need to utilize the suite. Indeed, there have been instances when patients with injuries that were suitable for treatment in the RAPTOR suite were taken to the operating theater. Retrospective discussions regarding the decision-making process often reveal that the clinicians on site felt more confident in the familiar environment of the operating theater. This issue is being addressed through an increased emphasis on education and training for new clinicians beginning work at our center. We are also in the process of conducting a retrospective review of the use of our hybrid suite with the goal of developing formal criteria that will assist clinicians in identifying when to activate the RAPTOR suite.

Finally, there will always be clinicians who are more comfortable treating traumatically injured patients in the traditional compartmental model of trauma care. Thus, it is imperative to develop a core group of clinicians with a passion for utilizing the hybrid suite to improve the delivery of trauma care. One strategy to reduce the reliance on personnel to operate the suite is to increase the skill set of clinicians that are passionate about traumatology. In the United States, there are surgeons who are completing a secondary vascular fellowship after their trauma fellowship to develop competency in catheter-based hemorrhage control [19]. While, at present, no common standard or credentialing exists for trauma surgeons interested in adding interventional techniques to their skill set, this may be the natural evolution of trauma fellowships [19].

8.5 Future Directions

If these challenges can be successfully addressed, it is exciting to consider the impact that hybrid suites could potentially have on the delivery of quality trauma care. Decades before the construction of the first hybrid suite, Griswold and Drye introduced the concept of saving critical time by bypassing the emergency department and moving patients with suspected cardiac injuries straight to the operating theater for an exploratory thoracotomy [20]. More recently, Martin et al. described a model of care that involves recognizing patients requiring immediate surgery (defined by their own criteria) and transporting them from the prehospital scene directly to a dedicated trauma operating room that is prepared for both resuscitation and surgical intervention [21]. A 10-year retrospective review of their experience demonstrated a remarkable door to intervention time of 13 min in patients requiring emergency surgery with a survival rate that was significantly better than that predicted by TRISS methodology. With access to radiological modalities in the RAPTOR suite, many have suggested that the future role of the omnicapable hybrid theater will be to serve as a "one stop shop" for the unstable trauma patient.

The fundamental barrier preventing this is the resource intensive nature of the RAPTOR suite. As alluded to, the successful operation of this suite requires the rapid mobilization of senior medical, nursing, and allied health staff from several disciplines. Despite the successful experience of Martin et al., only 33% of the patients that met the criteria to bypass the emergency department actually required immediate emergency surgery [21]. Given the relative infancy of hybrid suites in trauma care, as well as the economic and political potential costs of overtriage, more work must be done to define evidence-based criteria to guide the triage of patients to these suites.

Conclusion

Time to hemorrhage control is the crucial factor in the care of the critically ill, hemorrhaging patient. The hybrid suite represents a dedicated location where open and percutaneous procedures can be performed concurrently and thus offers great potential to expedite hemorrhage control. Harnessing the potential of hybrid suites requires a change from the traditionally compartmentalized model of trauma care to one that is more integrated. This transition will require passionate clinicians to broaden their skill set and champion further education and training among their colleagues. Finally, given the resource-intensive nature of hybrid suites, further work must be done to develop formal criteria that will assist clinicians in identifying which patients will benefit from management in this domain.

References

1. Champion HR, Bellamy RF, Roberts CP, Leppaniemi A. A profile of combat injury. J Trauma. 2003;54:S13–9.
2. Soreide K, Kruger AJ, Vardal AL, Ellingsen CL, Soreide E, Lossius HM. Epidemiology and contemporary patterns of trauma deaths: changing place, similar pace, older face. World J Surg. 2007;31:2092–103.
3. Bellamy RF. The causes of death in conventional land warfare: implications for combat casualty care research. Mil Med. 1984;149:55–62.
4. Rhee PM, Acosta J, Bridgeman A, Wang D, Jordan M, Rich N. Survival after emergency department thoracotomy: review of published data from the past 25 years. J Am Coll Surg. 2000;190:288–98.
5. Howell GM, Peitzman AB, Nirula R, Rosengart MR, Alarcon LH, Billiar TR, et al. Delay to therapeutic interventional radiology postinjury: time is of the essence. J Trauma. 2010;68:1296–300.
6. Hess JR, Brohi K, Dutton RP, Hauser CJ, Holcomb JB, Kluger Y, et al. The coagulopathy of trauma: a review of mechanisms. J Trauma. 2008;65:748–54.
7. MacLeod JB, Lynn M, McKenney MG, Cohn SM, Murtha M. Early coagulopathy predicts mortality in trauma. J Trauma. 2003;55:39–44.
8. Papakostidis C, Kanakaris N, Dimitriou R, Giannoudis PV. The role of arterial embolization in controlling pelvic fracture hemorrhage: a systematic review of the literature. Eur J Radiol. 2012;81:897–904.
9. Schnuriger B, Inaba K, Konstantinidis A, Lustenberger T, Chan LS, Demetriades D. Outcomes of proximal versus distal splenic artery embolization after trauma: a systematic review and meta-analysis. J Trauma. 2011;70:252–60.
10. Lee WA, Matsumura JS, Mitchell RS, Farber MA, Greenberg RK, Azizzadeh A, et al. Endovascular repair of traumatic thoracic aortic injury: clinical prac-

tice guidelines of the Society for Vascular Surgery. J Vasc Surg. 2011;53:187–92.

11. Hamill J, Holden A, Paice R, Civil I. Pelvic fracture pattern predicts pelvic arterial hemorrhage. Aust N Z J Surg. 2000;70:338–43.
12. Ertel W, Keel M, Eid K, Platz A, Trentz O. Control of severe hemorrhage using C-clamp and pelvic packing in multiply injured patients with pelvic ring disruption. J Orthop Trauma. 2001;15:468–74.
13. Eastridge BJ, Starr A, Minei JP, O'Keefe GE, Scalea TM. The importance of fracture pattern in guiding therapeutic decision-making in patients with hemorrhagic shock and pelvic ring disruptions. J Trauma. 2002;53:446–50; discussion 50–1.
14. Tai DK, Li WH, Lee KY, Cheng M, Lee KB, Tang LF, et al. Retroperitoneal pelvic packing in the management of hemodynamically unstable pelvic fractures: a level I trauma center experience. J Trauma. 2011;71:E79–86.
15. Thorson CM, Ryan ML, Otero CA, Vu T, Borja MJ, Jose J, et al. Operating room or angiography suite for hemodynamically unstable pelvic fractures? J Trauma Acute Care Surg. 2012;72:364–70; discussion 71–2.
16. Hauschild O, Aghayev E, von Heyden J, Strohm PC, Culemann U, Pohlemann T, et al. Angioembolization for pelvic hemorrhage control: results from the German pelvic injury register. J Trauma Acute Care Surg. 2012;73:679–84.
17. Fehr A, Beveridge J, D'Amours SD, Kirkpatrick AW, Ball CG. The potential benefit of a hybrid operating environment among severely injured patients with persistent hemorrhage: how often could we get it right? J Trauma Acute Care Surg. 2016;80:457–60.
18. Kirkpatrick AW, Vis C, Dube M, Biesbroek S, Ball CG, Laberge J, et al. The evolution of a purpose designed hybrid trauma operating room from the trauma service perspective: the RAPTOR (resuscitation with angiography percutaneous treatments and operative resuscitations). Injury. 2014;45:1413–21.
19. Holcomb JB, Fox EE, Scalea TM, Napolitano LM, Albarado R, Gill B, et al. Current opinion on catheter-based hemorrhage control in trauma patients. J Trauma Acute Care Surg. 2014;76:888–93.
20. Griswold RA, Drye JC. Cardiac wounds. Ann Surg. 1954;139:783–5.
21. Martin M, Izenberg S, Cole F, Bergstrom S, Long W. A decade of experience with a selective policy for direct to operating room trauma resuscitations. Am J Surg. 2012;204:187–92.

9 Damage Control Neurosurgery

Mark H. Wilson

Abstract

The principals of damage control surgery are as applicable to neurosurgery as they are to torso and limb injury—prevent secondary injury and stop the bleeding/relieve the pressure. This chapter will describe an up to date approach to intracranial injury and damage control neurosurgery techniques.

9.1 Introduction

The principals of damage control surgery are as applicable to neurosurgery as they are to torso and limb injury—prevent secondary injury and stop the bleeding/relieve the pressure. Definitive surgery (e.g. replacing cranial bone) can take place at the time if the patient's physiology and the surgeon's skill set allow; however, in damage control neurosurgery (DCNS), it may well be best to leave aspects for someone more experienced to complete the case when the patient's physiology is improved and consistent.

Neurotrauma is often considered "easy" surgery, and often, it is. However, time is usually of the essence and ensuring rapid resuscitation and progress to surgery is a skill set. The technical aspects of burr holes and turning a flap are also usually straightforward; hence, this is a skill set that should be in the possession of the general or trauma surgeon who, possibly because of remote location, may well face the need to urgently control intracranial haemorrhage and/or decompress. This chapter will outline these basic skills; however, practical experience from spending time in a neurosurgical centre or attending a specific trauma skills course should also be sort. This chapter will describe specific techniques and nuances that can help control bleeding and be of use to the neurosurgeon who is often operating in non-trauma situations.

9.2 Basic Principles

The final aim of all aspects of physiology in every living creature is to maintain brain oxygenation. Indeed, everything we do as clinicians drives towards maintaining aerobic respiration in this most fragile of tissues. Once central neurons have died, they do not come back. Hence time-critical meaningful interventions must be undertaken when neuronal tissue is threatened.

Primary brain injury is the injury that occurs at the moment of impact. There is no treatment. It is the domain of public health physicians and policy makers to pass laws regarding protective measures such as seatbelt and helmet regula-

M.H. Wilson
Neurotrauma Centre, Imperial College London, London, UK
e-mail: m.wilson@imperial.ac.uk

J. Duchesne et al. (eds.), *Damage Control in Trauma Care*,
https://doi.org/10.1007/978-3-319-72607-6_9

tions that reduce primary brain injury. Secondary brain injury refers to all injuries that occur after primary, for example, the loss of airway and resulting hypoxia, the hypotension and the expanding haematoma. All of these occur over a period of time, which therefore provides a window of opportunity in which interventions may reduce/stop progression. Many people class extradural haematoma as a primary brain injury, but it isn't. The skull fracture that occurred at the time of the impact is the primary injury. The clot subsequently develops, and it is only when it causes pressure resulting in parenchymal damage (ischemia) that a brain injury actually occurs.

Our job as physicians and surgeons is to minimise/stop secondary brain injury, through systemic resuscitation and direct surgical intervention.

9.3 Resuscitation

The basics of resuscitation are covered elsewhere in this book; however, two key principals are the maintenance of oxygenation and blood pressure.

Hypoxia following traumatic brain injury (TBI) is common. The phenomenon of Impact Brain Apnoea (IBA) is often forgotten but is well recognised in the animal literature [1]. The loss of airway through obstruction is also common secondary to loss of consciousness. Both of these phenomenon need rapid reversal by bystander intervention (jaw thrust +/− ventilation). Subsequent airway patency can be maintained by oro- or nasopharyngeal airways. If appropriate a more definitive endotracheal tube can be placed with the assistance of drugs. Ventilation to maintain a normal end tidal CO_2 (~4.5 kPa) can then be optimised.

Hypotension occurs from a number of causes. In multi-trauma, concomitant injuries such as pelvic/long bone fractures and vascular injury can cause hypovolemic shock. The priority is to stop the bleeding and to replace the loss. Spinal injuries (neurogenic shock) and cardiac injuries (cardiogenic shock) are less common causes. The hypoxia that commonly occurs in brain injury can cause a catecholamine surge and subsequent cardiovascular collapse, and hence, despite it being an old ATLS adage that brain injury can't, isolated head injuries themselves can cause shock. Approximately 13% of "Code Red"/hypotensive presentations may relate to this [2]. An episode of hypotension in the prehospital phase is definitely associated with a worse outcome [3, 4]. This does NOT however mean that it causes injury. It may do if there is high ICP, but equally hypertension could make bleeding worse. The ideal cerebral perfusion pressure is probably disease specific (extradural vs. subdural vs. diffuse axonal, etc.); however, profound hypotension is likely to do harm, and hence bleeding should be stopped and normal physiology restored.

9.4 Basic Types of Brain Injury

Figure 9.1 shows the main types of brain injury that can occur in isolation. An individual patient can have multiple types.

9.4.1 Blunt Injuries

An extradural or epidural haematoma usually occurs secondary to a skull fracture rupturing a middle meningeal artery branch. It is bound by suture margins but is outside the brain. The pressure can be relieved by a simple burr hole, but a craniotomy is required as a definitive procedure to remove residual clot and ensure no ongoing bleeding.

A subdural haematoma usually occurs from a shearing injury disrupting veins between the cortical surface and sagittal sinus. It is under the dura across the surface of the brain and hence is not bound by suture margins and can have more mass effect. When acute, the blood is usually thick clot, and hence a craniotomy and dura opening are required to remove any significant amount of clot.

Subarachnoid haemorrhage can occur when the pial vessels beneath the arachnoid release blood. This is a marker of a shearing injury (and

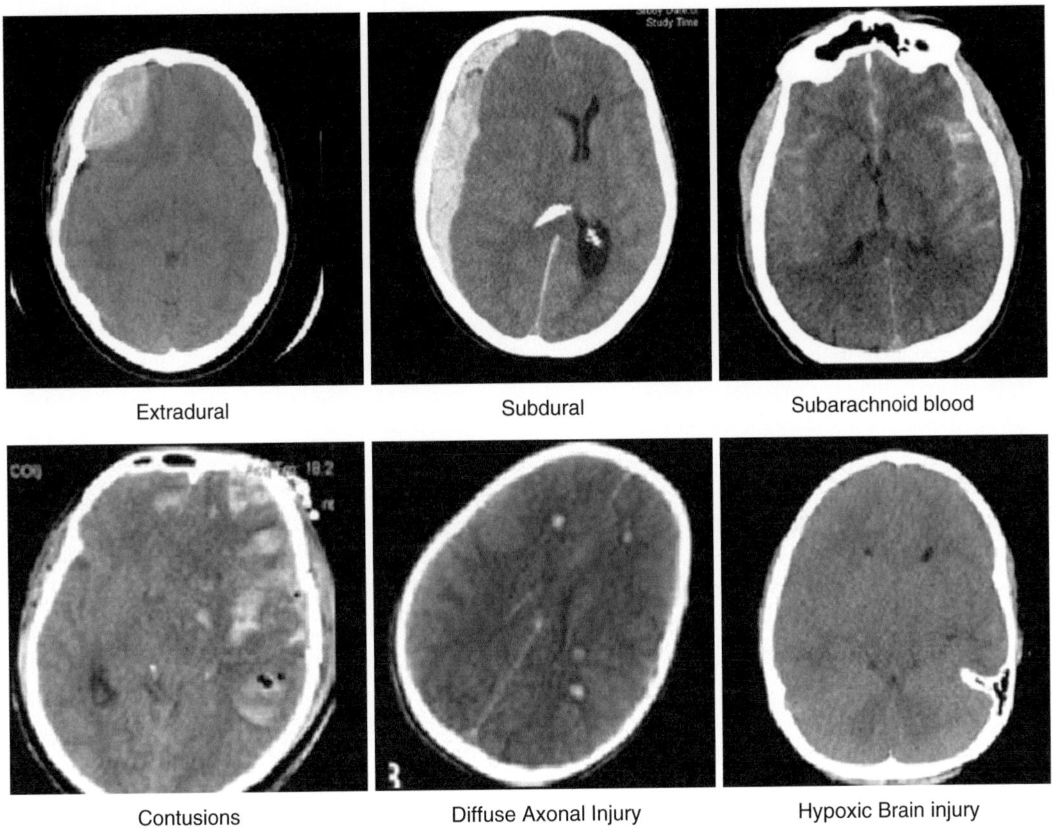

Fig. 9.1 A collection of CT images demonstrating the main types of TBI

there may be underlying diffuse axonal injury), but it does not normally require surgical intervention specifically.

A contusion is a bruise within the brain which can often evolve in the same way that any bruise can. They can coalesce to form a **haematoma**. Both of these are parenchymal brain injuries unlike the extra-axial bleeds described above.

Diffuse axonal injury is a neuronal injury caused by shearing, classically between the grey and white matters. It is associated with microhaemorrhages (better seen on MRI) and diffuses swelling. There is rarely neurosurgical intervention other than ICP monitoring and decompression if intracranial hypertension is refractory.

Hypoxia/diffuse brain swelling. This is seen when there has been a period of apnoea/airway obstruction. Neurosurgical intervention is not normally of benefit.

9.4.2 Penetrating Injuries

Penetrating injuries can be low velocity (e.g. knives) and high velocity (e.g. bullets/shrapnel). Clearly if something is protruding from the skull, it needs to be removed; however, deep small foreign bodies may well be best managed conservatively. See below.

9.4.3 Futility

It is important for a neurosurgeon or trauma surgeon, especially in a resource poor environment where overuse of resources results in others not receiving adequate treatment, to recognise when an injury is so severe it makes further treatment futile. Devastating neurology and a devastating scan usually mean the outcome is highly likely to be devastating.

9.5 Basics of Neurosurgery

9.5.1 Wound Debridement

The prevention of infection is paramount in neurosurgery, but not normally immediately life threatening. Hence wound debridement is not normally an immediate "damage control" procedure. However, it is important to do this early. Basic principles include removing foreign matter and large debris, washing copiously with saline, not exploring deep into brain and trying to create barriers (e.g. pericranial flap to replace lost dura; good skin closure).

9.5.2 Burr Hole Placement

Probably the more basic potential damage control procedure is burr hole placement to decompress an expanding extradural hematoma. This is a simple procedure and almost always will require a definitive craniotomy to follow. The procedure is straightforward if a CT scan has confirmed the location of the extradural hematoma. See "Targeted Burr Holes" below if no CT is available.

Procedure:

1. Position the patient with a sandbag behind the shoulder on the same side as the EDH.
2. Place the patients head on a horse shoe or donut ring and turn the head so the side with the EDH is parallel with the floor.
3. Confirm the location of the EDH—approximately 2/3 are temporal with the remainder usually being frontal or parietal. *Confirm the side again.* If temporal, the burr hole should be approximately 1 cm in front of the ear at a level of the top of the ear. If frontal it should be in the mid pupillary line approximately 10 cm back from the eye. If parietal it should be over the parietal eminence (Fig. 9.2).
4. Rapidly shave, mark and prep the skin.
5. Prepare as if you are going to do a trauma craniotomy (as you or someone else will have to)—see below.
6. Place some local anaesthetic with adrenaline to minimise skin bleeding.
7. Mark your burr hole incision 3.5 cm long to bone (the direction of which should be such that if extended it would be in the line of the trauma craniotomy).
8. Use a periosteal elevator or the other end of the knife to strip the periosteum off the skull.
9. Use a drill to create a burr hole. There are two types of drill: (1) the Hudson brace and (2) the perforator drill bit (Fig. 9.3). For both you should stand with one foot in front of the other so that you can apply pressure on the front foot immediately to withdraw the drill in the event of "plunging". The Hudson brace comprises a sharp drill bit for getting through the outer table and part of the inner table and a round burr to drill the remaining bit of inner table relatively safely. There is a large risk of plunging with this old system. Perforator drill bits can be attached to manual-, electric- and air-powered tools, and, because they contain a clutch mechanism which cuts out when the tip pierces the inner table, they are much safer.
10. Once the hole is drilled, remove any residual inner table with a blunt hook or toothed forceps, and extradural blood should come out. If it is thick clot, it could be removed with forceps/suction, but a trauma craniotomy is almost certainly needed. If the patient has a subdural, the dura should be diathermied and then opened in a cruciate manner elevating the dura with a sharp hook. This enables liquid chronic subdural to be evacuated but is unlikely to expel acute subdural blood.

9.5.3 Targeted Burr Holes

The term "exploratory burr holes" used to apply when a surgeon was unsure of where a hematoma was because of lack of CT. The procedure was to first do temporal burr holes (as that is where most clots are), then frontal/parietal. However, it is better to use the term "targeted burr holes". In most western environments, it is very rare to consider this procedure without imaging evidence; however, in a remote location with a patient with low Glasgow Coma Score (GCS) and a dilating pupil, it may be the only life-saving possibility.

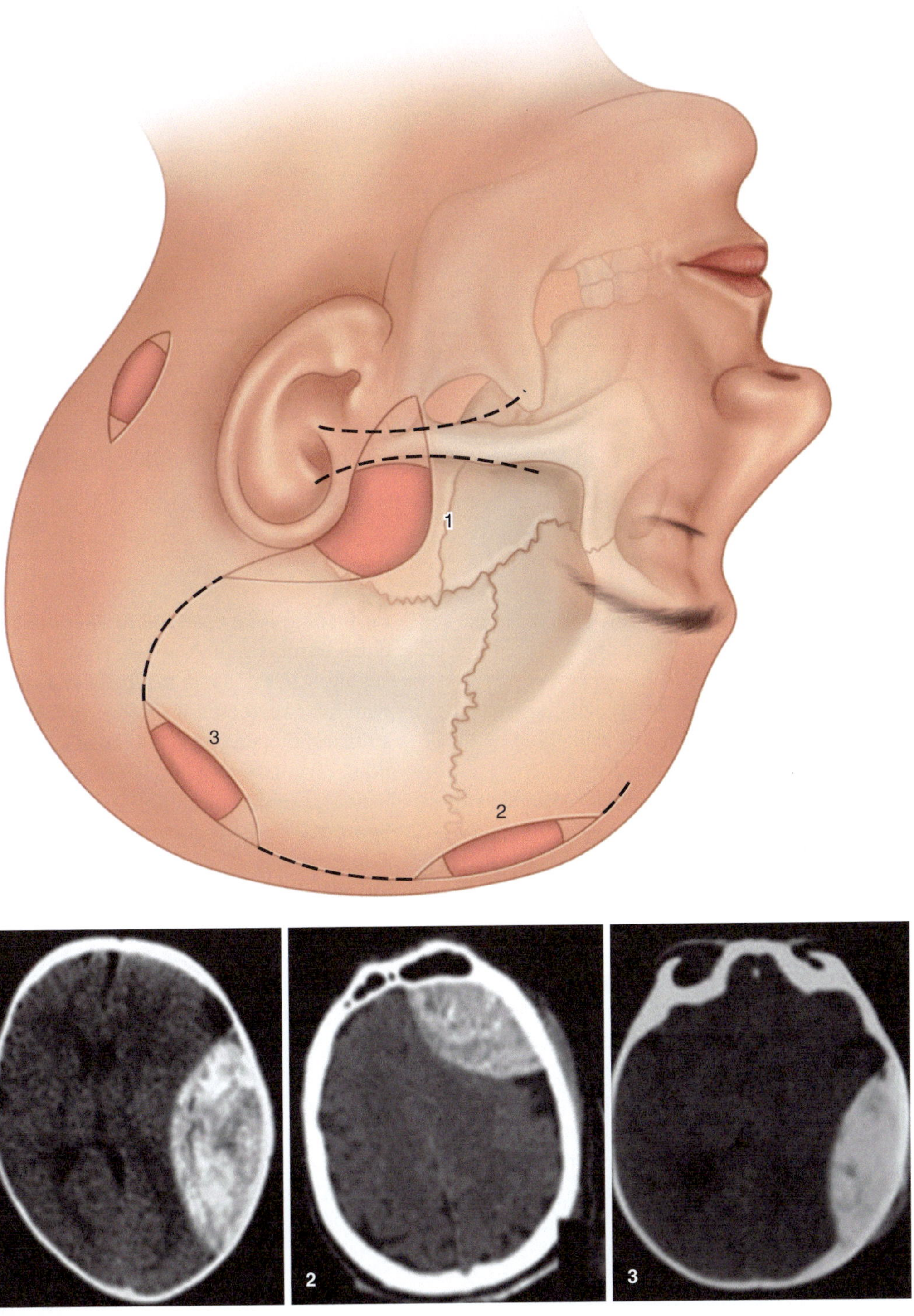

Fig. 9.2 Location of burr holes and a subsequent trauma cranial flap. 1 = temporal, 2 = frontal and 3 = parietal eminence

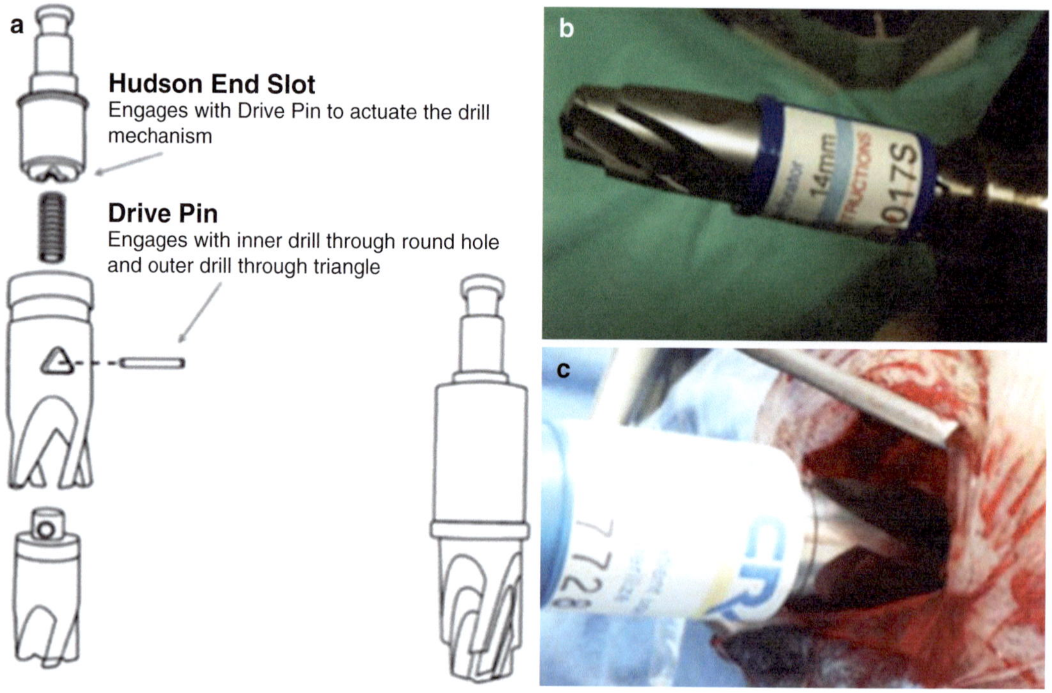

Fig. 9.3 The perforator drill bit—(**a**) a technical drawing and (**b**) a photograph with (**c**) a burr hole being performed. From [5]

In such a case, utilise the following to "target" where to perform the first burr hole:

1. The side of the injury—especially if there is a palpable skull fracture, this is likely to be the side of any extra-axial bleed.
2. The side of the dilating pupil—contralateral pupil dilatation is rare.
3. Temporal most likely (but look to see if there is another injury location).

9.5.4 Trauma Craniotomy

A trauma craniotomy is required to evacuate any significant amount of clot, extra or subdural. If the skull wound is large and the bone left out, it can also act to decompress swollen brain (a craniectomy). Described below is how to do a standard trauma flap (Fig. 9.1). This can be modified to be located over the main component of the hematoma when not temporal.

1. Positioning is key and follows the same principals as for burr holes above. Have the patient supine, sandbag under the ipsilateral shoulder with their head on a horseshoe or donut ring so that the operation site is parallel with the floor. Try not to kink neck veins (which increases venous bleeding).
2. Shave the head, mark out the burr holes and skin flap and prepare the skin with povo-iodine/chlorhexidine. Drape the patient.
3. Make an incision through the skin. Use clips to prevent bleeding from skin edges.
4. Reflect the galea and temporalis muscle forward en masse.
5. Clear the bone and mark out the craniotomy.
6. Usually burr holes are placed in the temporal region, at the frontal (10 cm from the pupil, 2–3 cm from the midline) and the parietal eminence (the widest part of the skull). If using a Gigli saw, you will need to perform more intermediary holes to enable easier cutting.

7. Once burr holes are placed, if using a Gigli, pass the guidewire and dural protector between two holes and connect the Gigli handles to cut. Repeat to free the bone segment.
8. If using a craniotome, ensure the gap between the dura and skull is cleared and then use a craniotome to open the skull.
9. If there is extradural, it should now be present. If there is not, then the dura should be opened.

9.5.5 Specific Techniques to Stop Haemorrhage

Be aware of where bleeding can come from.

9.5.5.1 Venous Bleeding

A common mistake is to turn the head too far over resulting in kinking of neck veins. This increases venous pressures and hence venous bleeding. This is especially common in children. When faced with excessive bleeding, ensure that the neck is in a more neutral position.

9.5.5.2 Bleeding from Skull Base

Skull base bleeding is common in extradurals. Use a bone nibbler to get down to the skull base and retract the inferior aspect of the temporal lobe to see if the bleeding source can be visualised. If it can be, use bone wax. If it can't then it may need temporary packing with haemostatic agents and mastoid/tonsil swabs.

9.5.5.3 Beware of the Fracture Over the Sinus

Be hyperaware of bilateral extra/subdurals when the patient has a fracture extending over the vertex (Fig. 9.4). Bleeding in such cases is often from the sagittal sinus. A craniotomy can be done in the normal way, but the rapid creation of hitch sutures may be required to tamponade bleeding coming down from the sinus.

Bone wax: Bone wax is a useful aid in bone bleeding. When performing a craniotomy, the bone edges can have a continuous ooze that cannot be controlled with diathermy. Soft bone wax applied directly and then pressed with a mastoid swab or pattie arrests bone bleeding.

Cellulose-based haemostatic agents: Sections of cellulose-based haemostatic agents can be cut to act as a matrix for clot to form on. These can be applied to non-bone oozing areas and with the addition of a mastoid swab/pattie and a couple of minutes, often bring haemostasis.

Tacking sutures: Hitch or tacking sutures are used to oppose dura to the inner table of the skull. Cellulose-based haemostatic material can be placed under the bone edge and the dura lifted onto it (Fig. 9.5). Hitch sutures can be anchored to overlying soft tissue or through obliquely

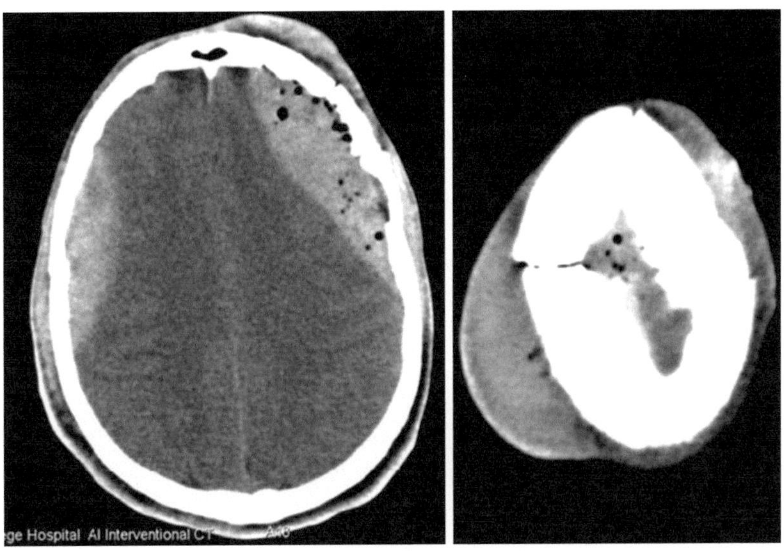

Fig. 9.4 Beware bilateral subdurals/extradurals. It can be caused by a fracture through the sagittal sinus. Check the top slice of the CT scan

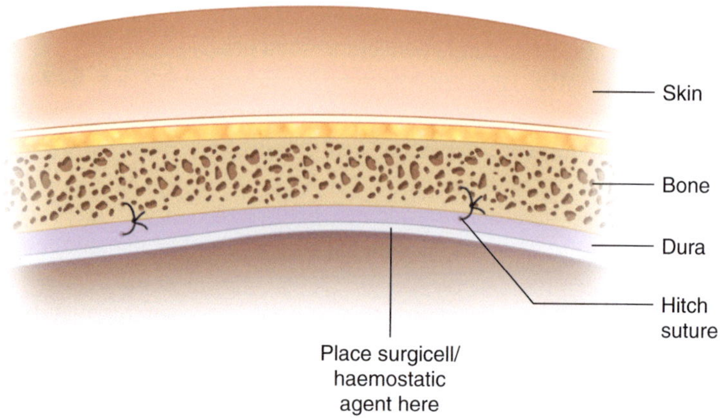

Fig. 9.5 Hitch or tacking sutures can pull dura next to the skull to tamponade bleeding from under the skull and minimise space for hematoma to accumulate

drilled holes in the bone edge. These holes can also be created quickly using a sharp towel clip biting the skull edge.

Haemostatic agents: A number of haemostatic agents are licenced for intracranial use (e.g. Flo Seal™). These should be applied to the bleeding region when dry (use suction to keep it dry), and then gentle pressure should be applied through a mastoid swab.

Packing: Packing is not normally required in neurosurgery; however, it may be used when confronted with uncontrollable bleeding. Packing of mastoid swabs using the remaining bone to tamponade bleeding can be used when all else fails. This is most likely to be needed when bleeding comes from an area that is not easily accessible, e.g. the skull base. If the patient survives, the packing can be removed at a second-stage operation.

9.5.6 Decompressive Craniectomy

Decompressive craniectomy is done when the brain is swollen or there is sufficient fear that the brain will swell. It is simply the same as a craniotomy with dural opening; however, the bone is not replaced. It is always best to ensure meticulous haemostasis and leave a drain in such cases.

The technique of bifrontal craniotomy for refractory intracranial pressure is beyond the scope of this book, however more information can be found out in the Rescue ICP protocol [6].

9.5.7 ICP Monitoring/External Ventricular Drain (EVD) Insertion

It is unlikely that a parenchymal ICP monitor will be available in an austere environment; however, the placement of both a parenchymal ICP monitor (purely enables ICP monitoring) and EVD placement (which also allows CSF withdrawal) is similar.

Both are usually placed on the side with the most injury or the right (non-dominant) at Kocher's point, approximately a centimetre anterior to the coronal suture and 3 cm from the midline (= approximately 10 cm from the pupil in the mid pupillary line). A simple ICP monitor is inserted with a 5 mm stab incision, twist drill through the skull, bolt insertion and then catheter threading. An EVD is placed by making a 2.5 cm incision, creating a burr hole, opening the dura and then inserting an external ventricular drain approximately 5 cm in the direction of the ipsilateral inner canthus and external auditory meatus (= perpendicular to the skull) (Fig. 9.6).

9.5.8 Management of Penetrating Injury

Penetrating injuries can be deep and isolated (e.g. bullet or fragments) or relatively low velocity and more superficial (such as knife injury).

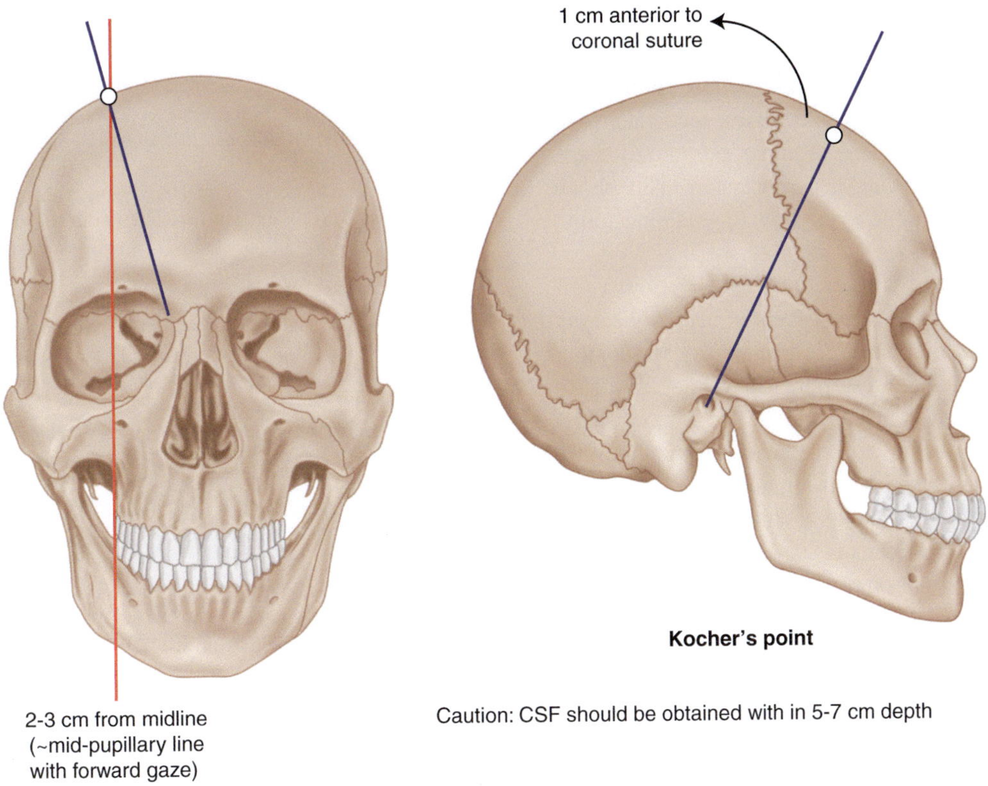

Fig. 9.6 Insertion of an external ventricular drain. See text for details

9.5.8.1 Low-Velocity Injuries, e.g. Knife Injuries

Penetrating injuries that still have components protruding or are superficial should be removed. This should be done in an operating theatre where haemorrhage control can be more easily established.

The approach should be planned with the skin incision incorporating the penetrating object (otherwise skin has to be pulled over it). Be aware of moving the object during the craniotomy. A high-speed drill may enable the bone surrounding the object to be removed to prevent movement of the penetrating component.

9.5.8.2 High-Velocity Injuries, e.g. Bullets

The energy transfer of high-velocity injuries results in many being fatal. If missile fragments remain deep in the brain substance, exploration to remove it is likely to cause more harm than benefit. Debriding the superficial wounds, controlling haemorrhage and decompressing to allow brain swelling are the mainstays of treatment.

9.5.8.3 Blast/Shrapnel Injuries

Blast injuries will often result in large quantities of dirty foreign material being embedded in brain substance and superficial tissues. These wounds need meticulous debridement and haemostasis control. The use of hydrogen peroxide can help both cleaning and haemostasis. Beware to remove any material (e.g. bone) that is not viable.

9.6 Damage Control Spinal Surgery

Acute spinal surgery is rarely required outside the civilian setting. The role of acute decompression for neurological injury is increasingly recognised but is still contested, and the benefits will depend on injury type. Spinal fixation enables easier nursing and transfer of patients, but there is no role for this acutely by the non-specialist. In the rare case where neurology is evolving secondary to spinal compression (e.g. from an extradural), there is a place for acute decompression. This should be kept as simple as possible (e.g. laminectomy).

Conclusion

The rapid management of neurological injuries can minimise secondary injury and neuron loss. This requires optimal physiological as well as surgical management. The role of surgery is principally to stop haemorrhage/remove hematoma that is causing pressure on the brain and debride wounds. Whilst this chapter outlines those principals, experience in a major trauma centre or on a specific neurotrauma course will enable those skills to be more rapidly and effectively deployed when needed.

References

1. Wilson MH, Hinds J, Grier G, Burns B, Carley S, Davies G. Impact brain apnoea—a forgotten cause of cardiovascular collapse in trauma. Resuscitation. 2016;105:52–8.
2. Mahoney EJ, Biffl WL, Harrington DT, Cioffi WG. Isolated brain injury as a cause of hypotension in the blunt trauma patient. J Trauma. 2003;55:1065–9.
3. Chesnut RM, Marshall LF, Klauber MR, et al. The role of secondary brain injury in determining outcome from severe head injury. J Trauma. 1993;34:216–22.
4. Murray GD, Butcher I, McHugh GS, et al. Multivariable prognostic analysis in traumatic brain injury: results from the IMPACT study. J Neurotrauma. 2007;24:329–37.
5. Wilson MH, Wise D, Davies G, Lockey D. Emergency Burr holes: 'how to do it'. Scand J Trauma Resusc Emerg Med. 2012;20:24–34.
6. Hutchinson PJ, Kolias AG, Timofeev IS, et al. Trial of Decompressive Craniectomy for traumatic intracranial hypertension. N Engl J Med. 2016;375:1119–30.

10 Damage Control Orthopaedics

Daniel Benz and Zsolt J. Balogh

Abstract

Musculoskeletal injuries represent the most common lesions requiring surgical intervention in polytrauma patients and in long-term survivors present challenging scenarios in terms of functional outcomes and quality of life (Balogh et al., Lancet 380(9847):1109–191, 2012; Banerjee et al., Injury 44(8):1015–212, 2013). More than 70% of all patients ith major trauma need at least one orthopaedic surgical procedure (Balogh, ANZ J Surg 80(3):119–21, 2010) and extremity injuries are associated with higher rates of blood transfusions, longer hospital stays and overall worse outcomes (Banerjee et al., Injury 44(8):1015–212, 2013; Pape et al., J Trauma 69(5):1243–514, 2010; Ringburg et al., J Trauma 70(4):916–22, 2011; Gabbe et al., Ann Surg 255(6):1009–15, 2012).

The term 'damage control orthopaedics' (DCO) represents a staged surgical approach to the management of selected polytrauma patients with orthopaedic injuries (Scalea et al., J Trauma 48(4):613–21, 2000; Giannoudis et al., Injury 40(Suppl 4):S47–52, 2009). The principle of DCO is to provide adequate skeletal stability of major fractures to prevent further bleeding/soft tissue damage, potential fat embolism and to permit better positioning of the multiple injured patient without the potential adverse effects of early definitive fixation (Pape et al., J Trauma 53(3):452–61, 2002; Roberts et al., Instr Course Lect 54:447–62, 2005). This abbreviated procedure allows for resuscitation following the initial hit of severe trauma and optimises patient physiology for later definitive fixation (Taeger et al., J Trauma 59(2):409–16, 2005).

In the context of improved trauma resuscitation and understanding of trauma physiology, the indications for DCO have developed since its initial description (Scalea et al., J Trauma 48(4):613–21, 2000). Today DCO may be implemented in the prevention of physiological deterioration in the critically injured patient (patient mode), in the management of complex periarticular injuries with critical soft tissue damage (limb mode) and in settings of inadequate surgical expertise, equipment or manpower (resource mode).

D. Benz, M.D. • Z.J. Balogh, M.D. (✉)
Division of Surgery, Department of Traumatology, John Hunter Hospital and University of Newcastle, Newcastle, NSW, Australia
e-mail: zsolt.balogh@hnehealth.nsw.gov.au; zsolt.balogh@newcastle.edu.au

10.1 Historical Perspective

Prior to the 1980s, polytrauma patients were often considered too unwell to withstand the physiological insult associated with internal fixa-

J. Duchesne et al. (eds.), *Damage Control in Trauma Care*,
https://doi.org/10.1007/978-3-319-72607-6_10

tion of associated major fractures. These patients were typically managed in a staged manner involving immediate resuscitation and emergency surgery for life-threatening injuries only [12]. Major fractures were often placed in traction for days to weeks [13] until patients were considered well enough to tolerate operative fracture fixation. This involved prolonged immobilisation, typically in recumbence, often resulting in pneumonia, deep vein thrombosis, muscle wasting and decubitus ulcers [14]. Additionally, lack of skeletal stability was thought to increase the incidence of thrombotic [15] and fat [16] pulmonary embolism.

Evidence put forward in the 1980s supported a move away from traction and bed rest towards early stabilisation of long bones, citing a reduction in the rates of pulmonary and late septic complications, hospital/intensive care unit stays and associated health-care costs [13, 15, 17, 18].

Bone and colleagues in 1989 [19] published a seminal prospective randomised study examining early versus delayed fixation of acute femoral fractures in 178 patients. Subjects were randomised to early (<24 h) or delayed (>48 h) fracture fixation. In patients with isolated femoral fractures and an ISS < 18, the timing of fixation had no effect on outcomes; however in multiple injured patients with an ISS > 18, early fixation led to a decrease in postoperative pulmonary morbidity. Patients who underwent 'early total care' (ETC) had markedly decreased incidence of acute respiratory distress syndrome (ARDS), pulmonary dysfunction, fat embolism syndrome, pulmonary emboli and pneumonia. These patients also had a mean ICU and total hospital LOS that was 5–10 days less, respectively, and an average cost of hospitalisation that was 50% lower than polytrauma patients managed with delayed fixation. Despite criticism regarding study design in terms of unequal pulmonary injuries between groups, limited details regarding resuscitation and limited statistical comparison, it clearly remains one of the most influential studies demonstrating the virtues of ETC.

Following Bone and colleagues' publication, conflicting evidence became apparent both supporting [20, 21] and demonstrating no benefit [22] with early fixation of major fractures in polytrauma. Additionally, some authors suggested that although early fixation may be beneficial, fixation within the first 24 h may actually be detrimental in certain patients, in particular those with associated pulmonary [23] or traumatic brain injuries [24, 25].

In the 1990s, the universal approach to ETC was challenged [23] as it was realised that providing definitive fixation of femoral shaft fractures with intramedullary nailing had detrimental physiological effects on the already compromised polytrauma patient [26]. The instrumentation of the medullary canal with reaming and nail insertion became known as a modifiable 'second hit' in the development of post-injury complications such as acute lung injury (ALI), ARDS and multiple organ failure (MOF) [1].

During the same period, Rotondo et al. in 1993 reported the benefits of 'damage control surgery', a staged surgical approach to the management penetrating abdominal trauma [27]. In a retrospective analysis, a subset of 46 patients, with major vascular and visceral abdominal injuries, showed increased survival with initial control of haemorrhage/contamination followed by intraperitoneal packing/rapid closure and subsequent delayed definitive re-exploration once patient physiology allowed.

During a period of conflicting evidence regarding the optimal timing of femoral fractures in polytrauma patients, Scalea et al. in 2000 reported on the use of external fixation as a temporising bridge to definitive intramedullary fixation, terming the approach 'damage control orthopaedics' [7]. The authors credited Rotondo and colleagues with applying the naval war term 'damage control' to the limited initial treatment of penetrating abdominal trauma. This work prompted a new era of publications and surgical education regarding the concept of DCO.

Scalea and colleagues examined the clinical course and outcomes of 43 adult trauma patients managed with early temporising external fixation and staged nailing (median 4 days, IQR 2.5–6) which were retrospectively compared to 281 patients who underwent primary femoral nailing. External fixation was selected only when the care of associated injuries or patient physiology at presentation precluded early intramedullary nailing (IMN). Despite significantly higher ISS (26.8 vs. 16.8, $P = 0.001$), shock on presentation, resuscitation requirements, AIS head ≥3, rates of laparotomy and ICU stays in the DCO cohort, only four deaths occurred (9% vs. <1%; $P = 0.001$), and minimal orthopaedic complications were recorded. No deaths occurred as a result of the fracture management option selected. Although the authors advocated for the early stabilisation of femoral fractures when appropriate, they considered a DCO approach with external fixation to be a safe alternative in a trauma patients unsuitable for prolonged traction and staged fixation or immediate stabilisation with IMN.

Preceding the initial description of DCO, Pape and colleagues at the Department of Orthopedics and Trauma Surgery, Hannover Medical School, Germany, had been performing staged fixation of femoral fractures in polytrauma patients at risk of post-traumatic complications for almost 10 years [9]. In 2002, the group published a retrospective cohort study examining the clinical outcomes of these patients prior to and after the implementation of DCO. Although some criticism has been raised in regard to patient selection, statistical analysis and conclusions drawn [28, 29], the overall incidence of ARDS and MOF decreased significantly over a 20-year period in which ETC and then DCO treatment protocols were implemented, regardless of the type of fixation selected. In addition, the relative incidence of ARDS decreased from 54.6% (ETC) to 26.4% (DCO) when primary IMN was performed and decreased from 97.4% (ETC) to 22.1% (DCO) when primary external fixation was implemented. The authors suggested these changes were due in part to a more appropriate treatment selection in respect to patient physiology and associated injuries. They concluded the introduction of DCO is likely to have had a positive impact in the treatment of polytrauma femoral shaft fractures and appeared to be an adequate alternative for patients at high risk of post-traumatic complications.

Prior to 2007, recommendations regarding the surgical approach to major fractures in polytrauma patients had been based on level II to III evidence. Although several prospective randomized studies considered fracture management in general [19, 30], no level I studies had investigated whether temporary fracture fixation (DCO) should be recommended for certain patient populations.

Pape and colleagues, in 2007 [31], published the first prospective, randomised, controlled analysis examining the development of systemic complications in polytrauma patients with femoral shaft fractures managed with initial temporary fracture stabilisation or immediate definitive stabilisation. One hundred sixty-five consecutive patients from ten level 1 trauma centres across Europe were included. Patients were categorised as stable, borderline, unstable or in extremis based on prior defined criterion [32, 33]. Unstable or those 'in extremis' were excluded. Stable and borderline patients were randomised to receive either initial (<24 h) intramedullary femoral nailing ($n = 94$) or external fixation ($n = 71$) and later conversion to an intramedullary nail (once deemed stable enough for surgery).

The study found that in stable patients, primary femoral nailing was associated with shorter ventilation times without an increase in postoperative complications, confirming the findings of previous studies that early fracture stabilisation is beneficial in stable patients [19]. In borderline patients, the odds of developing acute lung injury were 6.69 times greater ($P < 0.05$) when managed with initial femoral nailing, compared to a staged DCO approach. Importantly, however, no increase in the incidence of clinically significant adverse outcomes, such as ARDS, systemic inflammatory response syndrome (SIRS), pneumonia, sepsis or MOF, was seen.

These findings were further reinforced by the experience of centres that routinely provided ETC to patients with 'borderline' physiology and whose patients had fewer days on a ventilator, earlier discharge from intensive care and less infectious complications than did those enrolled in the trial by Pape et al. (2007) [34]. The publication by Pape and colleagues encouraged a new era of reflected ETC rather than the rigid application of DCO in physiologically uncompromised patients or those who had readily reversible acute physiological compromise.

Due to the lack of conclusive evidence-based guidelines for the implementation of DCO, more recently, patient selection based particularly on the physiologic level of resuscitation in conjunction with presenting injury characteristics has been used to determine whether DCO or ETC is undertaken. This approach known as 'risk-adapted DCO' [35] has demonstrated encouraging results in terms of perioperative morbidity and patient mortality [36–38].

Recently Nahm and colleagues [39] coined the term early appropriate care (EAC) to describe the preferential fixation of femoral fracture within 24 h as opposed to other extremity fractures which could be splinted and addressed later. With attention to resuscitation and medical optimisation of patients before and during surgery, femoral fixation in polytrauma patients within 24 h was associated with lower rates of pulmonary complications, DVT, sepsis, MOF (18.9% vs. 42.9%, $P < 0.037$) and shorter hospital and ICU length of stay ($P < 0.001$) than femoral fractures managed in a delayed fashion. The authors stated that provided aggressive resuscitation was implemented, EAC would provide a compromise between staged DCO and the fixation of all fractures with ETC.

10.2 Physiology

The major transfer of mechanical energy to the body is known to stimulate the immune system [1]. Cell death, haemorrhage, resuscitation, bacterial invasion and pain [40] all release proinflammatory elements resulting in both local and systemic side effects. Even in the absence shock, substantial soft tissue injury leads to cellular release of danger-associated molecular patterns (DAMPs) into the circulation, which activate innate immunity and may result in SIRS. While SIRS is essential to cope with injury, exaggerated or prolonged SIRS is thought to result in secondary/remote organ damage manifesting as MOF [41–43]. Up to 20% of major trauma patients experience MOF [44, 45] with mortality rates being reported between 4% and 50%. Although recent advances in trauma care have reduced the incidence and severity of MOF, it remains a significant cause of resource utilisation in the ICU population and leading cause of death in polytrauma. Additionally, patients with subclinical MOF may linger and progress to persistent inflammation, immunosuppression and catabolism syndrome (PICS) [46].

Fractures themselves contribute to the release of DAMPs and subsequent inflammatory cytokines into the circulation as well as the release of highly acidic lipid emboli that can lodge in vital organs causing fat embolism syndrome [26, 47]. The marrow of fractured long bones is known to be a potent source of proinflammatory cytokines, with concentrations of interleukin-6 in the marrow of fracture femora reported to be 1000 times higher than in those femora of patients undergoing major elective surgery. Interleukin-6 levels are known to increase further during intramedullary nailing [48]. Prolonged fracture manipulation and/or surgical intervention is therefore considered to further increase systemic delivery of inflammatory mediators which can be considered a preventable 'second hit' in the development of post-injury complications like ARDS and MOF.

In regard to orthopaedic trauma care, two main concepts of post-traumatic physiological response have emerged.

The one-hit theory postulates that a traumatic insult triggers an initial inflammatory response that, if exaggerated or dysfunctional, may progress from SIRS to ARDS and MOF directly [49–51]. The development of these complications is dependent on the extent of the initial injury and subsequent resuscitation [52]. In contrast, the two-hit theory postulates that the initial injury results in priming of the immune system, in particular neutrophils, which are then vulnerable to activation in the event of further inflammatory stimuli ('second hits') [49, 53]. Thus subsequent events such as surgical interventions, infection, periods of hypoxia, hypovolaemia and blood transfusions can trigger and worsen the hyperinflammation that leads to MOF [54–56]. Surgical interventions and their timing have generated particular interest as they represent a major modifiable risk factor for complications. This is the basis of 'damage control' surgery after trauma in which an initial more minor procedure (e.g. stabilisation of fractures with external fixation, haemostasis and decontamination at laparotomy) is performed allowing for optimisation of patient physiology [7, 27, 57, 58] and the abatement of the systemic inflammatory response [1] prior to major definitive surgical intervention.

Much literature has examined the perioperative changes in serum immune markers after trauma. Early evidence reported during the 1990s supported the shift from ETC to DCO in polytrauma patients with major orthopaedic injuries [59, 60].

A recent systematic review [53] aimed to evaluate whether trauma patients demonstrated a measurable 'second hit' phenomenon in immune markers with surgical intervention. Fifteen studies from 1996 to 2010 were included in the analysis. Limitations in the overall quality of studies were noted with only one randomised trial including 19 patients being identified [61]. All 15 studies totalled 563 subjects, and heterogeneity precluded combined statistical analysis. All available studies demonstrated a measurable rise in at least one serum marker after surgical intervention, generally 24–48 h post-op. IL-6 and IL-10 consistently showed an increase following major surgical procedures. The review also noted the magnitude and timing of surgery may modulate the immune response—in particular, delayed operations following 'damage control' did not produce the same increase in serum cytokines as primary fixation. Importantly however, the majority of studies did not provide clinical correlation to changes in immune markers. Those which did [62, 63] showed few associations with questionable clinical relevance. The review concluded that the 'second hit' phenomenon in serum cytokines can be demonstrated after surgery in trauma patients, but there is a paucity of research describing the clinical associations mirroring these changes.

In 2011, Xiao and colleagues [64] challenged several current clinical dogma regarding human response to severe injury, including the second hit phenomenon. By examining gene expression patterns of blood leucocytes, severe injury produced an unexpected 'genomic storm' manifesting as changes in innate and adaptive immunity that occur rapidly after injury. The absence of late episodes of new organ injury in the patient population argued strongly against evidence of any clinically relevant second inflammatory hit. Instead the initial magnitude and duration of these genomic changes were thought to discriminate patients who experienced complicated and uncomplicated recoveries.

It now seems clear that the dogma of a second hit effect by intramedullary nailing of femoral fractures has been overemphasised. It is likely that much of the 'second hit' phenomenon observed in the 1990s and 2000s was related to resuscitation techniques including the use of large volumes of crystalloid as opposed to the mode of fracture stabilisation [65]. This aligns with evidence emerging from general and trauma surgery, regarding strategies to deal with exsanguinating abdominal injury encapsulated in the philosophy of damage control resuscitation (DCR) [66, 67]. DCR has produced dramatic improvements in survival by combining strategies of permissive hypotension and haemostatic resuscitation with damage control surgery. To date, no large-scale study reappraising the changes in inflammatory mediators or effector cells in the era of DCR has been published.

10.3 Practical Application of DCO

10.3.1 Patient Mode

Despite a wealth of literature focusing on the application of DCO principles to avoid physiological exhaustion and early organ failure and to save critically injured patients lives, there are still no universally agreed criteria indicating its use in polytrauma.

Indeed, a retrospective comparative study of multiple injured patients with femoral fractures managed at two level 1 trauma centres in Australia and Germany reflects the difference in attitude between surgeons [68]. Despite no difference in patient demographics or ISS, the utilisation of ETC and DCO was 70% vs. 30% in Australia and 30% vs. 70% in Germany. Additionally, the median ISS for ETC was 34 and 25.5 for Australian and German hospitals, respectively. Interestingly, no difference in incidence of ARDS, MODS or mortality was seen between the Australian and German trauma population.

Most literature examining ETC and DCO has focused on femoral shaft fractures, almost invariably because these injuries occur typically via high-energy mechanisms and are frequently associated with multiple other injuries and mortality [7]. Adult femora are not amendable to splinting and require recumbence/traction prior to fixation, typically via intramedullary instrumentation which may augment the inflammatory response to trauma [52]. The principles of DCO however may also be successfully applied to fractures of other long bones [69], pelvic [70–73] and acetabular injuries [73, 74] and the thoracolumbar spine [75–81].

In contrast to ETC, DCO strategies should aim for rapid fracture stabilisation with minimal blood loss and soft tissue injury. DCO can frequently be performed on supine patients on standard radiolucent tables in conjunction with major lifesaving procedures of the head, chest and abdomen. Temporary stabilisation may also be performed in intensive care units when required. Although DCO has traditionally paralleled external fixation of femoral fractures [7], other modes of temporary stabilisation may be implemented. Percutaneous locked plating ('internal fixateur'), unreamed unlocked intramedullary nailing and skeletal traction are appropriate adjuncts to DCO arsenal in selected circumstances.

DCO is frequently oversimplified to the dilemma of nailing or externally fixing the femur fracture. The initial phase of staged care of multiple musculoskeletal injuries in the polytrauma patient must be more comprehensive. Priorities in the initial management of the multiple injured patient should also include the completion of unsalvageable traumatic amputations, the decompression of acute compartment syndrome via fasciotomy, acute revascularisation with temporary shunts when definitive repair is not possible/feasible, the reduction of dislocations and the irrigation/debridement and antimicrobial management of open fractures.

The timing of definitive fixation following DCO is controversial. Specifically delaying secondary major fracture fixation until the 5th day after injury has been suggested to avoid exacerbation of the systemic inflammatory response to injury [59, 62, 82, 83]. The clinical ramification of this is still controversial. Additionally, multiple injured patients are a diverse group, and clinical judgement on an individual patient basis is more appropriate rather than abiding by strict timeframes. Concerns regarding the risk of secondary infection with staged definitive fixation have also been addressed in the literature. Low infection rates after staged intramedullary nailing of femoral fractures have been reported between 1.7% and 3% after an average of 4.8–7 days of provisional external fixation [7, 84]. Infection risk in tibial fractures seems to be somewhat higher at 9% when staged fixation from external fixation to intramedullary nailing is undertaken [85]. However unlike femoral fractures, closed tibial fractures may be splinted as an alternative during immediate DCO.

To aid surgical decision regarding patient selection for DCO, Pape et al. have suggested multiple trauma patient with femoral shaft fractures be stratified into stable, borderline, unstable and 'in extremis' groups at the time of presentation [23, 32, 33, 86]. The classification system is based on clinical parameters in four separate categories: shock, coagulopathy, hypothermia and the presence/severity of associated injury to the pelvis, abdomen, chest and extremities. Much literature has previously focused on an algorithmic management approach based on these categories. However, the stable/borderline/unstable/in extremis concept is now somewhat dated and unhelpful since trauma resuscitation methods have advanced significantly over the last two decades and resuscitation is a dynamic process over time rather than a static snapshot of physiology. Resuscitation and timing of definitive fracture fixation cannot be addressed separately, and understanding patient physiology is key.

To this end, recent literature has focused on suitable physiological parameters to identify polytrauma patients adequately resuscitated and appropriate for early definitive fixation (EAC) of major fractures [36–38] from those requiring a staged DCO approach to definitive care. In addition, increasing evidence is reinforcing the understanding that early definitive fracture fixation of the femur, spine and pelvis in appropriately resuscitated patients leads to reduced rates of ARDS, MODS and ICU length of stay [38].

Parameters of acid-base balance in polytrauma provide prognosis regarding patient morbidity/mortality and are proportional to the magnitude of resuscitation requirements, including blood and blood products [87]. An inability to normalise acidosis during resuscitation is associated with ARDS [88–90], organ failure [89, 91, 92] and death [93–98]. Base excess (BE) has been shown to be superior to pH in the evaluation of trauma-induced acidosis [99] and when persistently raised should be considered a sign of inadequate resuscitation [100]. Serum lactate in particular is a valid indirect measure of tissue hypoperfusion and a predictor of postoperative morbidity in multiple trauma with associated long bone and pelvic fractures [88, 101].

O'Toole and colleagues [36] demonstrated that emphasising resuscitation before stabilisation of femoral fractures limited ARDS and mortality in polytrauma patients despite infrequent use of DCO. The group retrospectively reviewed 227 trauma patients (ISS > 17) with femoral fractures managed with intramedullary nailing after adequate resuscitation had been demonstrated by normalising lactate levels (approaching 2.5 mmol/L at the commencement of surgery) plus optimised ventilatory and hemodynamic parameters. DCO with primary external fixation was reserved for those few patients who did not respond to resuscitation. Despite infrequent use of DCO (12%), low rates of ARDS (1.5%) and death (2%) with primary fixation were seen. Subgroup analysis showed similarly low rates in those patients most severely injured (ISS > 28, thoracic AIS >2; ARDS 3.3%; death 1.7%) and those with significant lung injury (thoracic AIS > 2; ARDS 2%; death 2%). In the context of aggressive resuscitation, ARDS rates were significantly lower ($P < 0.001$) than similar studies in which DCO was utilised in up to 36% patients [32, 35]. The authors suggested the discrepancy in postoperative morbidity/mortality between centres to be due in part to differences in preoperative resuscitation or medical care provided to treat shock.

Consistent with this theme, Vallier et al. [38] found that in 1443 adult trauma patients with surgically managed femoral, acetabulum, pelvis and spine fractures, pH and base excess values were significantly lower at presentation ($P < 0.0001$) and rate of improvement with resuscitation slower ($P < 0.007$) in those who developed pneumonia or ARDS. Similarly, lactate values were greater with pulmonary complications ($P < 0.02$). Subsequent logistic predictive models found lactate to be the most specific predictor of postoperative complications. Based on these findings, the group prospectively evaluated an EAC protocol in which definitive fixation of femur, acetabulum, pelvis and spine fractures was performed within 36 hours, provided patient acidosis showed improvement to resuscitation as demonstrated by at least one of the following: lactate <4.0 mmol/L, pH ≥ 7.25 or base excess ≥ −5.5 mmol/L. In cases of persistent acidosis, DCO was undertaken. Three hundred thirty-five polytrauma patients were prospectively compared to the historical cohort of 1443 patients managed prior to EAC protocol implementation. Complications including infection/sepsis, DVT/PE, pneumonia, ARDS and organ failure occurred less (19.7% vs. 22.1%, $P = 0.17$), and overall hospital LOS was significantly shorter ($P = 0.018$) in patients managed with EAC [102].

Importantly, parameters of patient physiology, including serum lactate trend, should be monitored intraoperatively to determine whether a change in surgical tact is required in circumstances where patients manifest early signs of deterioration. Conversely it may be possible to extend the original surgical plan in patients who show physiological improvement.

Severe head injuries are common in the multiple injured patient. No firm guidelines exist regarding which of these injuries are safe to receive early definitive care of associated major fractures [52]. This typically remains a clinical decision between orthopaedic and neurosurgical teams. Early fracture stabilisation reduces persistent pain and is advocated to have positive effects on patient metabolism, muscle tone, body temperature and thereby cerebral function. Furthermore, unstabilised fractures can cause physiological deterioration as a result of unrestricted soft tissue damage, fat embolism and respiratory insufficiency [15, 19, 20, 103]. However, concerns surrounding additional cerebral injury from blood and intracranial pressure fluctuations, hypoxia, blood loss and fluid requirements during extensive fracture surgery often make neurosurgery hesitant to clear patients for theatre and may force the orthopaedic surgeon to implement DCO strategies in the short term [104, 105]. Although increased intraoperative fluid requirements and periods of hypotension can be expected [24, 25], current weight of evidence suggests no effect of definitive femoral fixation on neurological outcomes in patients with concurrent severe head injuries [87, 105].

Emphasis must be made that the goals of fracture stabilisation are to assist overall physiology of polytrauma patients and resuscitation should be tailored to maximise cerebral perfusion and oxygenation.

10.3.2 Limb Mode

DCO can be successfully implemented in the management of traumatic injuries involving complex articular injuries and critical local soft tissue compromise [10]. These indications are independent to those strategies outlined to prevent physiological compromise and patient mortality (patient mode).

The concept of temporary spanning fixation for complex periarticular injuries, especially those of the proximal and distal tibia, has become widely accepted [106, 107]. The ability to achieve immediate axial realignment of the limb and ligamentotaxis reduction substantially decreases the amount of injury-related swelling and oedema and promotes soft tissue recovery.

Staged fixation allows for additional imaging and preoperative planning in a controlled setting. Conversely, delayed reduction can result in an inability to disimpact displaced metaphyseal fragments resulting in more difficult delayed definitive reconstruction.

Limb mode DCO can also be implemented in the management of the mangled extremity. The use of spanning external fixation, vascular shunts, prophylactic fasciotomy and vacuum assisted wound closure techniques can provide a bridge to staged osseous reconstruction and soft tissue coverage procedures. When necessary, DCO techniques also provide time for sequential assessment of limb viability and informed discussion with patients prior to definitive amputation.

10.4 Resource Mode

In the context of natural disaster or conflict and in certain hospital settings, early total care may not be possible or safe. DCO strategies can be applied to avoid complications from inadequate resources or expertise and definitive surgery performed at a later stage.

Damage control for orthopaedic care has been successfully implemented in numerous situations of disaster and conflict [108, 109]. Musculoskeletal injuries in these settings are typically high energy and often compound and routinely represent only part of the scope of injury in the polytrauma patient [110]. External fixation of extremity injuries in particular is resource and time efficient, requires basic surgical expertise and can be performed without intraoperative fluoroscopy. These injuries often require serial wound evaluation and debridement and frequent dressing changes. External fixation provides ease of wound management for both patient and surgeon [111].

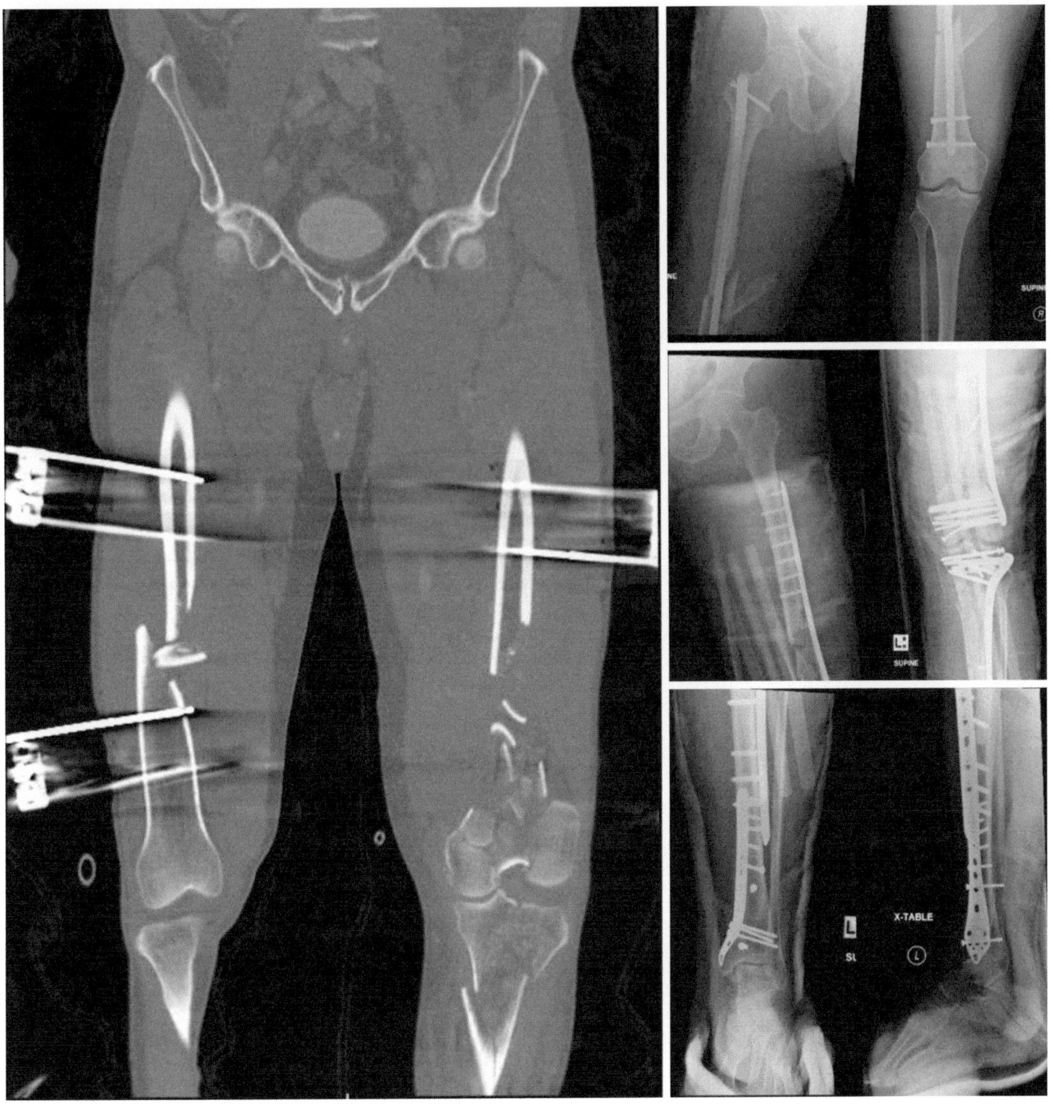

Fig. 10.1 A 64-year-old male was involved in a motorcycle accident sustaining multiple injuries including a right femoral shaft fracture and compound fractures of the left femur and left proximal tibia/fibula. A CT scan following damage control external fixation of both lower limb injuries, debridement and negative pressure dressings of associated compound wounds and 'on-table' bilateral diagnostic femoral angiograms excluding vascular injury. Postoperatively the patient developed rhabdomyolysis with acute kidney injury and bilateral pulmonary emboli. Following adequate resuscitation and therapeutic anticoagulation in the ICU, the patient returned to theatre after 9 days for definitive fixation. Postoperative radiographs demonstrating a right antegrade reamed femoral nail with proximal/distal locking, percutaneous LISS plate fixation of the left femur and inter-fragmentary/percutaneous LISS plate fixation of the left proximal tibia (note left distal tibia fixation also from a motorcycle accident 8 years prior)

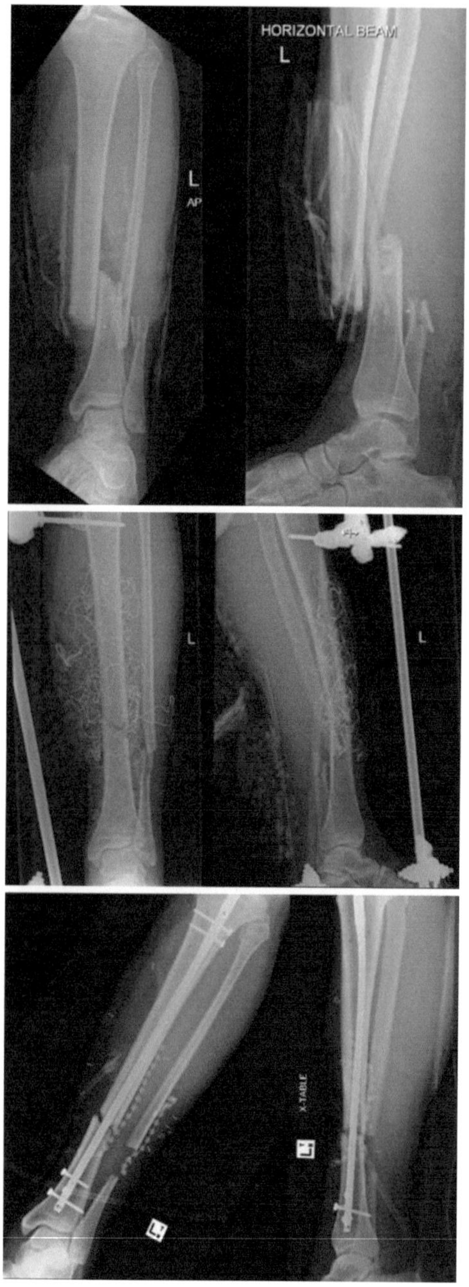

Fig. 10.2 A 28-year-old male was involved in a motorcycle accident sustaining multiple injuries including a compound left tibia/fibula fracture with extensive soft tissue loss and wound contamination. Following initial wound debridement and damage control external fixation in a regional hospital, the patient was transferred to a level 1 trauma centre for staged debridement and definitive intramedullary nail fixation. A large (200 × 40 mm) soft tissue defect was subsequently covered with a rectus abdominus free flap and split skin graft

Conclusion

Although the indications for the implementation of damage control orthopaedics have developed over the last two decades, the strategies of provisional fracture stabilisation and delayed definitive care remain invaluable to the modern-day orthopaedic trauma surgeon. Today, DCO may be successfully implemented in the management of unstable polytrauma patients ‘in extremis’ or those who do not respond to modern-day resuscitation techniques. Delaying definitive care in the context of complex periarticular and soft tissue injuries and in settings of resource or expertise scarcity remains a valid option.

Current indications for DCO:

1. Patient mode
   (a) Polytrauma patients ‘in extremis’
   (b) Unstable polytrauma patients not responding to resuscitation
2. Limb mode
3. Resource mode

References

1. Balogh ZJ, Reumann MK, Gruen RL, Mayer-Kuckuk P, Schuetz MA, Harris IA, et al. Advances and future directions for management of trauma patients with musculoskeletal injuries. Lancet. 2012;380(9847):1109–19.
2. Banerjee M, Bouillon B, Shafizadeh S, Paffrath T, Lefering R, Wafaisade A, et al. Epidemiology of extremity injuries in multiple trauma patients. Injury. 2013;44(8):1015–21.
3. Balogh Z. Traumatology in Australia: provision of clinical care and trauma system development. ANZ J Surg. 2010;80(3):119–21.
4. Pape HC, Probst C, Lohse R, Zelle BA, Panzica M, Stalp M, et al. Predictors of late clinical outcome following orthopedic injuries after multiple trauma. J Trauma. 2010;69(5):1243–51.
5. Ringburg AN, Polinder S, van Ierland MC, Steyerberg EW, van Lieshout EM, Patka P, et al. Prevalence and prognostic factors of disability after major trauma. J Trauma. 2011;70(4):916–22.
6. Gabbe BJ, Simpson PM, Sutherland AM, Wolfe R, Fitzgerald MC, Judson R, et al. Improved functional outcomes for major trauma patients in a regionalized, inclusive trauma system. Ann Surg. 2012;255(6):1009–15.

7. Scalea TM, Boswell SA, Scott JD, Mitchell KA, Kramer ME, Pollak AN. External fixation as a bridge to intramedullary nailing for patients with multiple injuries and with femur fractures: damage control orthopedics. J Trauma. 2000;48(4):613–21; discussion 21–3.
8. Giannoudis PV, Giannoudi M, Stavlas P. Damage control orthopaedics: lessons learned. Injury. 2009;40(Suppl 4):S47–52.
9. Pape HC, Hildebrand F, Pertschy S, Zelle B, Garapati R, Grimme K, et al. Changes in the management of femoral shaft fractures in polytrauma patients: from early total care to damage control orthopedic surgery. J Trauma. 2002;53(3):452–61; discussion 61–2.
10. Roberts CS, Pape HC, Jones AL, Malkani AL, Rodriguez JL, Giannoudis PV. Damage control orthopaedics: evolving concepts in the treatment of patients who have sustained orthopaedic trauma. Instr Course Lect. 2005;54:447–62.
11. Taeger G, Ruchholtz S, Waydhas C, Lewan U, Schmidt B, Nast-Kolb D. Damage control orthopedics in patients with multiple injuries is effective, time saving, and safe. J Trauma. 2005;59(2):409–16; discussion 17.
12. Wolff G, Dittmann M, Rüedi T, Buchmann B, Allgöwer M. Prevention of posttraumatic respiratory insufficiency by coordination of surgery and intensive care (author's transl). Unfallheilkunde. 1978;81(6):425–42.
13. Goris RJ, Gimbrère JS, van Niekerk JL, Schoots FJ, Booy LH. Early osteosynthesis and prophylactic mechanical ventilation in the multitrauma patient. J Trauma. 1982;22(11):895–903.
14. Reynolds MA, Richardson JD, Spain DA, Seligson D, Wilson MA, Miller FB. Is the timing of fracture fixation important for the patient with multiple trauma? Ann Surg. 1995;222(4):470–8; discussion 8–81
15. Seibel R, LaDuca J, Hassett JM, Babikian G, Mills B, Border DO, et al. Blunt multiple trauma (ISS 36), femur traction, and the pulmonary failure-septic state. Ann Surg. 1985;202(3):283–95.
16. Riska EB, von Bonsdorff H, Hakkinen S, Jaroma H, Kiviluoto O, Paavilainen T. Prevention of fat embolism by early internal fixation of fractures in patients with multiple injuries. Injury. 1976;8(2):110–6.
17. Johnson KD, Cadambi A, Seibert GB. Incidence of adult respiratory distress syndrome in patients with multiple musculoskeletal injuries: effect of early operative stabilization of fractures. J Trauma. 1985;25(5):375–84.
18. Riska EB, Myllynen P. Fat embolism in patients with multiple injuries. J Trauma. 1982;22(11):891–4.
19. Bone LB, Johnson KD, Weigelt J, Scheinberg R. Early versus delayed stabilization of femoral fractures. A prospective randomized study. J Bone Joint Surg Am. 1989;71(3):336–40.
20. Behrman SW, Fabian TC, Kudsk KA, Taylor JC. Improved outcome with femur fractures: early vs. delayed fixation. J Trauma. 1990;30(7):792–7; discussion 7–8.
21. Charash WE, Fabian TC, Croce MA. Delayed surgical fixation of femur fractures is a risk factor for pulmonary failure independent of thoracic trauma. J Trauma. 1994;37(4):667–72.
22. Pelias ME, Townsend MC, Flancbaum L. Long bone fractures predispose to pulmonary dysfunction in blunt chest trauma despite early operative fixation. Surgery. 1992;111(5):576–9.
23. Pape HC, Auf'm'Kolk M, Paffrath T, Regel G, Sturm JA, Tscherne H. Primary intramedullary femur fixation in multiple trauma patients with associated lung contusion–a cause of posttraumatic ARDS? J Trauma. 1993;34(4):540–7; discussion 7–8.
24. Jaicks RR, Cohn SM, Moller BA. Early fracture fixation may be deleterious after head injury. J Trauma. 1997;42(1):1–5; discussion -6.
25. Townsend RN, Lheureau T, Protech J, Riemer B, Simon D. Timing fracture repair in patients with severe brain injury (Glasgow coma scale score <9). J Trauma. 1998;44(6):977–82; discussion 82–3.
26. Giannoudis PV, Smith RM, Bellamy MC, Morrison JF, Dickson RA, Guillou PJ. Stimulation of the inflammatory system by reamed and unreamed nailing of femoral fractures. An analysis of the second hit. J Bone Joint Surg Br. 1999;81(2):356–61.
27. Rotondo MF, Schwab CW, McGonigal MD, Phillips GR, Fruchterman TM, Kauder DR, et al. 'Damage control': an approach for improved survival in exsanguinating penetrating abdominal injury. J Trauma. 1993;35(3):375–82; discussion 82–3.
28. Meek RN. The John border memorial lecture: delaying emergency fracture surgery--fact or fad. J Orthop Trauma. 2006;20(5):337–40.
29. Pape HC. Confusion regarding method of patient selection. J Trauma. 2006;60(3):685–6.
30. Anwar IA, Battistella FD, Neiman R, Olson SA, Chapman MW, Moehring HD. Femur fractures and lung complications: a prospective randomized study of reaming. Clin Orthop Relat Res. 2004;422: 71–6.
31. Pape HC, Rixen D, Morley J, Husebye EE, Mueller M, Dumont C, et al. Impact of the method of initial stabilization for femoral shaft fractures in patients with multiple injuries at risk for complications (borderline patients). Ann Surg. 2007;246(3):491–9; discussion 9–501.
32. Pape HC, Giannoudis P, Krettek C. The timing of fracture treatment in polytrauma patients: relevance of damage control orthopedic surgery. Am J Surg. 2002;183(6):622–9.
33. Pape HC, Giannoudis PV, Krettek C, Trentz O. Timing of fixation of major fractures in blunt polytrauma: role of conventional indicators in clinical decision making. J Orthop Trauma. 2005;19(8):551–62.
34. Nicholas B, Toth L, van Wessem K, Evans J, Enninghorst N, Balogh ZJ. Borderline femur fracture

patients: early total care or damage control orthopaedics? ANZ J Surg. 2011;81(3):148–53.
35. Rixen D, Grass G, Sauerland S, Lefering R, Raum MR, Yücel N, et al. Evaluation of criteria for temporary external fixation in risk-adapted damage control orthopedic surgery of femur shaft fractures in multiple trauma patients: "evidence-based medicine" versus "reality" in the trauma registry of the German trauma society. J Trauma. 2005;59(6):1375–94; discussion 94–5.
36. O'Toole RV, O'Brien M, Scalea TM, Habashi N, Pollak AN, Turen CH. Resuscitation before stabilization of femoral fractures limits acute respiratory distress syndrome in patients with multiple traumatic injuries despite low use of damage control orthopedics. J Trauma. 2009;67(5):1013–21.
37. Morshed S, Miclau T, Bembom O, Cohen M, Knudson MM, Colford JM. Delayed internal fixation of femoral shaft fracture reduces mortality among patients with multisystem trauma. J Bone Joint Surg Am. 2009;91(1):3–13.
38. Vallier HA, Wang X, Moore TA, Wilber JH, Como JJ. Timing of orthopaedic surgery in multiple trauma patients: development of a protocol for early appropriate care. J Orthop Trauma. 2013;27(10):543–51.
39. Nahm NJ, Como JJ, Wilber JH, Vallier HA. Early appropriate care: definitive stabilization of femoral fractures within 24 hours of injury is safe in most patients with multiple injuries. J Trauma. 2011;71(1):175–85.
40. Dutton RP. Resuscitative strategies to maintain homeostasis during damage control surgery. Br J Surg. 2012;99(Suppl 1):21–8.
41. Goris RJ, te Boekhorst TP, Nuytinck JK, Gimbrère JS. Multiple-organ failure. Generalized autodestructive inflammation? Arch Surg. 1985;120(10):1109–15.
42. Mollen KP, Anand RJ, Tsung A, Prince JM, Levy RM, Billiar TR. Emerging paradigm: toll-like receptor 4-sentinel for the detection of tissue damage. Shock. 2006;26(5):430–7.
43. Zhang Q, Raoof M, Chen Y, Sumi Y, Sursal T, Junger W, et al. Circulating mitochondrial DAMPs cause inflammatory responses to injury. Nature. 2010;464(7285):104–7.
44. Nast-Kolb D, Aufmkolk M, Rucholtz S, Obertacke U, Waydhas C. Multiple organ failure still a major cause of morbidity but not mortality in blunt multiple trauma. J Trauma. 2001;51(5):835–41; discussion 41–2.
45. Sauaia A, Moore FA, Moore EE, Norris JM, Lezotte DC, Hamman RF. Multiple organ failure can be predicted as early as 12 hours after injury. J Trauma. 1998;45(2):291–301; discussion -3.
46. Lord JM, Midwinter MJ, Chen YF, Belli A, Brohi K, Kovacs EJ, et al. The systemic immune response to trauma: an overview of pathophysiology and treatment. Lancet. 2014;384(9952):1455–65.
47. Giannoudis PV, Tzioupis C, Pape HC. Fat embolism: the reaming controversy. Injury. 2006;37(Suppl 4):S50–8.
48. Morley JR, Smith RM, Pape HC, MacDonald DA, Trejdosiewitz LK, Giannoudis PV. Stimulation of the local femoral inflammatory response to fracture and intramedullary reaming: a preliminary study of the source of the second hit phenomenon. J Bone Joint Surg Br. 2008;90(3):393–9.
49. Bose D, Tejwani NC. Evolving trends in the care of polytrauma patients. Injury. 2006;37(1):20–8.
50. Dewar D, Moore FA, Moore EE, Balogh Z. Postinjury multiple organ failure. Injury. 2009;40(9):912–8.
51. Evans JA, van Wessem KJ, McDougall D, Lee KA, Lyons T, Balogh ZJ. Epidemiology of traumatic deaths: comprehensive population-based assessment. World J Surg. 2010;34(1):158–63.
52. D'Alleyrand JC, O'Toole RV. The evolution of damage control orthopedics: current evidence and practical applications of early appropriate care. Orthop Clin North Am. 2013;44(4):499–507.
53. Easton R, Balogh ZJ. Peri-operative changes in serum immune markers after trauma: a systematic review. Injury. 2014;45(6):934–41.
54. Botha AJ, Moore FA, Moore EE, Kim FJ, Banerjee A, Peterson VM. Postinjury neutrophil priming and activation: an early vulnerable window. Surgery. 1995;118(2):358–64; discussion 64–5.
55. Bosse MJ, MacKenzie EJ, Riemer BL, Brumback RJ, McCarthy ML, Burgess AR, et al. Adult respiratory distress syndrome, pneumonia, and mortality following thoracic injury and a femoral fracture treated either with intramedullary nailing with reaming or with a plate. A comparative study. J Bone Joint Surg Am. 1997;79(6):799–809.
56. Ogura H, Tanaka H, Koh T, Hashiguchi N, Kuwagata Y, Hosotsubo H, et al. Priming, second-hit priming, and apoptosis in leukocytes from trauma patients. J Trauma. 1999;46(5):774–81; discussion 81–3.
57. Pachter HL, Feliciano DV. Complex hepatic injuries. Surg Clin North Am. 1996;76(4):763–82.
58. Hildebrand F, Giannoudis P, Kretteck C, Pape HC. Damage control: extremities. Injury. 2004;35(7):678–89.
59. Waydhas C, Nast-Kolb D, Trupka A, Zettl R, Kick M, Wiesholler J, et al. Posttraumatic inflammatory response, secondary operations, and late multiple organ failure. J Trauma. 1996;40(4):624–30; discussion 30–1.
60. Pape HC, Schmidt RE, Rice J, van Griensven M, das Gupta R, Krettek C, et al. Biochemical changes after trauma and skeletal surgery of the lower extremity: quantification of the operative burden. Crit Care Med. 2000;28(10):3441–8.
61. Hartsock LA, Barfield WR, Kokko KP, Liles LL, Wind T, Green J, et al. Randomized prospective clinical trial comparing reamer irrigator aspirator (RIA) to standard reaming (SR) in both minimally injured and multiply injured patients with closed femoral shaft

fractures treated with reamed intramedullary nailing (IMN). Injury. 2010;41(Suppl 2):S94–8.
62. Pape HC, van Griensven M, Rice J, Gänsslen A, Hildebrand F, Zech S, et al. Major secondary surgery in blunt trauma patients and perioperative cytokine liberation: determination of the clinical relevance of biochemical markers. J Trauma. 2001;50(6):989–1000.
63. Pape HC, Grimme K, Van Griensven M, Sott AH, Giannoudis P, Morley J, et al. Impact of intramedullary instrumentation versus damage control for femoral fractures on immunoinflammatory parameters: prospective randomized analysis by the EPOFF study group. J Trauma. 2003;55(1):7–13.
64. Xiao W, Mindrinos MN, Seok J, Cuschieri J, Cuenca AG, Gao H, et al. A genomic storm in critically injured humans. J Exp Med. 2011;208(13):2581–90.
65. Bates P, Parker P, McFadyen I, Pallister I. Demystifying damage control in musculoskeletal trauma. Ann R Coll Surg Engl. 2016;98(5):291–4.
66. Parker PJ. Damage control surgery and casualty evacuation: techniques for surgeons, lessons for military medical planners. J R Army Med Corps. 2006;152(4):202–11.
67. Jansen JO, Thomas R, Loudon MA, Brooks A. Damage control resuscitation for patients with major trauma. BMJ. 2009;338:b1778.
68. Andruszkow H, Dowrick AS, Frink M, Zeckey C, Krettek C, Hildebrand F, et al. Surgical strategies in polytraumatized patients with femoral shaft fractures - comparing a German and an Australian level I trauma centre. Injury. 2013;44(8):1068–72.
69. Suzuki T, Hak DJ, Stahel PF, Morgan SJ, Smith WR. Safety and efficacy of conversion from external fixation to plate fixation in humeral shaft fractures. J Orthop Trauma. 2010;24(7):414–9.
70. Goldstein A, Phillips T, Sclafani SJ, Scalea T, Duncan A, Goldstein J, et al. Early open reduction and internal fixation of the disrupted pelvic ring. J Trauma. 1986;26(4):325–33.
71. Latenser BA, Gentilello LM, Tarver AA, Thalgott JS, Batdorf JW. Improved outcome with early fixation of skeletally unstable pelvic fractures. J Trauma. 1991;31(1):28–31.
72. Riemer BL, Butterfield SL, Diamond DL, Young JC, Raves JJ, Cottington E, et al. Acute mortality associated with injuries to the pelvic ring: the role of early patient mobilization and external fixation. J Trauma. 1993;35(5):671–5; discussion 6–7.
73. Vallier HA, Cureton BA, Ekstein C, Oldenburg FP, Wilber JH. Early definitive stabilization of unstable pelvis and acetabulum fractures reduces morbidity. J Trauma. 2010;69(3):677–84.
74. Plaisier BR, Meldon SW, Super DM, Malangoni MA. Improved outcome after early fixation of acetabular fractures. Injury. 2000;31(2):81–4.
75. Cengiz SL, Kalkan E, Bayir A, Ilik K, Basefer A. Timing of thoracolomber spine stabilization in trauma patients; impact on neurological outcome and clinical course. A real prospective (rct) randomized controlled study. Arch Orthop Trauma Surg. 2008;128(9):959–66.
76. Dimar JR, Carreon LY, Riina J, Schwartz DG, Harris MB. Early versus late stabilization of the spine in the polytrauma patient. Spine (Phila Pa 1976). 2010;35(21 Suppl):S187–92.
77. Frangen TM, Ruppert S, Muhr G, Schinkel C. Respiratory failure in thoracic spine injuries. Does the timing of dorsal stabilization have any effect on the clinical course in multiply injured patients? Orthopade. 2007;36(4):365–71.
78. Kerwin AJ, Griffen MM, Tepas JJ, Schinco MA, Devin T, Frykberg ER. Best practice determination of timing of spinal fracture fixation as defined by analysis of the National Trauma Data Bank. J Trauma. 2008;65(4):824–30; discussion 30–1.
79. McHenry TP, Mirza SK, Wang J, Wade CE, O'Keefe GE, Dailey AT, et al. Risk factors for respiratory failure following operative stabilization of thoracic and lumbar spine fractures. J Bone Joint Surg Am. 2006;88(5):997–1005.
80. Schinkel C, Frangen TM, Kmetic A, Andress HJ, Muhr G, Registry GT. Timing of thoracic spine stabilization in trauma patients: impact on clinical course and outcome. J Trauma. 2006;61(1):156–60; discussion 60.
81. Stahel PF, Flierl MA, Moore EE, Smith WR, Beauchamp KM, Dwyer A. Advocating "spine damage control" as a safe and effective treatment modality for unstable thoracolumbar fractures in polytrauma patients: a hypothesis. J Trauma Manag Outcomes. 2009;3:6.
82. Pape H, Stalp M, v Griensven M, Weinberg A, Dahlweit M, Tscherne H. Optimal timing for secondary surgery in polytrauma patients: an evaluation of 4,314 serious-injury cases. Chirurg. 1999;70(11):1287–93.
83. Harwood PJ, Giannoudis PV, van Griensven M, Krettek C, Pape HC. Alterations in the systemic inflammatory response after early total care and damage control procedures for femoral shaft fracture in severely injured patients. J Trauma. 2005;58(3):446–52; discussion 52–4.
84. Nowotarski PJ, Turen CH, Brumback RJ, Scarboro JM. Conversion of external fixation to intramedullary nailing for fractures of the shaft of the femur in multiply injured patients. J Bone Joint Surg Am. 2000;82(6):781–8.
85. Bhandari M, Zlowodzki M, Tornetta P, Schmidt A, Templeman DC. Intramedullary nailing following external fixation in femoral and tibial shaft fractures. J Orthop Trauma. 2005;19(2):140–4.
86. Pape HC, Regel G, Dwenger A, Sturm JA, Tscherne H. Influence of thoracic trauma and primary femoral intramedullary nailing on the incidence of ARDS in multiple trauma patients. Injury. 1993;24(Suppl 3):S82–103.

87. Dalal SA, Burgess AR, Siegel JH, Young JW, Brumback RJ, Poka A, et al. Pelvic fracture in multiple trauma: classification by mechanism is key to pattern of organ injury, resuscitative requirements, and outcome. J Trauma. 1989;29(7):981–1000; discussion -2.
88. Crowl AC, Young JS, Kahler DM, Claridge JA, Chrzanowski DS, Pomphrey M. Occult hypoperfusion is associated with increased morbidity in patients undergoing early femur fracture fixation. J Trauma. 2000;48(2):260–7.
89. Davis JW, Parks SN, Kaups KL, Gladen HE, O'Donnell-Nicol S. Admission base deficit predicts transfusion requirements and risk of complications. J Trauma. 1996;41(5):769–74.
90. Eberhard LW, Morabito DJ, Matthay MA, Mackersie RC, Campbell AR, Marks JD, et al. Initial severity of metabolic acidosis predicts the development of acute lung injury in severely traumatized patients. Crit Care Med. 2000;28(1):125–31.
91. Guyette F, Suffoletto B, Castillo JL, Quintero J, Callaway C, Puyana JC. Prehospital serum lactate as a predictor of outcomes in trauma patients: a retrospective observational study. J Trauma. 2011;70(4):782–6.
92. Manikis P, Jankowski S, Zhang H, Kahn RJ, Vincent JL. Correlation of serial blood lactate levels to organ failure and mortality after trauma. Am J Emerg Med. 1995;13(6):619–22.
93. Abramson D, Scalea TM, Hitchcock R, Trooskin SZ, Henry SM, Greenspan J. Lactate clearance and survival following injury. J Trauma. 1993;35(4):584–8; discussion 8–9.
94. Claridge JA, Crabtree TD, Pelletier SJ, Butler K, Sawyer RG, Young JS. Persistent occult hypoperfusion is associated with a significant increase in infection rate and mortality in major trauma patients. J Trauma. 2000;48(1):8–14; discussion -5.
95. Davis JW, Kaups KL. Base deficit in the elderly: a marker of severe injury and death. J Trauma. 1998;45(5):873–7.
96. Hindy-François C, Meyer P, Blanot S, Marqué S, Sabourdin N, Carli P, et al. Admission base deficit as a long-term prognostic factor in severe pediatric trauma patients. J Trauma. 2009;67(6):1272–7.
97. McNelis J, Marini CP, Jurkiewicz A, Szomstein S, Simms HH, Ritter G, et al. Prolonged lactate clearance is associated with increased mortality in the surgical intensive care unit. Am J Surg. 2001;182(5):481–5.
98. Randolph LC, Takacs M, Davis KA. Resuscitation in the pediatric trauma population: admission base deficit remains an important prognostic indicator. J Trauma. 2002;53(5):838–42.
99. Davis JW, Kaups KL, Parks SN. Base deficit is superior to pH in evaluating clearance of acidosis after traumatic shock. J Trauma. 1998;44(1):114–8.
100. Duchesne JC, McSwain NE, Cotton BA, Hunt JP, Dellavolpe J, Lafaro K, et al. Damage control resuscitation: the new face of damage control. J Trauma. 2010;69(4):976–90.
101. Grey B, Rodseth RN, Muckart DJ. Early fracture stabilisation in the presence of subclinical hypoperfusion. Injury. 2013;44(2):217–20.
102. Vallier HA, Moore TA, Como JJ, Wilczewski PA, Steinmetz MP, Wagner KG, et al. Complications are reduced with a protocol to standardize timing of fixation based on response to resuscitation. J Orthop Surg Res. 2015;10:155.
103. Rüedi T, Wolff G. Prevention of post-traumatic complications through immediate therapy in patients with multiple injuries and fractures. Helv Chir Acta. 1975;42(4):507–12.
104. Brundage SI, McGhan R, Jurkovich GJ, Mack CD, Maier RV. Timing of femur fracture fixation: effect on outcome in patients with thoracic and head injuries. J Trauma. 2002;52(2):299–307.
105. Giannoudis PV, Veysi VT, Pape HC, Krettek C, Smith MR. When should we operate on major fractures in patients with severe head injuries? Am J Surg. 2002;183(3):261–7.
106. Watson JT. High-energy fractures of the tibial plateau. Orthop Clin North Am. 1994;25(4):723–52.
107. Watson JT, Moed BR, Karges DE, Cramer KE. Pilon fractures. Treatment protocol based on severity of soft tissue injury. Clin Orthop Relat Res. 2000;375:78–90.
108. Bar-On E, Lebel E, Kreiss Y, Merin O, Benedict S, Gill A, et al. Orthopaedic management in a mega mass casualty situation. The Israel Defence forces field Hospital in Haiti following the January 2010 earthquake. Injury. 2011;42(10):1053–9.
109. Rowley DI. The management of war wounds involving bone. J Bone Joint Surg Br. 1996;78(5):706–9.
110. Owens BD, Kragh JF, Macaitis J, Svoboda SJ, Wenke JC. Characterization of extremity wounds in operation Iraqi freedom and operation enduring freedom. J Orthop Trauma. 2007;21(4):254–7.
111. Lebel E, Blumberg N, Gill A, Merin O, Gelfond R, Bar-On E. External fixator frames as interim damage control for limb injuries: experience in the 2010 Haiti earthquake. J Trauma. 2011;71(6):E128–31.

11 Open Damage Control Vascular Surgery

Joseph M. White and Todd E. Rasmussen

Abstract

Damage control vascular surgery incorporates strategies to achieve rapid control of hemorrhage while mitigating ischemia by establishing adequate end-organ perfusion in an abbreviated initial intervention. Vascular damage control surgery functions in concert with damage control resuscitation focused on the correction of physiologic derangements and metabolic acidosis, the correction of coagulopathy, appropriate blood product transfusion, and active patient warming measures to ameliorate hypothermia. Ultimately, the patient's physiology dictates the technical feasibility of vascular intervention and determines operative planning with respect to injury management. Surgeon experience and technical familiarity with vascular injury and location of the vascular injury are significant factors that alter patient outcomes.

J.M. White, M.D., F.A.C.S.
The Department of Surgery, Uniformed Services University of the Health Sciences, Walter Reed National Military Medical Center, Bethesda, MD, USA

Todd E. Rasmussen, M.D., F.A.C.S. (✉)
Walter Reed National Military Medical Center, Bethesda, MD, USA

F. Edward Hebert School of Medicine—"America's Medical School", Uniformed Services University of the Health Sciences, Bethesda, MD, USA
e-mail: todd.rasmussen@usuhs.edu

11.1 Introduction

Damage control vascular surgery incorporates strategies to achieve rapid control of hemorrhage while mitigating ischemia by establishing adequate end-organ perfusion in an abbreviated initial intervention. Vascular damage control surgery functions in concert with damage control resuscitation focused on the correction of physiologic derangements and metabolic acidosis, the correction of coagulopathy, appropriate blood product transfusion, and active patient warming measures to ameliorate hypothermia. Ultimately, the patient's physiology dictates the technical feasibility of vascular intervention and determines operative planning with respect to injury management. Surgeon experience and technical familiarity with vascular injury and location of the vascular injury are significant factors that alter patient outcomes.

The military has extensive experience with damage control vascular surgery strategies. Hemorrhage has been identified as a leading cause of preventable death on the modern battlefield [1–4]. Analysis from the recent wars in Iraq and Afghanistan has demonstrated that hemorrhage was the underlying physiologic insult in 90% of potentially survivable battlefield injuries [1]. The current incidence of wartime vascular injury on the modern battlefield has significantly increased compared to past conflicts [5–16]. Because of this increased incidence, the military offers a unique perspective with regard to damage

J. Duchesne et al. (eds.), *Damage Control in Trauma Care*,
https://doi.org/10.1007/978-3-319-72607-6_11

control techniques and strategies. Reports from DeBakey, Hughes, and Rich [5–11] laid the foundation for the characterization of wartime vascular injury and demonstrated the feasibility regarding the management of complex, often devastating, injuries. Subsequent reports have continued to define and describe additional surgical adjuncts and implementation of strategies across the continuum of the modern battlefield. The Golden Hour Offset Surgical Treatment Team (GHOST-T) initiative positions forward surgical treatment and resuscitative teams within a 60-min medical evacuation radius from combat elements. These small units provide combat support and perform damage control surgery and resuscitation. Following the completion of damage control maneuvers, patients are rapidly transported to the next echelon of military medical care.

Rapid hemorrhage control and alleviation of end-organ ischemia are the central tenets to damage control vascular surgery. Hemorrhage control techniques include intracavitary packing for solid organ injury and pelvic packing following severe pelvic fractures. These techniques have an important role in initial trauma laparotomy. Peripheral vascular hemorrhage control includes the use of tourniquets, ligation of bleeding vessels, and primary amputation of the mangled extremity. Mitigation of end-organ ischemia focuses on the use of temporary vascular shunts (TVS) and revascularization strategies. Endovascular capabilities have extended the therapeutic options for vascular trauma with adjuncts that include resuscitative balloon occlusion of the aorta (REBOA), primary stenting for central vascular injuries, and coil embolization techniques. REBOA has demonstrated clinical feasibility and is an effective means of proactive aortic control for patients in end-stage hemorrhagic shock [17–23]. An extended discussion regarding endovascular principles and procedures is beyond the scope of this chapter, and a more detailed description can be found in the endovascular damage control surgery section. This chapter on open damage control vascular surgery will focus on hemorrhage control techniques, temporary revascularization strategies, revascularization operations, and specific technical considerations regarding vascular injury management.

11.2 Hemorrhage Control

11.2.1 Tourniquets

Death from compressible hemorrhage remains a significant cause of mortality during modern combat operations [2, 3, 24]. The tourniquet has become a ubiquitous lifesaving tool in the military. Minimal training and familiarity are required for effective utilization of an extremity tourniquet making it an ideal prehospital intervention. Combat medics operating in a forward, austere environment deploy tourniquets in the prehospital setting to reduce hemorrhage from compressible extremity injury. The tourniquet is associated with improved combat casualty survival and low complication rates [25–33]. Kragh et al. [25] reviewed 232 combat casualties with major limb trauma and reported on 428 tourniquets applied on 309 injured limbs. This report demonstrated a significant mortality reduction following early prehospital tourniquet application compared to delayed use once the patient had reached a military treatment facility (MTF) (mortality of 11–24%, respectively). Early use of tourniquets prior to the onset of hemorrhagic shock was associated with improved survival and no limb loss demonstrating the safety and efficacy of tourniquet application. Additionally, tourniquet duration was not associated with increased morbidity. A subsequent report form Kragh et al. [30] reviewed the military's experience from 2001 to 2010 with a retrospective review of tourniquet use during combat operations. In total, 4297 combat casualties were identified, and tourniquets were applied in 1272 casualties. Interestingly, the additional experience with tourniquets, as well as an understanding of the efficacy, resulted in an increase in the use of tourniquets from 4% in 2001 to 40% in 2010. Survival rates with tourniquet use also increased from 2004 to 2010 despite the simultaneous increase in injury severity. Beekley et al. [31] reviewed data from 3444 injured casualties during Operation Iraqi Freedom in

2004. One hundred sixty-five patients were identified with a major vascular injury to an extremity, traumatic amputations, or annotation of a prehospital tourniquet placement. Of this cohort, 67 (40%) patients arrived to the Role 3 combat support hospital with a tourniquet in place. Tourniquet use resulted in effective hemorrhage control on arrival to the MTF. In summary, tourniquets have demonstrated clear clinical utility in the prehospital phase of casualty care preventing life-threatening extremity hemorrhage when applied early, and the use of tourniquets has revealed an overall low complication profile. Tourniquets remain a critical prehospital adjunct for the mitigation of exsanguinating hemorrhage from compressible extremity hemorrhage.

The civilian literature reflects similar trends regarding the efficacy and safety of tourniquet use in vascular injury. Inaba et al. [34] retrospectively reported on 87 civilian trauma patients at the Level 1 trauma center that had a tourniquet applied in the prehospital setting, emergency room, or operating room. Eighty-one percent of patients demonstrated a major vascular injury. One identified difference in military versus civilian trauma management indicated that civilian patients exist in a system with more constant and rapid transport times [34]. Therefore, the overall incidence and implementation of tourniquets are reduced compared to military trauma which occurs in more austere environments. Interestingly, the civilian literature prehospital tourniquet rate varies from 5.6% to 50.6% depending on the study [34, 35]. In the face of explosive blast injuries as the primary mechanism of injury and increased wartime experience, the military rate of prehospital tourniquet application is 40% [30].

11.2.2 Ligation

Selective vessel ligation remains a viable and appropriate damage control option. In patients who present in extremis with severe physiology derangement, ligation offers rapid hemorrhage control and does not necessarily exclude future revascularization options. Patient physiology and surgeon experience contribute to the surgical plan significantly. At times, initial ligation, followed by rapid casualty evacuation to a higher echelon of care, allows for reexploration and TVS placement for central vascular injuries. Conversely, selective peripheral vascular injury ligation remains an acceptable method of hemorrhage control.

In a review of vascular surgery procedures in recent combat, ligation and reconstruction were observed in nearly equal proportions for the treatment of battlefield vascular trauma [16]. This fact represents the utility of vessel ligation as a damage control maneuver. Burkhardt et al. [36] reported outcomes after a selective approach to revascularization for the distal lower extremity. This report reviewed 1332 patients with combat-related vascular injuries and characterized the management of 135 tibial-level disruptions or occlusions. Selective revascularization of isolated tibial-level arterial injury was the predominant technical approach reported, and 83% of limb salvage patients were managed without arterial reconstruction. Arterial ligation remains an effective damage control option in the context of single tibial-vessel injury. However, patients with complete or persistent ischemia should be considered for revascularization.

11.2.3 Primary Amputation

Primary amputation should be considered for non-salvageable extremity injury with complex, multi-system trauma in a damage control setting. Additionally, for patients in extremis who are unable to tolerate an attempt at temporary revascularization, primary amputation is an appropriate option. Stannard et al. [15] reviewed 1203 service personnel injured in combat and identified 110 vascular injuries. The overall amputation rate among all patients with extremity vascular injury was 47%.The patient cohort included in this analysis underwent damage control maneuver after sustaining significant limb trauma with a high mangled extremity severity score (MESS). Blast ordinance is the most common mechanism of injury in modern combat. Due to the destructive nature of these weapons, extremity injury frequently presents as a non-salvageable limb. The decision for a primary amputation is often straightforward in these cases. However, civilian reports have demonstrated that the incorporation of a multidisciplinary decision-making process offers the patient significant insight following the injury [35, 37].

11.3 Temporary Revascularization

11.3.1 Temporary Vascular Shunt

Utilization of a temporary vascular shunt (TVS) during damage control maneuvers is a well-described method to accomplish restoration of flow and end-organ perfusion in vascular trauma [38–48]. Shunts for arterial injury allow for temporary preservation of distal end-organ perfusion (Fig. 11.1). If the TVS is placed in the peripheral arterial distribution, the end organ at risk is the extremity itself. Shunting of venous injury provides necessary drainage of blood and subsequent reduction of venous hypertension that compounds tissue ischemia and bleeding.

Rasmussen et al. [39] described a contemporary wartime experience with TVS as a damage control adjunct during Operation Iraqi Freedom at Balad Air Base, Iraq. This report included 30 TVS inserted for arterial (87%) and venous injury (13%). TVS patency was reported for proximal or central vascular injuries at 86% and distal or peripheral shunting at 12%. No systemic heparin was used following shunt insertion, and no shunt complications were reported. Limb salvage, determined by early preservation of a viable limb, occurred in 92% of the casualties. Utilization of a TVS represents a damage control adjunct that is safe and effective with respect to establishing distal perfusion and extending the window of opportunity for limb salvage. Chambers et al. [40] reviewed 582 traumatic injuries in 293 combat casualties treated by a Marine Corps forward resuscitative surgical system team from 2004 to 2005. This reviewed identified 66 casualties that sustained a major vascular injury. Of these, 29 arterial and venous injuries were managed with a TVS representing 44% shunt utilization. Shunt patency was reported at 78%, and limb salvage was achieved in 85% of injured patients.

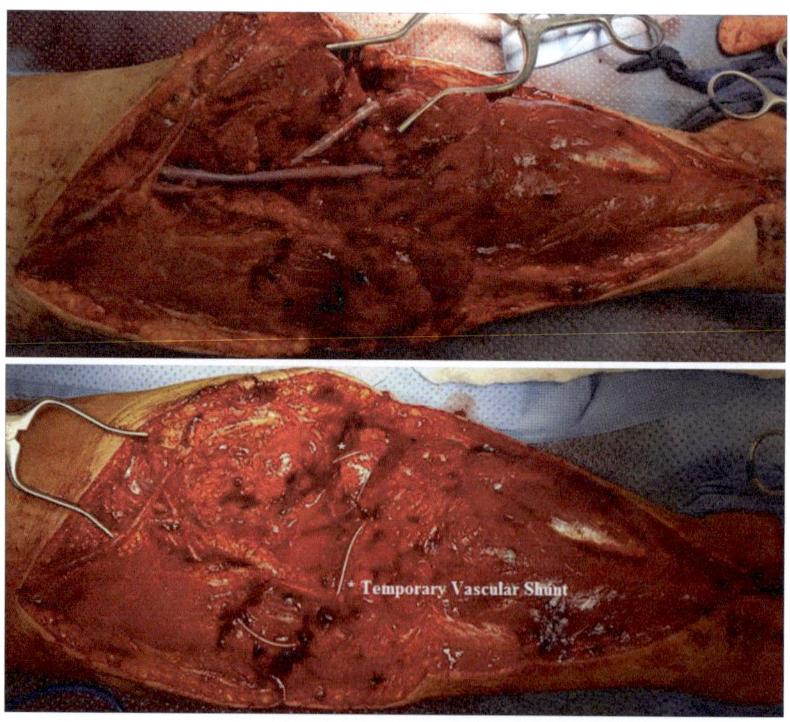

Fig. 11.1 Utilization of a temporary vascular shunt (TVS) for damage control management of severe ulnar and radial artery injury. Following resuscitation and physiologic improvement, the patient underwent brachial artery to radial artery bypass with the reversed greater saphenous vein (rGSV) and an interposition bypass from the proximal ulnar artery to distal ulnar artery with rGSV

Taller et al. [41] reported on 610 combat trauma patients treated over a 7-month period in Iraq. In total, 37 patients sustained 73 major traumatic vascular injuries with 26 TVS inserted for limb salvage. Regarding shunt placement, 36% of the injuries were initially managed with TVS insertion in the prehospital setting. Reported TVS patency was 96%, and early limb salvage was achieved in all patients who underwent temporary revascularization with TVS. Gifford et al. [42] published a retrospective database review incorporating the Balad Vascular Registry, Walter Reed Vascular Registry, and Joint Theater Trauma System (now consolidated into the Department of Defense Trauma Registry). Failure of limb salvage was the primary endpoint. Two groups were established for analysis, the TVS group and a matched control group, in which no TVS was utilized. In the TVS group, 61 injured US troops sustained 64 arterial injuries (64 arterial stents inserted) and 25 concomitant venous injuries (14 venous stents inserted). In the control group, 60 injured patients sustained 61 arterial injuries and 23 concomitant venous injuries. After propensity score adjustment, there was a trend suggesting a reduced risk of amputation with TVS; however the primary endpoint of limb salvage was 78% in the TVS group and 77% in the control group. Associated orthopedic injury, an elevated mangled extremity severity score, and venous ligation were identified as independent risk factors for amputation. The military's experience with TVS suggests that this damage control adjunct is an effect technique to temporarily provide distal perfusion. In a porcine model of limb ischemia, early TVS insertion protected the injured extremity from further ischemic insult and reduced circulating markers of tissue injury [43]. Preservation of perfusion allows for an attempt at limb salvage.

The civilian experience with TVS demonstrates similar technical success and efficacy. Subramanian et al. [44] reported on the 10-year experience of a Level I trauma center, in a large retrospective review of TVS. This report included 786 patients treated for vascular injury. Indications for shunt placement included significant physiology derangement requiring the need for a damage control treatment strategy and utilization of the TVS at the initial operation in preparation for a staged, definite vascular repair. In total, 73 patients had 108 TVS inserted. This represents 9% TVS usage in the management of vascular trauma compared to 44% in a wartime application. Shunt patency was reported at 91%, and the limb salvage rate was 74%. The multicenter shunt study group reported on the use of temporary vascular shunts performed at several high-volume Level I trauma centers [45]. This report detailed the largest multicenter aggregate of patients in the civilian literature who underwent damage control vascular surgery with TVS. This retrospective study identified 213 vascular injuries (201 patients) requiring TVS in a cohort of 7385 patients (2.7% aggregate shunt insertion rate). Of the 213 TVS, 95% of the shunts were used for arterial injuries. Shunting of the extremity occurred in 75% of patients, and the superficial femoral artery was the most common location for shunt placement (24%), followed by the popliteal artery (19%) and brachial artery (13%). This civilian report demonstrated excellent TVS patency with shunt thrombosis recorded at only 5.6% and minimal TVS complications with TVS dislodgement at 1.4%. TVS were implemented in a damage control treatment strategy in 63% of patients and used in concomitant orthopedic and vascular injury in the remaining 36% of patients. A 96% limb salvage rate was achieved. Systemic heparin was only used in 22% on shunted patients. The use of heparin was not associated with a reduced incidence of shunt thrombosis. This report demonstrated no independent predictors for shunt thrombosis. Granchi et al. [46] described the long-term effectiveness of TVS without systemic heparinization. In this report, 19 patients demonstrated TVS patency with no shunt thrombosis reported, and the average shunt dwell time was greater than 10 h. Overall limb salvage was reported at 89%. In the severely injured patient, multiple simultaneous injury is common. Frequently, these additional injuries represent a contraindication to therapeutic anticoagulation or, at least, limit the ability to anticoagulated. Review of available data suggests that anticoagulation is not required during shunting.

Insertion of a TVS requires technical familiarity as well as experience with the relative arterial and venous system anatomy at risk. Generally, proximal or central vascular control and distal or peripheral vascular control must be achieved at the location of injury. Once vascular control has been established, the surgeon must assess distal perfusion. Typically, the injured vessel can be forward-bled and back-bled to confirm uninterrupted flow. If flow is not visualized, balloon thromboembolectomy catheters are passed to remove thrombus. The shunt is subsequently inserted into the distal or peripheral vascular bed and allowed to back-bleed. Next, the TVS is inserted into the proximal or central vessel. Flow is generally confirmed with continuous-wave Doppler. The shunt is secured into position with heavy silk suture to prevent dislodgement. Table 11.1 describes several commercially available vascular shunts.

11.3.2 Temporary Synthetic Conduit

Autologous vein remains the standard bypass conduit for traumatic vascular injuries. Devastating combat blast injuries can render an ischemic limb with no suitable autologous conduit. The use of prosthetic graft for reconstruction of military and civilian vascular injuries has demonstrated feasibility as a damage control adjunct allowing for reestablishing distal perfusion in some scenarios (Fig. 11.2). Feliciano et al. [47] reported on 206 patients with 236 polytetrafluoroethylene (PTFE) grafts inserted in traumatic vascular wounds. PTFE was found to be an acceptable conduit for interposition grafting of segmental arterial defects; however long-term follow-up and determination of long-term patency were lacking. This early study demonstrated the feasibility of using synthetic conduit in repair of vascular trauma. Vertrees et al. [48] described 95 emergent bypasses performed for military vascular injuries. Fourteen bypasses were constructed with polytetrafluoroethylene (PTFE).

Table 11.1 Commercially available Temporary Vascular Shunt (TVS): manufactured lengths, diameters and features

Temporary vascular shunt	Available lengths	Available diameter	Features
Argyle (CR Bard, Murray Hill, NJ)	6″ in-line configuration 11″ looped configuration	8, 10, 12, 14 French	– Smooth beveled ends facilitate easy insertion – Radiopaque line permits location verification
Javid (IMPRA, Tempe, AZ)	27.5 cm looped configuration	17 French tapered to 10 French	– Soft, kink-resistant, and tapered – Extra length allows looping to facilitate visual inspection of the carotid artery
Sundt (Integra NeuroSciences, Plainsboro, NJ)	10 cm in-line configuration 30 cm looped configuration	3 mm tapered to 4 mm 3 mm tapered to 5 mm 4 mm tapered to 5 mm	– Stainless steel spring reinforcement to minimize kinking and occlusion – Ends have cone-shaped bulbs to facilitate fixation – The 1 cm section of non-reinforced shunt is available
Pruitt-Inahara (LeMaitre Vascular, Burlington, MA)	15 cm (9F) in-line configuration 31 cm (9F) looped configuration 25 cm (8F) looped configuration	8, 9 French	– Dual-lumen devices with balloons at both the distal and proximal ends – T-Port stopcock allows for angiography, heparin, or vasodilator infusions

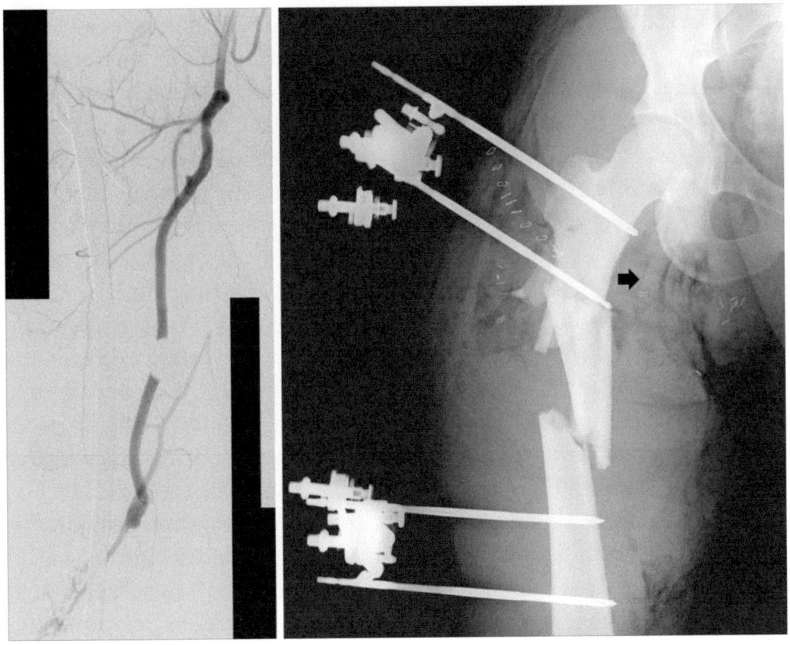

Fig. 11.2 This combat casualty sustained a devastating penetrating injury to the right lower extremity with injuries to the femoral vessels and femur. The patient was initially managed with temporary bypass using polytetrafluorethylene (PTFE) and external fixation of the femur fracture. The black arrow identifies the PTFE conduits for the femoral artery and vein injuries. The angiogram depicts the definitive common femoral artery reconstruction and bypass (tunneled anterolateral) with the autologous greater saphenous vein

Indications for the use of PTFE included major vessel segmental loss (79%), pseudoaneurysm (7%), and vein graft disruption (14%). This study reported 79% of prosthetic grafts maintained short-term patency allowing for patient stabilization, continued medical evacuation, and eventual definitive revascularization with autologous conduit. Four PTFE grafts (29%) required explantation for presumed infection. No prosthetic graft disruptions were reported, and no patients required amputation due to prosthetic graft failure. Secondary hemorrhage related to prosthetic vascular graft anastomotic disruption was reviewed by Greer et al. [49]. Combat-related vascular injuries are frequently associated with heavy contamination and soft tissue devastation resulting in a high risk of infection [50, 51]. This report included 181 US casualties sustaining arterial injury treated with bypass grafting for limb salvage identified. Autologous venous conduit was used in 97% of arterial repairs. Only six patients (3%) underwent reconstruction with prosthetic conduit. Anastomotic disruption was reported in 6% of repairs; all disruptions occurred at the arterial vein graft anastomosis. Infection was the cause of the disruption process. Watson et al. [52] identified 3569 vascular injuries in US service personnel. Four hundred thirty-five (12%) were managed with interposition bypass graft reconstruction with 410 autologous vein grafts and 25 expanded polytetrafluorethylene (PTFE) grafts. This retrospective cohort comparison demonstrated that PTFE had similar effectiveness and durability when compared to autologous conduit. However, the use of prosthetic conduit resulted in higher rates of complications. The utilization of synthetic conduit has demonstrated technical and clinical success regarding limb preservation following severe low extremity injury. When feasible, temporary synthetic conduit should be explanted and autologous bypass completed.

11.4 Revascularization

Definitive revascularization has a limited role in damage control vascular surgery, often because of the time, technical experience, and operative support required for such measures. Primary repair of minor vascular trauma can be performed rapidly without physiologic consequences. In 1946, DeBakey [5] commented that "therapeutic measures designed to save the limb are applicable, at best, in not more than 20% of cases" on the battlefield. Hughes and Rich [6–11] demonstrated the feasibility of complex vascular repair as an option for combat-related vascular injuries. During modern combat, nearly 50% of vascular injuries sustained in battle are now managed with repair or bypass which confirms that the window of opportunity for limb salvage has been extended [16, 53, 54]. Advanced methods of flow preservation and elaborate revascularization have been successfully performed in a forward, austere environment in conjunction with damage control resuscitation [12, 13, 55]. Fox et al. [55] reported on 16 combat casualties that underwent 20 vascular reconstructions for upper and lower extremity major vascular injuries for limb salvage. Routine fasciotomy and stabilization of concomitant orthopedic injury were performed. Damage control resuscitation resulted in physiologic recovery and avoided the lethal triad of hypothermia, coagulopathy, and progressive acidosis. Reported median operative time was 4.5 h for revascularization. This report documented the technical success of 19 saphenous vein bypass grafts and 1 synthetic bypass graft performed for definitive revascularization. Fasciotomies remain a critical adjunct when considering revascularization [56].

11.5 Specific Damage Control Vascular Surgery Considerations

11.5.1 General Principles

The fundamental principles regarding the management of vascular injury include adequate exposure, proximal and distal control, debridement to viable tissue, shunting, revascularization, or ligation. Damage control vascular decisions must account for patient physiology, concomitant injuries, anatomic location of the injured vessels, and available resources. Frequently, the most challenging aspect in the management of vascular injury relates to the anatomic exposure. Primary repair, construction of an anastomosis, and shunt placement are generally considered a straightforward technical exercise. However, in the context of devastating tissue destruction, concomitant injuries, hematoma formation, and significantly distorted anatomic landmarks, the identification and subsequent exposure of these vascular injuries can be challenging for even an experienced surgeon. The following sections will discuss general diagnostic considerations and vessel-specific exposures. It is important to note that the patient's physiology dictates the surgical plan and should be considered prior to implementing temporary or definitive revascularization.

11.5.2 Carotid Artery

Penetrating cervical trauma involving the carotid artery remains a challenging vascular injury. The modern incidence of wartime cervical vascular injury is 8% [16]. Injury to the carotid injury can result in life-threatening exsanguinating hemorrhage, significant cervical hematoma formation with airway compromise, and devastating neurologic complications. Hemorrhage and occlusion are indications for intervention. When feasible, contrast CTA should be performed. CTA facilitates the triage process, improves operative planning, and records baseline neurologic imaging. The patient's physiologic status determines the surgical plan with respect to revascularization. TVS has a clear utility during damage control maneuvers and also during the definitive revascularization allowing for continued cerebral perfusion to potentially ischemic neurons.

Exposure of the carotid artery is through an incision at the anterior margin of the sternocleidomastoid muscle, ipsilateral to the injury. The platysma muscle is divided and the sternocleidomastoid muscle reflected posterolaterally. The internal jugular vein is mobilized laterally following ligation of the common facial vein thereby exposing the carotid artery bifurcation. If feasible, the common carotid artery is exposed proximal to the hematoma or injured segment of the vessel and controlled with a vessel loop secured by a Rummel tourniquet. In the absence of uncontrolled hemorrhage, there is no need to tighten down the Rummel tourniquet. The dissection proceeds distal into the zone of injury. If bleeding is encountered, the Rummel tourniquet can be cinched down, or a vascular clamp can be placed. Back bleeding from the internal carotid artery is a favorable sign and can be controlled with a small clamp or a vessel loop. It is important to recognize that distal thrombosis of the internal carotid artery results in poor or no back bleeding. If this is encountered, carefully passing a 2–3 French embolectomy catheter can remove the thrombus and restore appropriate back bleeding. Aggressive catheter manipulation can result in a carotid-cavernous fistula; therefore, great care should be practiced.

Following vascular control of the proximal common carotid artery and distal internal carotid artery, the injury is explored. A TVS should be placed to maintain perfusion while the injury is explored and options considered. With respect to TVS placement, the shunt should be placed into the internal carotid artery and secured with a vessel loop allowing back bleeding through the shunt. In order to secure the proximal shunt, in sequence, the shunt is placed in the common carotid artery through the Rummel tourniquet. As the shunt advances into the common carotid artery, the Rummel tourniquet is tightened down fully securing the shunt in place. Repair of carotid artery injuries typically requires placement of an interposition greater saphenous vein graft, although primary repair or vein patch angioplasty can be performed for less severe injuries. To perform the interposition graft over the TVS, the proximal end is removed using the DeBakey clamp to occlude the common carotid artery. The vein graft is placed over the shunt (i.e., shunt in the vein graft lumen). The proximal shunt is reinserted into the common carotid artery and secured with the Rummel device using the previously described sequence. After flow is restored in the shunt, the distal vein graft anastomosis is performed using 6-0 Prolene suture to the edge of the normal internal carotid. Next, the proximal anastomosis to the common is started also with 6-0 Prolene suture. When the anastomosis is nearly completed, the shunt is removed through the remaining anastomotic opening, first removing the distal TVS from the internal carotid artery observing back bleeding followed by the proximal extent of the TVS observing appropriate forward bleeding. The anastomosis is completed. Alternatively, the reconstruction can be performed without a shunt; however, this exposes the ipsilateral hemisphere to prolonged ischemia. Regardless of whether or not a shunt is used, the mean arterial pressure should be kept above 90 mmHg during the repair to optimize cerebral perfusion. If no other life-threatening injuries are present, a small amount of systemic heparin (50u/kg) is recommended along with generous flushing of the repair with heparinized saline to prevent platelet aggregation and clot formation. Ligation of the internal carotid artery is an acceptable damage control maneuver to stop hemorrhage but has an acute stroke rate of 30–50%.

11.5.3 Subclavian Artery

Management of injury to the subclavian artery requires technical familiarity with exposure of the involved portion of the vessel. The central right subclavian artery is approached through a median sternotomy, while the central left subclavian artery is approached through a high left anterolateral thoracotomy. The mid-subclavian artery can be exposed through a supraclavicular approach following division of the clavicular head of sternocleidomastoid muscle and scalene fat pad, identification of the phrenic nerve, and subsequent division of the anterior scalene muscle. The supraclavicular approach can be a meticulous, time-consuming dissection given the critical associated structures in the surgical field. Alternatively, the mid- and distal subclavian arteries can be exposed and controlled through a combined supraclavicular and infraclavicular incisions. There is no requirement to obtain proximal vascular control within the surgical field of injury; using separate incisions through non-traumatized tissues can expedite rapid vascular control. In a hemodynamically unstable patient, initial proximal control obtained via sternotomy or thoracotomy will allow for more rapid vascular control than use of the more time-consuming supraclavicular approach. Because of the technical challenges with exposure, the utility of temporary vascular shunts in this injury pattern is limited. Additionally, interposition graft using 6–8 mm PTFE or Dacron is sometimes required for subclavian artery repair. Endovascular intervention for this injury pattern allows for rapid definitive repair without the morbidity of the surgical approach.

11.5.4 Axillary Artery

Control of the proximal axillary artery is best accomplished through an ipsilateral supraclavicular incision (proximal control via the subclavian artery), although the axillary artery itself is exposed through an infraclavicular approach. The infraclavicular exposure includes division of the clavipectoral fascia and the blunt separation of the fibers of the pectoralis major muscle. The axillary vein is the first structure encountered in the axillary sheath. The axillary artery lies deep to the vein; mobilization and caudal retraction of the axillary vein will expose the first segment of the axillary artery. The pectoralis minor muscle can be retracted laterally or divided. Repair of the axillary artery most commonly involves an interposition graft using reversed saphenous vein. TVS are of significant utility for delayed reconstruction in the damage control setting.

11.5.5 Brachial Artery

The brachial artery and median nerve travel within the brachial sheath and are exposed through a medial incision in the upper arm in the bicipital groove. The median nerve is the most superficial structure encountered upon entering the brachial sheath. The ulnar nerve runs posterior to the artery which is surrounded by paired deep brachial veins. Repair of the brachial artery is most commonly accomplished using primary repair, reversed saphenous vein interposition graft, or TVS allowing for delayed reconstruction. Although it may be possible to ligate the brachial artery distal to the origin of the profunda brachii artery and maintain a viable arm and hand, this proposition is based on intact collateral circulation. Unfortunately, collaterals from the shoulder and profunda brachii artery are often damaged in the setting of penetrating blast wounds, and therefore maintenance of flow through the brachial artery with a TVS or definitive vascular repair is advised. Ligation or primary amputation is an acceptable damage control maneuver if there is not time for shunting or the patient is in extremis.

11.5.6 Thoracic and Abdominal Aorta

Management of penetrating injury to the thoracic and abdominal aorta is rare given the prehospital lethality of this injury. Wartime estimates reported a combined incidence of aortic injury at 2.9% [16]. Initial management of thoracic hemorrhage in the setting of penetrating trauma is directed by chest tube location and output in conjunction with the patient's physiology. The descending thoracic aorta is approached through the left anterior-lateral thoracotomy. An initial left thoracotomy can be extended into the right chest extending across the sternum (i.e., "clamshell" thoracotomy). Aortic control proximal and distal to the injury or hematoma must be obtained including isolation or control of any intercostal arteries in this segment. Aortic clamps are used to arrest flow in this segment, and the hematoma is entered with debridement of the injured aorta. An adequate length of the aorta must be debrided to allow placement of a large-caliber synthetic conduit (20 mm–26 mm Dacron graft) positioned end to end to the proximal and distal segments of the uninjured aorta. Endovascular management of blunt aortic injury to the thoracic aorta (i.e., partial aortic transection or pseudoaneurysm formation) in a patient who has demonstrated temporary physiologic stability allows for definitive repair without the morbidity of thoracotomy and improved outcomes [57].

Blunt and penetrating injuries to the abdominal aorta present as a central, zone I retroperitoneal hematoma. The surgical management of zone I retroperitoneal hematomas should be based upon the distribution of the hematoma. Supra-mesocolic, zone I retroperitoneal hematomas are best approached via a left medial-visceral rotation (Mattox maneuver) which exposes the supraceliac, paravisceral, and infrarenal segments of the abdominal aorta. Infra-mesocolic, zone I retroperitoneal hematomas can be approached via a standard transabdominal, transperitoneal approach with transverse colon cranial retraction and small bowel evisceration or with a right medial-visceral rotation (Cattell-Braasch maneuver) exposing the infrarenal aorta and inferior vena cava. Proximal and distal aortic control is paramount during surgical management. Proximal control is rapidly obtained in the supraceliac position and obtained through the gastrohepatic ligament by retracting the esophagus to the left and dividing the diaphragmatic crus. Alternatively, the Mattox maneuver exposes the supraceliac aorta from the lateral position, enabling proximal control as well. The iliac vessels or distal aorta are subsequently controlled, providing isolation before entering the hematoma. Repair techniques for the aorta and its branch vessels range from primary pledgetted closure to replacement with a Dacron interposition graft and depend upon the degree of injury.

11.5.7 Inferior Vena Cava

Intracavitary injury to the inferior vena cava (IVC) can result in massive hemorrhage and hemodynamic instability. The inferior vena cava is approached in the abdomen by performing the Cattell-Braasch and extended Kocher maneuvers. Mobilization of the liver is required to visualize the retro-hepatic vena cava. The lumbar venous tributaries into the injured segment of the IVC should be controlled to allow for comprehensive isolation. Because repair of the IVC is likely to require intermittent occlusion (i.e., sponge sticks or vascular clamps) or ligation in extreme cases, central venous access should be established above the diaphragm to allow effective volume resuscitation. If temporary occlusion of the IVC results in significant hypotension, the adjacent abdominal aorta may be temporarily occluded to support central pressures while continued resuscitation takes place. Repair of longitudinal injuries to the IVC can be accomplished with a running venorrhaphy provided that the residual lumen is not narrowed more than 50%. In instances where longitudinal repair will result in greater than 50% stenosis of the IVC, patch angioplasty or resection and interposition graft using ePTFE or Dacron is preferable. Ligation of the infrarenal IVC is acceptable as a damage control maneuver, although this carries a significant risk of mortality and major morbidity in the form of decreased cardiac preload and significant lower extremity edema. If infrarenal IVC ligation is needed, bilateral lower extremity fasciotomies must be completed in order to reduce the risk for compartment syndrome. Suprarenal occlusion of the IVC is generally not compatible with survival and should be considered a measure of last resort [58].

11.5.8 Common, External, and Hypogastric Iliac Arteries

Iliac artery injuries generally present as a zone III or pelvic hematoma with or without extremity ischemia. Exploration of the zone III hematoma should be performed following proximal control of the infrarenal abdominal aorta and the contralateral common iliac artery, if feasible. The distal external iliac artery should be identified as it exits the pelvis at the inguinal ligament at a position free from the hematoma formation. The hypogastric (internal iliac) artery may not be initially controlled or visualized before exploring the hematoma. The inability to initially control all bleeding from the hematoma necessitates preparation including multiple suction devices, Fogarty occlusion balloons, direct tamponade strategies or devices, and alerting anesthesia regarding the need for continued resuscitation during exploration. After proximal and distal control of the common and external iliac arteries is obtained, the hematoma is entered which facilitates exposure and clamping of the hypogastric artery and the injured vessel(s). Common and external artery injuries can be controlled and managed with a TVS as needed or repaired with interposition grafting using saphenous vein or prosthetic conduit (6–8 mm ePTFE or Dacron). In an unstable patient or a patient where there is significant contamination of the surgical field, shunt placement with delayed definitive repair or reconstruction is appropriate. If the primary injury is to the hypogastric artery, it can be ligated. Bleeding from associated iliac veins may be severe and difficult to expose. The common or external iliac artery may be divided if necessary to facilitate exposure of the iliac vein, followed by subsequent repair of the artery. Endovascular adjuncts, such as selective embolization of a bleeding hypogastric artery, are an option, particularly in blunt trauma with associated pelvic fracture.

11.5.9 Common and Superficial Femoral Artery

Injury to the common femoral artery is often fatal as hemorrhage control at this anatomic location is often difficult. Additionally, injury to the common femoral artery and superficial femoral artery represents the second most common anatomic location for wartime vascular trauma [16]. Surgeon experience and familiarity in damage control maneuvers for rapid vascular control of the femoral vessels are critical. Exposure of the common femoral artery is obtained through a longitudinal incision above the artery approximately 2 cm lateral to the pubic tubercle at the inguinal ligament. A technical point in exposing the common femoral artery is extending the incision cranial enough so that the inguinal ligament can be identified first in a consistent and familiar manner. Shunting with a TVS can be performed in conjunction with damage control maneuvers. However, distal common femoral artery injuries at the bifurcation of the superficial femoral artery and profunda artery represent a unique challenge with respect to maintaining forward perfusion to both structures. Every attempt should be made to maintain flow into the profunda femoris artery, although the feasibility of this will depend upon the pattern of injury and surgeon experience with more complicated vascular reconstruction. Alternatively, proximal control can be obtained in the retroperitoneum (i.e., external iliac artery) through the cranial extension of the groin incision or by using a limited transverse-oblique incision in the lower abdomen cranial to the inguinal ligament. After a transverse-oblique skin incision, the external and internal oblique aponeuroses are divided. The transversus abdominus muscle and transversalis fascia are opened allowing entrance into the retroperitoneum. The plane between peritoneum and retroperitoneum is developed, and the peritoneal contents are reflected cephalad, exposing the external iliac vessels along the medial border of the psoas muscle. Proximal vascular control is obtained at the external iliac artery.

Exposure of the distal superficial femoral artery is performed through a medial thigh incision and the adductors of the leg (i.e., adductor magnus). Exposure is facilitated by placing a lift or "bump" below the knee which allows the superficial femoral artery, sartorius muscle, and adductors to be suspended improving separation. Entry into the fascia of the lower thigh is performed at the anterior margin of the sartorius muscle which is subsequently reflected posteriorly. Exposure is facilitated with the surgeon seated looking across the dissection field with lights positioned directly over the shoulder if they do not have a headlight available. When exposing the superficial femoral artery, it is important to recognize the femoral vein which is in close proximity to the artery. Repair of superficial femoral artery injury is best performed by reversed saphenous vein interposition graft from the uninjured leg. Shunting of the superficial femoral artery is appropriate during damage control procedures.

11.5.10 Profunda Femoris Artery

The profunda femoris artery provides perfusion to the musculature of the thigh. Exposure of the proximal profunda femoris artery is obtained through a longitudinal incision used to expose the common femoral artery. Mid- and distal segments of the profunda femoris artery are exposed through a vertical incision made parallel to the lateral border of the sartorius muscle. The sartorius muscle is retracted medially and the rectus femoris is retracted laterally to expose the mid- and distal segments. Proximal profunda injuries should be repaired with reversed saphenous vein interposition graft. This is especially important if there is question about the integrity of the superficial femoral or popliteal vessels. In the setting of a compromised superficial femoral artery, flow through the profunda femoris is critical to allow healing of subsequent lower extremity wounds and amputations. In a patient who sustains a devastating blast injury with a non-salvageable lower extremity (i.e., above-knee traumatic amputation), the superficial femoral artery can be used as a conduit in order to maintain the integrity of the profunda femoris artery. If patency of the superficial femoral artery can be confirmed, ligation of mid- and distal profunda femoris arterial injuries is acceptable.

11.5.11 Popliteal Artery

Popliteal artery and vein injuries were identified in 9% of traumatic injuries during the wars in Iraq and Afghanistan [16]. Injuries in the popliteal space are exposed through a medial incision. The dissection is extended from cephalad to caudad at the medial aspect of the knee and is facilitated by a lift or "bump" under the calf of the leg with the knee flexed. When exposing caudal portion of the popliteal space, the bump is placed under the thigh. Natural dissection planes exist in exposing the above-knee popliteal artery with the exception of the need to divide the fibers of the adductor magnus which envelop the distal superficial femoral artery (Hunter's canal). Similarly, a natural dissection plane exists into the popliteal space for the below-knee popliteal artery; however, added exposure can be accomplished by division of the gastrocnemius and soleus muscle fibers from the medial tibial condyle thereby allowing a lengthy exposure of the below-knee popliteal artery and the origins of the anterior tibial artery and the tibial-peroneal trunk. To completely expose the popliteal space, the medial attachment of the pes anserinus (conjoined tendons of the sartorius, semitendinosus, semimembranosus, and gracilis) to the medial condyle of the tibia can be divided. When feasible, the pes anserinus should be reconstructed given its significant role in medial knee stabilization. Weitlaner retractors, cerebellar retractors, and flexible Adson-Beckman or Henly popliteal retractors with detachable side blades are necessary to expose the popliteal space. Typically, the medial head of the gastrocnemius can be retracted down using one of these devices and does not need to be divided. TVS are of significant utility in damage control management of popliteal artery injuries. Reconstruction generally incorporates the use of autologous greater saphenous vein when feasible.

11.5.12 Tibial Arteries

Peripheral vascular injury to the lower extremity continues to represent the most common injury pattern encountered throughout military history [5–16]. During modern warfare, tibial-level vascular injuries are present in 21% of wounded casualties. The recommended approach to tibial artery injury is one of selective repair. Because of their distal location and redundant nature, isolated and multiple tibial artery injuries can be ligated without adverse outcomes. As long as one tibial artery remains uninjured and patent to the ankle, no additional tests or repairs are required. This selective approach to tibial repair has been shown to be effective, confirming that although tibial injuries can be ligated, there is a distinct injury pattern which requires repair [36]. TVS can be inserted into tibial vessels although shunt patency is lower than that in more proximal vessels. The anterior tibial artery is exposed through an anterolateral longitudinal incision midway between the tibia and fibula. The fascia along the lateral border of the anterior tibialis muscle is divided, and the plane between the anterior tibialis and extensor digitorum longus muscles is developed. The anterior tibial artery lies deep along the interosseous membrane. Exposure of the posterior tibial artery in the deep compartment of the leg is through a medial incision with a lift or "bump" under the knee or thigh. A longitudinal incision is made 2 cm posterior to the posterior margin of the tibia. Division of the tibial attachments of the soleus muscle in the proximal and mid-leg and posterior retraction of the soleus exposes the artery. Reconstruction of a peroneal artery injury is rarely required, and ligation is adequate. Importantly, tibial reconstruction is technically more challenging and time-consuming because of the smaller size of the vessels. Like other vascular repairs, tibial reconstruction should not be undertaken if the patient has other life-threatening injuries or is in extremis.

11.6 Summary

Vascular damage control surgery emphasizes immediate hemorrhage control and mitigation of ischemia (and subsequent complications related to end-organ ischemia) with restoration of perfusion.

References

1. Eastridge BJ, Mabry RL, Seguin P, Cantrell J, Tops T, Uribe P, Mallett O, Zubko T, Oetjen-Gerdes L, Rasmussen TE, Butler FK, Kotwal RS, Holcomb JB, Wade C, Champion H, Lawnick M, Moores L, Blackbourne LH. Death on the battlefield (2001–2011): implications for the future of combat casualty care. J Trauma Acute Care Surg. 2012;73(6 Suppl 5):S431–7.
2. Holcomb JB, McMullin NR, Pearse L, Caruso J, Wade CE, Oetjen-Gerdes L, Champion HR, Lawnick M, Farr W, Rodriguez S, Butler FK. Causes of death in US special operations forces in the global war on terrorism 2001–2004. Ann Surg. 2007;245:986–91.
3. Bellamy RF. The cause of death in conventional land warfare: implications for combat casualty care research. Mil Med. 1984;149:55–62.
4. Kelly JF, Ritenour AE, McLaughlin DF, et al. Injury severity and causes of death from operation Iraqi freedom and operation enduring freedom: 2003–2004. J Trauma. 2008;64(suppl):s21–7.
5. DeBakey ME, Simeone FA. Battle injuries of the arteries in world war II. Ann Surg. 1946;123:534–79.
6. Hughes CW. The primary repair of wounds of major arteries; an analysis of experience in Korea in 1953. Ann Surg. 1955;141:297–303.
7. Hughes CW. Acute vascular trauma in Korean war casualties; an analysis of 180 cases. Surg Gynecol Obstet. 1954;99:91–100.
8. Jahnke EJ Jr, Hughes CW, Howard JM. The rationale of arterial repair on the battlefield. Am J Surg. 1954;87:396–401.
9. Rich NM, Hughes CW. Vietnam vascular registry: a preliminary report. Surgery. 1969;65:218–26.
10. Rich NM, Baugh JH, Hughes CW. Popliteal artery injuries in Vietnam. Am J Surg. 1969;118:531–14.
11. Rich NM, Baugh JH, Hughes CW. Acute arterial injuries in Vietnam: 1,000 cases. J Trauma. 1970;10:359–69.
12. Woodward EB, Clouse WD, Eliason JE, et al. Penetrating femoropopliteal injury during modern warfare: experience of the balad vascular registry. J Vasc Surg. 2007;47:1259–65.
13. Clouse WD, Rasmussen TE, Peck MA, et al. In-theater management of vascular injury: 2 years of balad vascular registry. J Am Coll Surg. 2007;204:625–32.
14. Rasmussen TE, Clouse WD, Jenkins DH, et al. Echelons of care and the management of wartime vascular injury: a report from the 332nd EMDG/air force theater hospital, Balad Air Base, Iraq. Persp Vasc Surg Endovasc Ther. 2006;18(2):91–9.
15. Stannard A, Brown K, Benson C, Clasper J, Midwinter M, Tai NR. Outcome after vascular trauma in a deployed military trauma system. Br J Surg. 2011;98(2):228–34.
16. White JM, Stannard A, Burkhardt GE, Eastridge BJ, Blackbourne LH, Rasmussen TE. The epidemiology of vascular injury in the wars in Iraq and Afghanistan. Ann Surg. 2011;253(6):1184–9.
17. White JM, Cannon JW, Stannard A, Markov NP, Rasmussen TE. Endovascular balloon occlusion of the aorta is superior to resuscitative thoracotomy with aortic clamping in a porcine model of hemorrhagic shock. Surgery. 2011;150(3):400–9.
18. Stannard A, Eliason JL, Rasmussen TE. Resuscitative endovascular balloon occlusion of the aorta (REBOA) as an adjunct for hemorrhagic shock. J Trauma. 2011;71(6):1869–72.
19. Markov NP, Percival TJ, Morrison JJ, Ross JD, Scott DJ, Spencer JR, Rasmussen TE. Physiologic tolerance of descending thoracic aortic balloon occlusion in a swine model of hemorrhagic shock. Surgery. 2013;153(6):848–56.

20. Scott DJ, Eliason JL, Villamaria C, Morrison JJ, Houston R 4th, Spencer JR, Rasmussen TE. A novel fluoroscopy-free, resuscitative endovascular aortic balloon occlusion system in a model of hemorrhagic shock. J Trauma Acute Care Surg. 2013;75(1):122–8.
21. Brenner ML, Moore LJ, DuBose JJ, Tyson GH, McNutt MK, Albarado RP, Holcomb JB, Scalea TM, Rasmussen TE. A clinical series of resuscitative endovascular balloon occlusion of the aorta for hemorrhage control and resuscitation. J Trauma Acute Care Surg. 2013;75(3):506–11.
22. Morrison JJ, Ross JD, Houston R, Watson JD, Sokol KK, Rasmussen TE. Use of resuscitative endovascular balloon occlusion of the aorta in a highly lethal model of noncompressible torso hemorrhage. Shock. 2014;41(2):130–7.
23. Morrison JJ, Galgon RE, Jansen JO, Cannon JW, Rasmussen TE, Eliason JL. A systematic review of the use of resuscitative endovascular balloon occlusion of the aorta in the management of hemorrhagic shock. J Trauma Acute Care Surg. 2016;80(2):324–34.
24. Mabry RL, Holcomb JB, Baker AM, Cloonan CC, Uhorchak JM, Perkins DE, Canfield AJ, Hagmann JH. United States Army rangers in Somalia: an analysis of combat casualties on an urban battlefield. J Trauma. 2000;49(3):515–28; discussion 528–9.
25. Kragh JF Jr, Walters TJ, Baer DG, Fox CJ, Wade CE, Salinas J, Holcomb JB. Practical use of emergency tourniquets to stop bleeding in major limb trauma. J Trauma. 2008;64(Suppl 2):S38–9.
26. Kragh JF Jr, Walters TJ, Baer DG, Fox CJ, Wade CE, Salinas J, Holcomb JB. Survival with emergency tourniquet use to stop bleeding in major limb trauma. Ann Surg. 2009;249(1):1–7.
27. Kragh JF Jr, Littrel ML, Jones JA, Walters TJ, Baer DG, Wade CE, Holcomb JB. Battle casualty survival with emergency tourniquet use to stop limb bleeding. J Emerg Med. 2011;41(6):590–7.
28. Kragh JF Jr, O'Neill ML, Walters TJ, Jones JA, Baer DG, Gershman LK, Wade CE, Holcomb JB. Minor morbidity with emergency tourniquet use to stop bleeding in severe limb trauma: research, history, and reconciling advocates and abolitionists. Mil Med. 2011;176(7):817–23.
29. Kragh JF Jr, Cooper A, Aden JK, Dubick MA, Baer DG, Wade CE, Blackbourne LH. Survey of trauma registry data on tourniquet use in pediatric war casualties. Pediatr Emerg Care. 2012;28(12):1361–5.
30. Kragh JF Jr, Dubick MA, Aden JK, McKeague AL, Rasmussen TE, Baer DG, Blackbourne LH. U.S. military use of tourniquets from 2001 to 2010. Prehosp Emerg Care. 2015;19(2):184–90.
31. Beekley AC, Sebesta JA, Blackbourne LH, Herbert GS, Kauvar DS, Baer DG, Walters TJ, Mullenix PS, Holcomb JB, 31st Combat Support Hospital Research Group. Prehospital tourniquet use in operation Iraqi freedom: effect on hemorrhage control and outcomes. J Trauma. 2008;64(2 Suppl):S28–37; discussion S37.
32. King DR, van der Wilden G, Kragh JF Jr, Blackbourne LH. Forward assessment of 79 prehospital battlefield tourniquets used in the current war. J Spec Oper Med. 2012;12(4):33–8.
33. Lairet JR, Bebarta VS, Burns CJ, Lairet KF, Rasmussen TE, Renz EM, King BT, Fernandez W, Gerhardt R, Butler F. Prehospital interventions performed in a combat zone: a prospective multicenter study of 1,003 combat wounded. J Trauma Acute Care Surg. 2012;73(2 Suppl 1):S38–2.
34. Inaba K, Siboni S, Resnick S, Zhu J, Wong MD, Haltmeier T, Benjamin E, Demetriades D. Tourniquet use for civilian extremity trauma. J Trauma Acute Care Surg. 2015;79(2):232–7.
35. Fortuna G, DuBose JJ, Mendelsberg R, Inaba K, Haider A, Joseph B, Skarupa D, Selleck MJ, O'Callaghan TA, Charlton-Ouw K, Lower Extremity Vascular Repairs Outcome Group. Contemporary outcomes of lower extremity vascular repairs extending below the knee: a multicenter retrospective study. J Trauma Acute Care Surg. 2016;81(1):63–70.
36. Burkhardt GE, Cox M, Clouse WD, Porras C, Gifford SM, Williams K, Propper BW, Rasmussen TE. Outcomes of selective tibial artery repair following combat-related extremity injury. J Vasc Surg. 2010;52(1):91–6.
37. Liang NL, Alarcon LH, Jeyabalan G, Avgerinos ED, Makaroun MS, Chaer RA. Contemporary outcomes of civilian lower extremity arterial trauma. J Vasc Surg. 2016;64(3):731–6.
38. Eger M, Golcman L, Goldstein A, Hirsch M. The use of a temporary shunt in the management of arterial vascular injuries. Surg Gynecol Obstet. 1971;132:67–70.
39. Rasmussen TE, Clouse WD, Jenkins DH, Peck MA, Eliason JL, Smith DL. The use of temporary vascular shunts as a damage control adjunct in the management of wartime vascular injury. J Trauma. 2006;61(1):8–12; discussion 12–5.
40. Chambers LW, Green DJ, Sample K, Gillingham BL, Rhee P, Brown C, Narine N, Uecker JM, Bohman HR. Tactical surgical intervention with temporary shunting of peripheral vascular trauma sustained during operation Iraqi freedom: one unit's experience. J Trauma. 2006;61(4):824–30.
41. Taller J, Kamdar JP, Greene JA, Morgan RA, Blankenship CL, Dabrowski P, Sharpe RP. Temporary vascular shunts as initial treatment of proximal extremity vascular injuries during combat operations: the new standard of care at echelon II facilities? J Trauma. 2008;65(3):595–603.
42. Gifford SM, Eliason JL, Clouse WD, Spencer JR, Burkhardt GE, Propper BW, Dixon PS, Zarzabal LA, Gelfond JA, Rasmussen TE. Early versus delayed restoration of flow with temporary vascular shunt reduces circulating markers of injury in a porcine model. J Trauma. 2009 Aug;67(2):259–65.

43. Gifford SM, Aidinian G, Clouse WD, Fox CJ, Porras CA, Jones WT, Zarzabal LA, Michalek JE, Propper BW, Burkhardt GE, Rasmussen TE. Effect of temporary shunting on extremity vascular injury: an outcome analysis from the global war on terror vascular injury initiative. J Vasc Surg. 2009;50(3):549–55; discussion 555–6.
44. Gifford SM, Eliason JL, Clouse WD, Spencer JR, Burkhardt GE, Propper BW, Dixon PS, Zarzabal LA, Gelfond JA, Rasmussen TE. Early versus delayed restoration of flow with temporary vascular shunt reduces circulating markers of injury in a porcine model. J Trauma. 2009;67(2):259–65.
45. Subramanian A, Vercruysse G, Dente C, Wyrzykowski A, King E, Feliciano DV. A decade's experience with temporary intravascular shunts at a civilian level 1 trauma center. J Trauma. 2008;65:316–26.
46. Inaba K, Aksoy H, Seamon MJ, Marks JA, Duchesne J, Schroll R, Fox CJ, Pieracci FM, Moore EE, Joseph B, Haider AA, Harvin JA, Lawless RA, Cannon J, Holland SR, Demetriades D, Multicenter Shunt Study Group. Multicenter evaluation of temporary intravascular shunt use in vascular trauma. J Trauma Acute Care Surg. 2016;80(3):359–64; discussion 364–5.
47. Granchi T, Schmittling Z, Vasquez J, Schreiber M, Wall M. Prolonged use of intraluminal arterial shunts without systemic anticoagulation. Am J Surg. 2000;180(6):493–6; discussion 496–7
48. Feliciano DV, Mattox KL, Graham JM, Bitondo CG. Five-year experience with PTFE grafts in vascular wounds. J Trauma. 1985;25(1):71–82.
49. Vertrees A, Fox CJ, Quan RW, Cox MW, Adams ED, Gillespie DL. The use of prosthetic grafts in complex military vascular trauma: a limb salvage strategy for patients with severely limited autologous conduit. J Trauma. 2009;66(4):980–3.
50. Greer LT, Patel B, Via KC, Bowman JN, Weber MA, Fox CJ. Management of secondary hemorrhage from early graft failure in military extremity wounds. J Trauma Acute Care Surg. 2012;73(4):818–24.
51. Sohn VY, Arthurs ZM, Herbert GS, Beekley AC, Sebesta JA. Demographics, treatment, and early outcomes in penetrating vascular combat trauma. Arch Surg. 2008;143(8):783–7.
52. Watson JD, Houston R, Morrison JJ, Gifford SM, Rasmussen TE. A retrospective cohort comparison of expanded polytetrafluorethylene to autologous vein for vascular reconstruction in modern combat casualty care. Ann Vasc Surg. 2015;29(4):822–9.
53. Fox CJ, Patel B, Clouse WD. Update on wartime vascular injury. Perspect Vasc Surg Endovasc Ther. 2011;23(1):13–25.
54. Chambers RW, Rhee P, Baker BC, et al. Initial experience of US marine corps forward resuscitative surgical system during operation Iraqi freedom. Arch Surg. 2005;140:26–32.
55. Fox CJ, Gillespie DL, Cox ED, Kragh JF Jr, Mehta SG, Salinas J, Holcomb JB. Damage control resuscitation for vascular surgery in a combat support hospital. J Trauma. 2008;65(1):1–9.
56. Percival TJ, White JM, Ricci MA. Compartment syndrome in the setting of vascular injury. Perspect Vasc Surg Endovasc Ther. 2011;23(2):119–24.
57. Kauvar DS, White JM, Johnson CA, Jones WT, Rasmussen TE, Clouse DW. Endovascular versus open management of blunt traumatic aortic disruption at two military trauma centers: comparison of in-hospital variables. Mil Med. 2009;174(8):869–73.
58. Sullivan PS, Dente CJ, Patel S, et al. Outcome of ligation of the inferior vena cava in the modern era. Am J Surg. 2009;199:500–6.

Endovascular Techniques in Hemorrhage Control and Resuscitation

12

Joe DuBose and Todd E. Rasmussen

Abstract

Advances in endovascular technologies have demonstrated their promise as potential damage control adjuncts. Resuscitative endovascular balloon occlusion of the aorta (REBOA) and other novel devices may provide solutions to some of the significant challenges of hemorrhage from non-compressible sites. This chapter outlines available endovascular tools for utilization and discusses their potential and present limitations.

Early hemorrhage control is a basic tenet of damage control surgery and remains a common challenge of modern trauma care. Over the past decade, a number of significant innovations have contributed to an improved ability to both diagnose bleeding sources and promote early hemorrhage control. The adoption of improved strategies for resuscitation and the introduction of novel systemic hemostatic adjuncts have also contributed to enhanced capabilities in mitigating the risk of death due to hemorrhage.

There remains, however, a need to control the source of hemorrhage through manual means. At accessible locations, bleeding sources can initially be controlled with either direct pressure or peripheral tourniquet utilization. An enhanced understanding of the impact of hemorrhage at non-compressible sites, however, has raised awareness of a need to develop and refine techniques that afford rapid control of hemorrhage at these locations.

Specific endovascular solutions have emerged as potentially important therapeutic adjuncts in this regard. The use of interventional procedures in trauma is not new to the realm of trauma care, and their use appears to have increased steadily over the past 10 years. A recent analysis of the National Trauma Data Bank (NTDB) reported that 8.1% of acute arterial injuries in 2003 were treated with endovascular therapy, compared to only 2.1% in 1994. This analysis demonstrated that this increased utilization is occurring after a variety of injury mechanisms, with nearly an equal number of blunt (55%) and penetrating (45%) injuries treated via endovascular means [1]. A more recent study, also using NTDB data, reported that 16% of traumatic vascular injuries were treated with endovascular therapy, including 20% who were hypotensive at the time of

J. DuBose, M.D., F.A.C.S., F.C.C.M. (✉)
R Adams Cowley Shock Trauma Center, University of Maryland, Baltimore, MD, USA

Uniformed Services University of the Health Sciences, Bethesda, MD, USA

T.E. Rasmussen, M.D., F.A.C.S.
F. Edward Hebert School of Medicine—"America's Medical School", Uniformed Services University of the Health Sciences, Bethesda, MD, USA

Walter Reed National Military Medical Center, Bethesda, MD, USA

J. Duchesne et al. (eds.), *Damage Control in Trauma Care*,
https://doi.org/10.1007/978-3-319-72607-6_12

intervention. The investigators reporting these findings also noted a decreased mortality that was associated with the increased use of endovascular intervention following traumatic injury [2]. These data suggest that, with advancements in both imaging and device technology, the use of endovascular techniques has become an integral part of treatment algorithms for an expanding subset of traumatically injured patients.

This chapter is designed to outline the contemporary utilization of endovascular techniques in the setting of hemorrhage control during damage control surgery, with an emphasis on early control of bleeding at non-compressible sites as a damage control adjunct. We will outline newly developed and refined approaches, highlighting the available data from both translational science and clinical utilization in the treatment of bleeding patients.

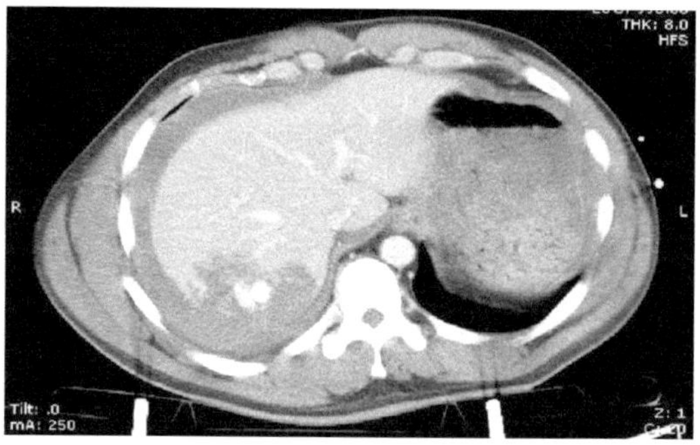

Fig. 12.1 Hepatic injury computed tomographic injury image demonstrating active extravasation with contrast blush from the liver. This patient went on to receive hepatic embolization of this bleeding source and did not require operative intervention

12.1 Angiography for Diagnosis and Treatment of Hemorrhage

The utilization of angiography and embolization for the diagnosis and treatment of traumatic hemorrhage has increased significantly over the past several decades. Initial reports of the successful application of these approaches were published in the 1970s. These early reports demonstrated that catheter-based therapy could effectively be utilized to assist in the timely management of hemorrhage from pelvic and renal sources [3, 4]. Shortly thereafter, similar success was described at other locations, including a 1977 report of intercostal bleeding successfully controlled by endovascular embolization [5]. Later case reports suggested angioembolization alone or in combination with surgical therapy for highly lethal pelvic hemorrhage was both a feasible and effective damage control adjunct [6–8]. Interventionalists in Brooklyn proved pioneers in advancing endovascular therapy for trauma, reporting good outcomes in several series of splenic and pelvic hemorrhage [9–11]. These successes were followed by the increasing adoption of algorithms that effectively incorporated endovascular adjuncts as routine elements of hemorrhage control for patient with both pelvic and solid organ bleeding sources. In one study documenting a continued evolution in this regard, Roudsari et al. reported the use of angioembolization for pelvic and liver injuries to have increased from 30% to 50% in 1996 to 100% in 2010 at a busy American College of Surgeons Level 1 designated trauma center [12] (Fig. 12.1).

As endovascular control of splenic, hepatic, pelvic, carotid, and intercostal artery injuries has occurred for decades, so too has a continued evolution in advancement in support of hemorrhage control with endovascular modalities. Advancements in technology have resulted in the present availability of a host of hemostatic adjuncts that can be delivered in a precise manner directly at the site of injury. Current capabilities vary from simple Gelfoam utilization to a variety of endovascular coil and plug devices that can be used to promote focal hemorrhage control in these locations. The use of angioembolization techniques is currently well established, with a proven track record in the treatment of pelvic and solid organ bleeding after injury [13–18].

Despite continued improvement in devices and techniques, however, it is important to recognize that controversy regarding optimal embolization utilization remains. Patient selection continues to be an active area of investigation regarding the ideal role of angioembolization after trauma. Patient physiology appears to play a significant role in the current utilization of this adjunct at most centers, but the specific parameters that should be utilized have not been well studied in a prospective, randomized fashion. Associated radiographic findings—including significant hematoma and active contrast extravasation or "blush"—also likely guide the employment of embolization in most environments, but the importance of these imaging findings in guiding optimal patient selection for endovascular intervention remains controversial. For these and other reasons, and despite extensive experience on the topic, ideal selection criteria for endovascular embolization remain a matter of active investigation. The available data has, however, afforded the development of several reasonable algorithms for use by leading trauma organizations, including the Western Trauma Association (WTA), the Eastern Association for the Surgery of Trauma (EAST), and the American Association for the Surgery of Trauma (AAST).

While available treatment algorithms provide some reasonable guidance on the utilization of angioembolization for traumatic hemorrhage, it is also important to appreciate that the optimal technique for the conduct of this intervention is not well defined. A variety of hemostatic adjuncts can be employed to promote the arrest of hemorrhage using endovascular means—including coils, nitinol plugs, and Gelfoam. The relative permanency of occlusion achieved is related to the adjunct chosen, with coils and plugs providing lasting occlusion of a treated vessel and Gelfoam facilitating more temporary hemorrhage control to promote clot formation locally. The available options provide alternatives that can be individualized to the clinical situation, but the optimal agent or approach for specific scenarios remains an area of active study.

Another key area of controversy regarding the delivery of endovascular hemostatic adjuncts involves the level of angioembolization. The relative ease with which embolization can be achieved at the level of an origin artery must be weighed against the regional sparing of organ tissue that can be achieved with more distal "selective" or "super-selective" embolization approaches. While all providers would likely agree that treatment focally at the specific site of hemorrhage is the most ideal, the complexity and time that may be associated with achieving this pinpoint hemostasis of a bleeding pelvic vessel or solid organ injury site requires consideration of other pressing needs in a multi-injured trauma patient. Defining the optimal approach is challenging, as the variety of variables that must be considered makes focused study of this issue problematic.

Perhaps the greatest limitation of angioembolization utilization is that of expedient availability. Even at major trauma centers with advanced capabilities, there appear to be discrepancies in availability of this adjunct during hours of peak trauma intake [19]. One novel solution being explored is to expand the skillset of trauma responders, who are most commonly present at the bedside when victims of significant injury arrive—even in the middle of the night and on weekends [20, 21]. Additional study is required, however, to determine the extent of training required to incorporate embolization into the skillset of the trauma/acute care surgeon.

12.2 Stent Grafting

When employed for the treatment of vascular injury, endovascular stenting is often considered a definitive repair modality. It is important to recognize, however, that endovascular endoluminal stent grafts can also be utilized effectively as a viable damage control adjunct that is a bridge to subsequent open repair. Stent grafts can be used temporarily to cover partial- or full-thickness injuries, particularly at sites of major vascular injury that cannot be easily or rapidly accessed with traditional open surgical exposure. Placing a stent across a full-thickness injury may save the physiologically devastated patient prolonged illness by decreasing blood loss and ensuing coagulopathy. In this fashion, the utilization of an endoluminal stent graft can be considered an "internal shunt" that restores in-line flow, mitigates the danger of distal ischemia, and affords the marshaling of optimal resources for open vascular repair or interposition vessel replacement should they be deemed optimal for long-term patient outcome.

As stent grafts have evolved, their use in the treatment of blunt thoracic aortic injury (BTAI) has emerged as a signature success story for the traumatic application of endovascular technologies. Significant BTAI remains a relatively infrequent but potentially rapidly lethal sequel of significant trauma. The advent of thoracic endovascular aortic repair (TEVAR) utilizing endovascular stent grafts has resulted in both improved morbidity and mortality among patients who survive to reach care after BTAI (Fig. 12.2a, b). Although appropriate patient selection remains paramount to success, the clear success of TEVAR has dramatically altered the standard of care for BTAI patients in the modern era.

In a landmark 2008 report, Demetriades and colleagues of the American Association for the Surgery of Trauma (AAST) BTAI study group [22] documented significant improvements in BTAI care associated with the transition from open to endovascular repair. In their examination of 193 patients with BTAI, they found that TEVAR was associated with significantly decreased transfusion requirements and lower mortality compared to open repair modalities. A more contemporary multi-institutional study on the topic demonstrated similar findings, noting a significantly lower PRBC requirement (mean 5.9 vs. 3.1 units, $p < 0.002$) in the first 24 h, lower overall mortality (8.6% vs. 19.7%, $p = 0.021$), and lower aortic-related mortality (13.1% vs. 2.5%, $p = 0.003$) among TEVAR-treated patients compared to counterparts repaired using open techniques [23].

Initial experience with TEVAR, however, highlighted significant concerns with newer endovascular approaches. One of the important findings of the 2008 report of the AAST BTAI study group was the significant rate of TEVAR-related complications that were observed [22]. In this early study of the topic, Demetriades and his group found that 18.4% patients undergoing TEVAR had some form of stent graft-specific complication, most notably endoleak at 13.6%. Advances in endovascular technologies have, in recent years however, dramatically decreased complication rates related to TEVAR. The introduction of two Federal Drug Administration (FDA)-approved devices specifically for TEVAR after BTAI in 2005 heralded considerable engineering advances for trauma applications. There are now a number of major device manufacturers who have developed TEVAR devices optimal for BTAI use, and an improved ability to avoid traditional adverse

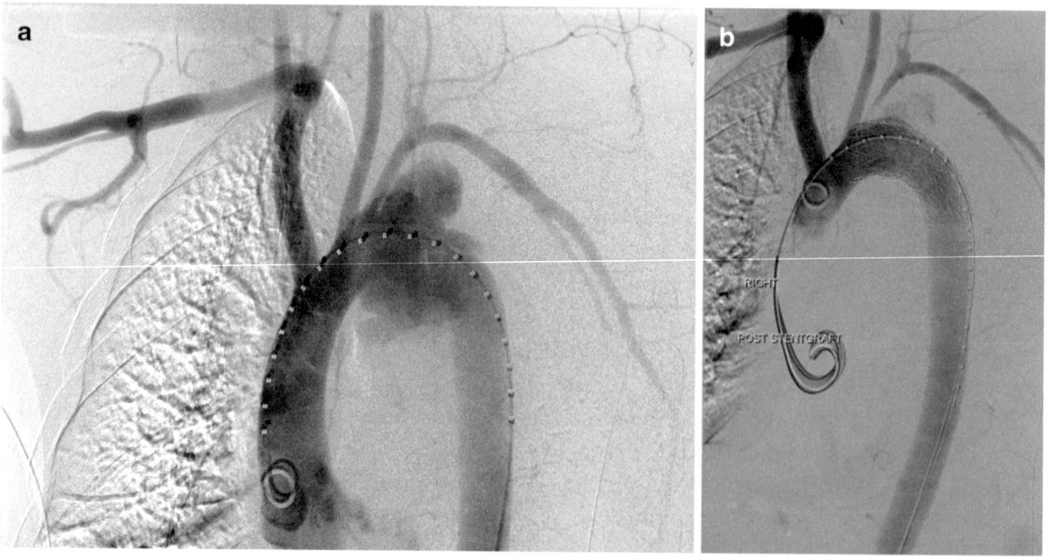

Fig. 12.2 (**a**, **b**) Pre (**a**)- and post (**b**)-repair angiographic images documenting treatment of a grade III (pseudoaneurysm) blunt thoracic aortic injury (BTAI)

events following TEVAR has been documented with their utilization [23]. Beyond limitations specific to device evolution, other traditional concerns following aortic repair after BTAI have included paralysis, stroke, and left upper extremity ischemia when coverage of the left subclavian artery (LSCA) is required for optimal TEVAR. Like the access and device-related issues of decades past, these complications appear to have significantly decreased over time [24–31].

In order to guide the optimal management of BTAI, the development of a functional grading system to guide the selection of therapy was required. Azizzadeh and colleagues were among the first to describe such a system for BTAI [31], designing the current system utilized by the Society of Vascular Surgery (SVS) for description of these injuries. This system has been utilized to develop the SVS clinical practice guidelines presently employed for BTAI care at many centers. The SVS guidelines suggest that the majority of grade I BTAI patients can be managed nonoperatively—as was documented in a large contemporary multicenter study (76.6%) [23]. According to the effort by DuBose et al. [23], the majority of grade II, III, and IV injuries are currently treated via either TEVAR or open repair (72.1%, 87.0%, 75%, respectively).

Growing awareness regarding the natural history of BTAI, however, has supported the examination of several alternate grading systems and algorithms for treatment. Both the Vancouver simplified grading system [32] and the alternate classification scheme proposed by Starnes et al. [33] have suggested that additional elements of CTA discernable BTAI data may be of importance in guiding therapy. Specifically, these groups have examined the impact of specific aortic lesion dimensions in dictating the need for treatment versus medical management alone. A group of investigators at R Adams Cowley Shock Trauma Center [34] has also proposed that associated secondary signs of injury may also be important for consideration—specifically the presence of extensive mediastinal hematoma and large left hemothorax. Despite these reports, there remains a substantial need for collaborative long-term study of these patients to compare the natural history of both untreated injuries and patients treated with TEVAR or open repair. The optimal type of treatment and timing of intervention remain matters of active investigation. Long-term outcomes following TEVAR must also be better elucidated. An ongoing prospective registry sponsored by the Aortic Trauma Foundation and the American Association for the Surgery of Trauma is designed to provide some of these answers in the near future.

The emergent nature of high-grade BTAI treatment requires the application of damage control thought processes to afford optimal outcomes. Immediate assessment of the patient with suspected blunt thoracic aortic injury (BTAI) includes imaging studies if hemodynamics allow. Once the diagnosis is confirmed, aggressive beta-blockade is highly recommended in the absence of contraindications. The decision regarding endovascular versus open repair is made largely on the position of the lesion relative to arch vessels. Traditionally, a proximal landing zone of 2 cm was considered acceptable, although newer devices have been used successfully with a proximal neck length, or "landing zone" of 1 cm or less. Aortic injuries are usually shorter than lesions due to aortic disease, negating the need for extensive coverage of the distal thoracic aorta and the need for a preoperative spinal drain to mitigate the risk of subsequent paralysis associated with extensive coverage of the thoracic aorta with a stent graft.

Fortunately, the most commonly encountered variant of BTAI is located distal to the left subclavian artery, with the lesion typically isolated to the proximal descending thoracic aorta. More extensive injuries to the thoracic aorta that are within proximity to major branch vessels, however, present a more significant clinical challenge. The most common branch vessel requiring coverage to achieve effective seal of the injury site with an endograft is the left subclavian artery (LSCA). Expanding experience has demonstrated, however, that coverage of this vessel by TEVAR can be performed routinely with minimal associated morbidity [23]. Close observation is usually sufficient following LSCA coverage, in the event that symptoms of subclavian steal or arm ischemia develop—a rare occurrence in trauma settings. If, however, these symptoms do manifest, a carotid-subclavian bypass may be required. Despite the excellent toleration of LSCA coverage in trauma settings, it is important to emphasize, however, that there are specific situations where a bypass procedure may be required prior to TEVAR for BTAI. Chief among these is the patient with prior cardiac surgery and the use of the left internal mammary artery for coronary artery bypass. Coverage of the LSCA in these patients invites potential major coronary malperfusion and a high risk of cardiac complications and arrest. It is also useful to determine pre-procedure the patency of the vertebral artery on the left and the role of this vessel in cerebral perfusion. Left vertebral artery dominance compared to the right suggests that coverage of the LSCA may result in cerebral malperfusion when left vertebral artery outflow is compromised. As an adjunct during emergent TEVAR for BTAI, intraoperative neuromonitoring can provide immediate information regarding cerebral flow after coverage of the LSCA. Cerebral angiography may also be performed if needed to gather this information.

Despite the need for further study, the success of TEVAR for BTAI to date has paved the way for collaborative efforts between trauma surgeons and endovascular providers in exploring other anatomical sites where endovascular stent grafts may potentially be of benefit in emergent settings. To determine the current use of endoluminal stent grafts after trauma, a recent study by Branco and colleagues [35] reviewed the recorded rate of endovascular stent graft use among trauma patients from the American College of Surgeons National Trauma Databank. These researchers found that, compared to the 0.3% rate of utilization in 2002, there was a significant increase in endovascular technology utilization for trauma by 2010 (to 9.0%, $p < 0.001$). Of important note, the most dramatic changes in utilization occurred among injured vessels located at sites associated with anatomically challenging open exposures—including iliac and axillo-subclavian locations (Figs. 12.3a, b and 12.4a, b). When outcomes were compared between matched patients who underwent endovascular and open procedures, patients undergoing endovascular procedures had significantly lower in-hospital mortality (12.9% vs. 22.4%, $p < 0.001$) and decreased rates of sep-

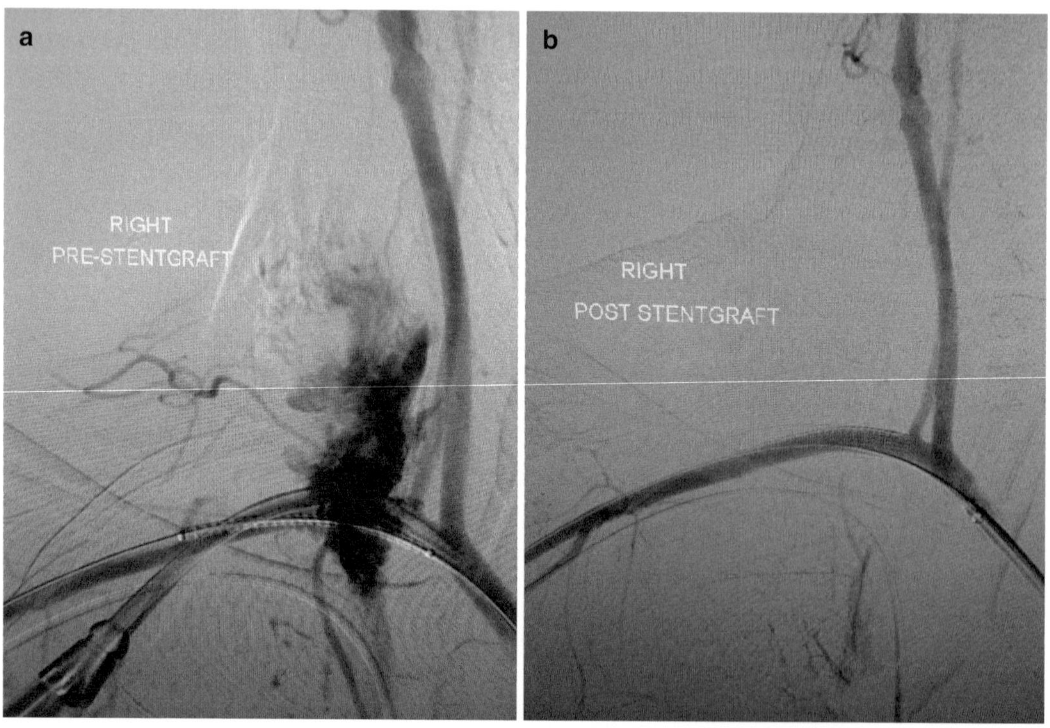

Fig. 12.3 (**a**, **b**) Pre (**a**)- and post (**b**)-repair angiographic images documenting stent graft repair of a left subclavian injury due to penetrating mechanism

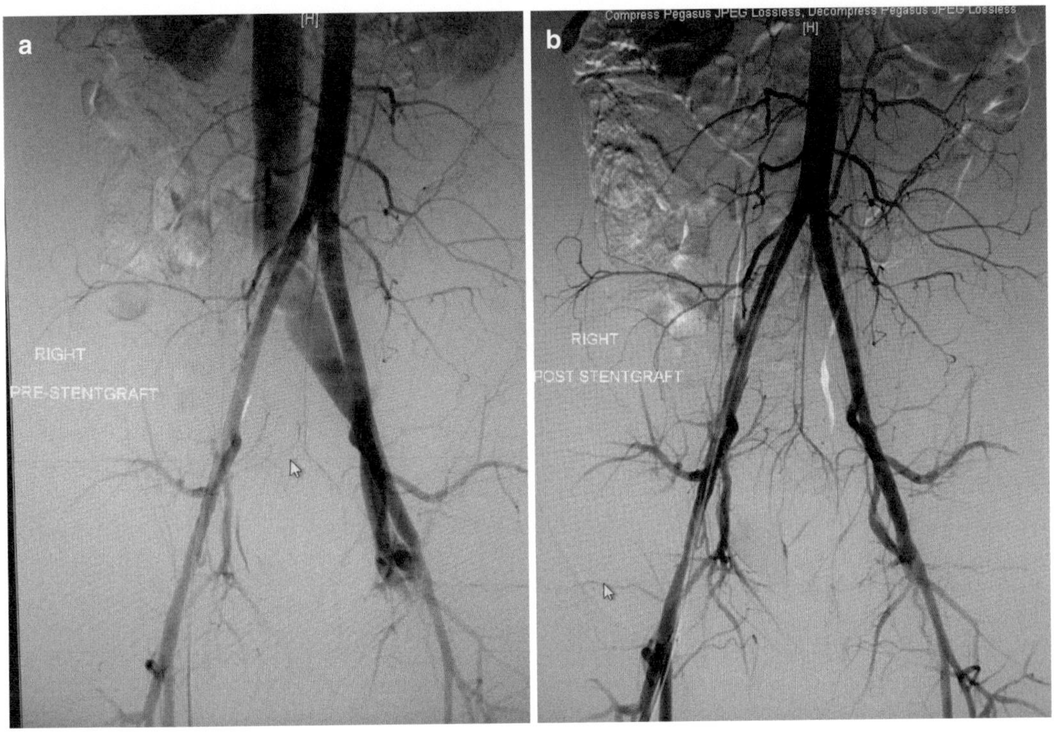

Fig. 12.4 (**a**, **b**) Pre (**a**)- and post (**b**)-repair angiographic images documenting endovascular stent graft coverage of a distal external iliac artery injury from gunshot with associated arteriovenous fistula (filling of iliac vein fistula apparent on image (**a**), absent after stent graft coverage of injury (**b**)

sis after intervention (7.5% vs. 5.4%, $p = 0.025$). Similar investigations have demonstrated findings reflective of increased utilization of endovascular approaches to hemorrhage control and blood vessel injury—associated with improved outcomes over historical controls [36].

Endovascular stent placement for intra-abdominal arteries may also be considered an important damage control adjunct in specific scenarios. Endograft repair of blunt abdominal aortic injury, although a rare entity, represents a repair alternative that does not mandate the exposure traditionally required for open repair. Particularly in the setting of associated bowel injury and contamination, the use of endoluminal endograft repair of the abdominal aorta and other visceral vessels may mitigate the risk of infection of traditional open repair conduit sites. The literature on this topic is not extensive at present, however, with most of the available reports limited to case reports and small case series where endovascular stents, aortic extension cuffs, or aortic endograft limb extensions have been used in cases of blunt and penetrating trauma [37, 38]. Indications for the use of such modalities might include not only cases with associated gross contamination from hollow viscus injury that can jeopardize aortic grafts due to risk of infection but also the initial management of injuries difficult to expose by open exploration due to prior operation or other operative challenges. In this fashion, endovascular interventions can be used as a stabilizing measure for these critically ill patients and a bridge to possible subsequent open definitive repair.

In the abdominal aorta, major injuries near the visceral and renal branch vessels have not traditionally been amenable to easy or rapid endograft placement (Fig. 12.5). Continued endovascular technologic advancements including fenestrated or branched grafts are presently only used in the United States in the context of trials for elective aortic surgery. These adjuncts have, however, been utilized with some success in other

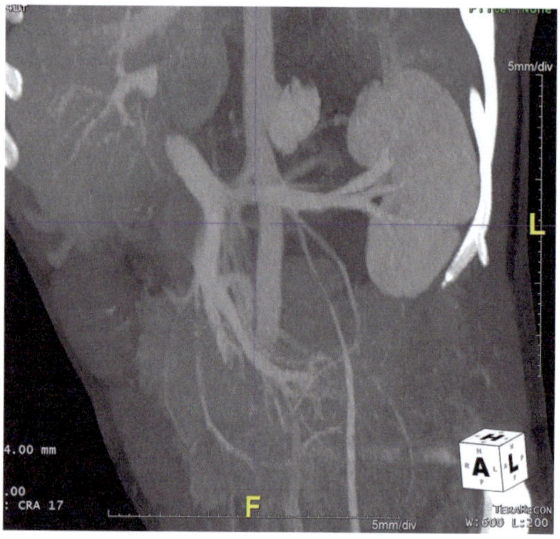

Fig. 12.5 Computed tomographic reconstruction of a gunshot wound to the abdominal aorta. Proximal vascular occlusion balloon was utilized to control the injury prior to open repair

countries. In the near future, newer devices may be available for off-label use for the injured aorta or abdominal branch vessels. Additionally, the chimney technique, in which the branch vessels are stented along with the aorta, may be an option for select patients. This latter technique is time-consuming, however, and requires significant expertise [38].

12.3 Resuscitative Endovascular Balloon Occlusion of the Aorta (REBOA)

Resuscitative endovascular balloon occlusion of the aorta (REBOA) is a new and exciting adjunct to the management of patients in profound shock (Fig. 12.6). Technically the principle of REBOA is not novel, as the use of an intra-aortic occlusive balloon placed through an open approach was first described for controlling major hemorrhage in the Korean War [39]. Reports in the literature of use for control of bleeding during pelvic surgery, hepatobiliary surgery, orthopedic surgery, postpartum hemorrhage, and repair of ruptured abdominal aortic aneurysm suggest that REBOA has the potential to be a life-saving measure after significant hemorrhage from a variety of causes.

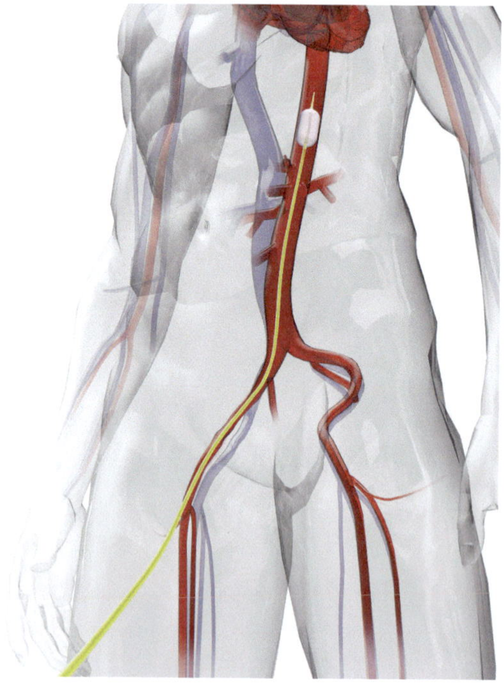

Fig. 12.6 An artist rendition of resuscitative endovascular occlusion of the aorta (REBOA) balloon placement in aortic zone 1 (descending thoracic aorta)

A growing body of translational literature also appears to support the potential of REBOA following hemorrhage, with physiologic parameters such as serum lactate, pH, pCO2, and central, cerebral, and coronary perfusion in animal models of hemorrhagic shock having been shown to improve with REBOA utilization [40].

The use of REBOA to obtain proximal aortic control at the level of the diaphragm prior to entering the abdomen may have a role in early control of intra-abdominal hemorrhage after trauma. Currently, indications for REBOA include persistent, refractory hypotension due to hemorrhage below the diaphragm, including severe pelvic and/or junctional hemorrhage. For patients arriving in arrest from blunt mechanisms without evidence of severe great vessel injury, thoracotomy with open cardiac massage has been largely replaced by REBOA with closed chest compression at several leading trauma centers [41]. The location of balloon placement and inflation is determined by source of hemorrhage. Placement can be performed in the resuscitation area using portable or

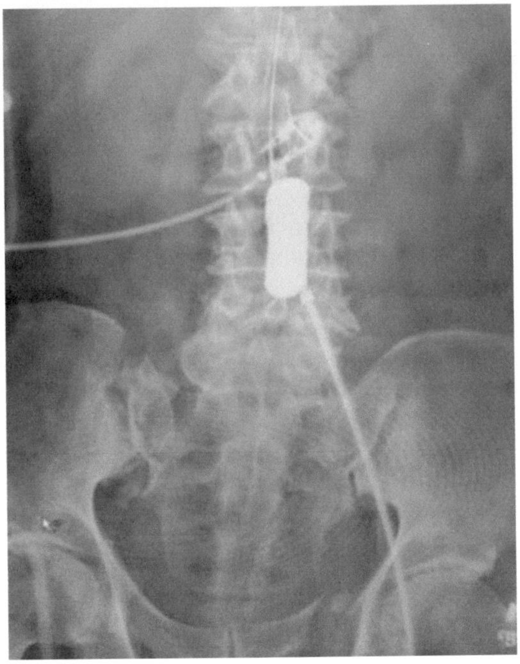

Fig. 12.7 REBOA balloon inflated in aortic zone 3 (infrarenal aorta)

digital x-ray. Transportation to definitive treatment can occur with the REBOA in place.

The duration of aortic occlusion varies considerably due to patient physiology, availability of resources, and time to definitive hemostasis. Recent evidence suggests that patients may survive zone 1 occlusion (just above the level of the diaphragm, between the left subclavian and celiac arteries) for up to 150 min [42], while anecdotal experience suggests patients can tolerate zone 3 occlusion (Fig. 12.7) (between the lowest renal artery and aortic bifurcation) for several hours without complication. While no consensus on optimal occlusion times yet exists, most providers experienced with REBOA utilization recommend minimizing occlusion times to the bare minimum required to reach expedient definitive hemorrhage control. The authors suggest that zone 1 occlusion times of less than 30 min and zone 3 of less than 60 min should be aggressively pursued until better evidence on the topic can be collected, with the overall being to deflate and remove the devices as rapidly as possible. To facilitate the shortest possible occlusion time, an emphasis on moving the patient after REBOA expediently to an environment where definitive hemorrhage control can be achieved—either the operating room or the interventional suite—is required.

For those patients who may experience delays to definitive hemorrhage control, regardless of the reason, two specific approaches for extending effective utilization of the of REBOA have been proposed. The first is intermittent occlusion, or temporarily deflating the REBOA balloon to provide intermittent momentary perfusion of distal tissue beds until definitive hemorrhage control can be achieved. This technique has been described as a potential means for extending the duration of aortic occlusion with REBOA in Japan [42, 43]. This practice may, however, create hemodynamic shifts resulting from rapid washout of ischemic metabolites during short periods of perfusion that undermine the body's autoregulatory mechanisms and may be detrimental to patient survival. Vasodilated ischemic tissue beds create a low-resistance, high-capacitance system that results in a profound loss of aortic afterload and cardiac output when occlusion is lifted—only to be immediately reversed again when occlusion is reapplied. Animal studies have demonstrated that this approach does not reduce ischemic injury or improve survival compared to complete occlusion of the same duration [43].

As an alternative approach to providing distal perfusion, early partial aortic occlusion has been studied in animal models and is starting to be described in human trauma patients [41, 43–46]. After control of major hemorrhage has been achieved (i.e., tourniquets applied, abdomen packed, chest opened), slow reintroduction of systemic circulation is begun as hemodynamically tolerated [47]. Low volume distal blood flow is maintained until definitive hemorrhage control has been completed and the patient is hemodynamically stable enough to tolerate full reintroduction of distal blood flow. In the setting of REBOA use, partial occlusion requires a dedicated provider to monitor the patient's vital signs and titrate aortic occlusion accordingly. The transition from complete endovascular aortic occlusion to partial REBOA requires additional attention to maintain proper balloon positioning as the loss of frictional forces between the aortic wall and the deflating balloon, combined with increased proximal blood pressure, can lead to catheter migration or prolapse [41]. Partial REBOA has been demonstrated in animal models to reduce the effects of distal ischemia and proximal overpressure injury compared to complete REBOA [46, 48], but its application in human patients is only just beginning [41, 44].

Beyond concerted efforts to limit aortic occlusion time, REBOA utilization also requires significant vigilance for other complications specific to the conduct of the procedure. Chief among these may be access-related complications resulting in distal limb ischemia. A Japanese series published by Saito et al. reported on REBOA use in 24 blunt injury patients treated at a single center [49]. This report demonstrated that AO could effectively increase mean systolic blood pressure in patients with hemoperitoneum and pelvic ring fracture, but the authors also highlighted that 12.5% (3 of 14) of patients in their series required amputations due to ischemic limb complications after access. Among these three, two amputations were directly associated with severe extremity or pelvic injury, and one was the result of an iatrogenic vascular injury complication occurring following multiple percutaneous access attempts in an obese patient. Importantly, the largest prospective series recording REBOA utilization in the United States has not demonstrated any ischemic complications resulting in amputation in North America to date [50].

Over the past several years, REBOA has increasingly been discussed as a potential adjunct to damage control and trauma resuscitation. Brenner and colleagues [51] published the first clinical series of REBOA utilization in the United States following trauma in 2013, demonstrating successful utilization following both blunt and penetrating mechanisms of injury. More recent reports of the use of REBOA demonstrate its potential benefit. Two institutions at the forefront of clinical use demonstrated a survival benefit for patients undergoing REBOA ($n = 24$) compared to emergency department thoracotomy (EDT) ($n = 72$) ($p = 0.003$) [52]. Furthermore, death from hemorrhage occurred more frequently in the resuscitation area in EDT patients than REBOA patients (69.2% vs. 29.7%, $p < 0.001$), and there were no ICU deaths from hemorrhage in patients who received a REBOA. The timeline of the study also showed a paradigm shift away from EDT and toward REBOA in select patients. The most recent multi-institutional report from the AAST AORTA trial also shows some promising results [50]. The initial report from this ongoing prospective registry documented 46 patients who underwent REBOA and compared their outcomes to 68 patients who received EDT with aortic cross-clamp. There was no difference in survival or in aortic occlusion time between the two groups. The initial AAST report did demonstrate, however, that the establishment of appropriate arterial access continues to require open cutdown with common femoral artery exposure in 50%. Despite the need for this more invasive access approach, however, only minor access complications of REBOA occurred, and all three were treated at the time of operative intervention for sheath removal [50].

The potential use of REBOA as a prehospital damage control adjunct has also been discussed, and this practice is already occurring in the United Kingdom and Japan. Emergency medicine physicians and medics are preforming the procedure at the roadside for patients in extremis from non-compressible torso hemorrhage. As a matter of fact, emergency medicine physicians have been performing REBOA in trauma patients for over a decade in Japanese emergency departments. Both Japan and the United Kingdom have access to smaller-diameter REBOA devices, which may improve the safety profile and expand the spectrum of users. In the United States, FDA-approved devices were traditionally not well suited for the trauma population. Over the last year, however, a lower-profile device has been approved by the FDA for trauma use (ER-REBOA™, Prytime Inc.). To date experience with this device has been encouraging but has only yielded anecdotal technical and/or clinical success.

As REBOA continues to be utilized and evaluated, clinical algorithms will mature and further specify which patients are most likely to benefit from the procedure. Currently, patients suffering from both blunt and penetrating mechanisms are suitable candidates for REBOA, and this procedure can be performed in the resuscitation area, operating room, in conjunction with thoracotomy and cardiac massage, and/or prior to further imaging and/or angioembolization.

A growing body of translational research regarding REBOA use suggests that the use of this adjunct may result in improved physiology compared to EDT. Clinical research is also growing but at present demonstrates that survival and outcomes may or may not be affected relative to emergency thoracotomy. This data has demonstrated to date, however, that major complications documented abroad have not occurred with its use in select US and Canadian centers. In addition, ongoing standardization of training efforts for acute care surgeons suggests that this subset of providers can learn this procedure after a brief but formal training course and apply this skillset safely and effectively in the clinical setting [53].

Conclusion

Endovascular technologies offer exciting new options for inclusion in damage control approaches after trauma. There do, however, remain questions about optimal patient selection, ideal technique, and long-term outcomes regarding these modalities. Ongoing research promises to better elucidate the optimal utilization of endovascular adjuncts for bleeding trauma patients in the context of damage control interventions.

References

1. Reuben BC, Whitten MG, Sarfati M, Kraiss LW. Increasing use of endovascular therapy in acute arterial injuries: analysis of the National Trauma Data Bank. J Vasc Surg. 2007;46(6):1222.
2. Avery LE, Stahfield KR, Corcos AC, Scifres AM, Ziembicki JA, Varcelotti J, Peitzman AB, Billiar TR, Sperry JL. Evolving role of endovascular techniques for traumatic vascular injury: a changing landscape. J Trauma Acute Care Surg. 2012;72(1):41–6.
3. Gerlock AJ. Hemorrhage following pelvic fracture controlled by embolization: case report. J Trauma. 1975;15(8):740–2.
4. Chuang VP, Reuter SR, Walter J, Foley WD, Bookstein JJ. Control of renal hemorrhage by selective arterial embolization. Am J Roentgenol Radium Therapy, Nucl Med. 1975;125(2):300–6.
5. Barbaric ZL, Luka NL. Angiographic demonstration and transcatheter embolic control of posttraumatic intercostal arterial hemorrhage. Surgery. 1977;81(4):409–12.
6. Ayella RJ, DuPriest RW Jr, Khaneja SC, Maekawa K, Soderstrom CA, Rodriguez A, Cowley RA. Transcatheter embolization of autologous clot in the management of bleeding associated with fractures of the pelvis. Surg Gynecol Obstet. 1978;147(6):849–52.
7. Maull KI, Sachatello CR. Current management of pelvic fractures: a combined surgical-angiographic approach to hemorrhage. South Med J. 1976;69(10):1285–9.
8. van Urk H, Perlberger RR, Muller H. Selective arterial embolization for control of traumatic pelvic hemorrhage. Surgery. 1978;83(2):133–7.
9. Panetta T, Sclafani SJ, Goldstein AS, Phillips TF, Shaftan GW. Percutaneous transcatheter embolization for massive bleeding from pelvic fractures. J Trauma. 1985;25(11):1021–9.
10. Sclafani SJ, Weisberg A, Scalea TM, Phillips TF, Duncan AO. Blunt splenic injuries: nonsurgical treatment with CT, arteriography, and transcatheter arterial embolization of the splenic artery. Radiology. 1991;181(1):189–96.
11. Sclafani SJ, Shaftan GW, Scalea TM, Patterson LA, Kohl L, Kantor A, Herskowitz MM, Hoffer EK, Henry S, Dresner LS, et al. Nonoperative salvage of computed tomography-diagnosed splenic injuries: utilization of angiography for triage and embolization for hemostasis. J Trauma. 1995;39(5):818–25; discussion 826–7.
12. Roudsari BS, Psoter K, Padia SA, Kogut MJ, Kwan SW. Utilization of angiography and embolization for abdominopelvic trauma: 14 years' experience at level 1 trauma center. AJR. 2014;202:W580–5.
13. Ierardi AM, Piacentino F, Fontana F, Petrillo M, Floridi C, Bacuzzi A, Cuffari S, Elabbassi W, Novario R, Carrafiello G. The role of endovascular treatment of pelvic bleeding in emergency settings. Eur Radiol. 2015;25(7):1854–64.
14. Niola R, Pinto A, Sparano A, Ignarra R, Romano L, Maglione F. Arterial bleeding in pelvic trauma: priorities in angiographic embolization. Curr Probl Diagn Radiol. 2012;41(3):93–101.
15. Velmahos GC, Toutouzas KG, Vassiliu P, Sarkisvan G, Chan LS, Hanks SH, Berne TV, Demetriades D. A prospective study on the safety and efficacy of angiographic embolization for pelvic and visceral injuries. J Trauma. 2002;53(2):303–8;discussion 308.
16. Misselbeck TS, Teicher EJ, Cippolle MD, Pasquale MD, Shah KT, Dangleben DA, Badelling MM. Hepatic angioembolization in trauma patients: indications and complications. J Trauma. 2009;67(4):769–73.

17. Ierardi AM, Duka E, Lucchina N, Floridi C, De Martino A, Donat D, Fontana F, Carrafiello G. The role of interventional radiology in abdominopelvic trauma. Br J Radiol. 2016;5:20150866. [Epub ahead of print].
18. Zarzaur BL, Kozar R, Myers JG, Claridge JA, Scalea TM, Neideen TA, Maung AA, Alarcon L, Corcos A, Kerwin A, Coimbra R. The splenic injury outcomes trial: an American Association for the Surgery of Trauma multi-institutional study. J Trauma Acute Care Surg. 2015;79(3):335–42. Ogura T1, Lefor AT, Nakano M, Izawa Y, Morita H. Nonoperative management of hemodynamically unstable abdominal trauma patients with angioembolization and resuscitative endovascular balloon occlusion of the aorta. J Trauma Acute Care Surg. 2015 Jan;78(1):132-5.
19. Schwartz DA, Medina M, Cotton BA, Rahbar E, Wade CE, Cohen AM, Beeler AM, Burgess AR, Holcomb JB. Are we delivering two standards of care for pelvic trauma? Availability of angioembolization after hours and on weekends increases time to therapeutic intervention. J Trauma Acute Care Surg. 2014;76(1):134–9.
20. Brenner M, Hoehn M, Teeter W, Stein D, Scalea T. Trading scalpels for sheaths: catheter-based treatment of vascular injury can be effectively performed by acute care surgeons trained in endovascular techniques. J Trauma Acute Care Surg. 2016;80(5):783–6.
21. Holcomb JB, Fox EE, Scalea TM, Napolitano LM, Albarado R, Gill B, Dunkin BJ, Kirkpatrick AW, Cotton BA, Inaba K, DuBose JJ, Cohen AA, Azizzadeh A, Brenner M, Cohen MJ, Wade CE, Lumsden AB, Andrassy R, Rhee PM, Bass BL, Mattox KL, Britt LD, Eastman AB, Hoyt DB, Rasmussen TE. Current opinion on catheter-based hemorrhage control in trauma patients. J Trauma Acute Care Surg. 2014;76:888–93.
22. Demetriades D, Velmahos G, Scalea T, et al. Operative repair or endovascular stent/graft in blunt traumatic thoracic aortic injuries: results of an AAST multicenter study. J Trauma. 2008;64:561–70.
23. DuBose JJ, Leake SS, Brenner M, Pasley J, O'Callaghan T, Luo-Owen X, Trust MD, Mooney J, Zhao FZ, Azizzadeh A, Aortic Trauma Foundation. Contemporary management and outcomes of blunt thoracic aortic injury: a multicenter retrospective study. J Trauma Acute Care Surg. 2015;78(2):360–9.
24. Mattox KL, Wall MJ. Historical review of blunt injury to the thoracic aorta. Chest Surg Clin N Am. 2000;10:167–82.
25. Fabian TC, Richardson JD, Groce MA, et al. Prospective study of blunt aortic injury: multicenter trial of the American Association for the Surgery of Trauma. J Trauma. 1997;42:374–80.
26. Demetriades D, Velmahos GC, Scalea TM, et al. Diagnosis and treatment of blunt thoracic aortic injuries: changing perspectives. J Trauma. 2008;64:1415–9.
27. Arthurs ZM, Starnes BW, Sohn VY, Singh N, Martin MJ, Andersen CA. Functional and survival outcomes in traumatic blunt thoracic aortic injuries: an analysis of the National Trauma Databank. J Vasc Surg. 2009;49:988–94.
28. Lee WA, Matsumura J, Mitchell RS, et al. Endovascular repair of traumatic thoracic aortic injury: clinical practice guidelines of the Society for Vascular Surgery. J Vasc Surg. 2011;53:187–92.
29. Piffaretti G, Benedetto F, Menegolo M, et al. Outcomes of endovascular repair for blunt thoracic aortic injury. J Vasc Surg. 2013;58:1483–9.
30. Khoynezhad A, Azizzadeh A, Donayre CE, Matsumoto A, Velazquez O, White R. RESCUE investigators. Results of a multicenter, prospective trial of thoracic endovascular aortic repair for blunt thoracic aortic injury (RESCUE trial). J Vasc Surg. 2013;57(4):899–905.
31. Azizzadeh A, Ray HM, Dubose JJ, Charlton-Ouw KM, Miller CC, Coogan SM, Safi HJ, Estrera AL. Outcomes of endovascular repair for patients with blunt traumatic aortic injury. J Trauma Acute Care Surg. 2014;76(2):510–6.3.
32. Lamarche Y, Berger FH, Nicolaou S, Bilawich AM, Louis L, Inacio JR, Janusz MT, Evans D. Vancouver simplified grading system with computed tomographic angiography for blunt aortic injury. J Thorac Cardiovasc Surg. 2012;144(2):347–54, 354.e1.
33. Starnes BW, Lundgren RS, Gunn M, Quade S, Hatsukami TS, Tran NT, Mokadam N, Aldea G. A new classification scheme for treating blunt aortic injury. J Vasc Surg. 2012;55(1):47–54.
34. Rabin J, DuBose J, Sliker CW, O'Connor JV, Scalea TM, Griffith BP. Parameters for successful non operative management of traumatic aortic injury. J Thorac Cardiovasc Surg. 2014;147(1):143–9.
35. Branco BC, DuBose JJ, Zhan LX, Hughes JD, Goshima KR, Rhee P, Mills JL Sr. Trends and outcomes of endovascular therapy in the management of civilian vascular injuries. J Vasc Surg. 2014;60(5):1297–307.
36. Branco BC, Boutrous ML, DuBose JJ, Leake SS, Charlton-Ouw K, Rhee P, Mills JL, Azizzadeh A. Outcome comparison between open and endovascular management of axillosubclavian arterial injuries. J Vasc Surg. 2016;63(3):702–9.
37. Shalhub S, Starnes BW, Tran NT, Hatsukami TS, Lundgren RS, Davis CW, Quade S, Gunn M. Blunt abdominal aortic injury. J Vasc Surg. 2012;55(5):1277–85.
38. Willis M, Neschis D, Menaker J, Lilly M, Scalea T. Stent grafting for a distal thoracic aortic injury. Vasc Endovasc Surg. 2011;45(2):187–90.
39. Hughes C. Use of intra-aortic balloon catheter tamponade for controlling intra-abdominal hemorrhage in man. Surgery. 1954;36(1):65–8.
40. White JM, Cannon JW, Stannard A, Markov NP, Spencer JR, Rasmussen TE. Endovascular balloon

occlusion of the aorta is superior to resuscitative thoracotomy with aortic clamping in a porcine model of hemorrhagic shock. Surgery. Mosby, Inc. 2011;150(3):400–9.

41. Ho rer TM, Cajander P, Jans A, Nilsson KF. A case of partial aortic balloon occlusion in an unstable multi-trauma patient. Trauma. 2016;18(2):150–4.
42. Ogura T, Lefor A, Nakano M, Izawa Y, Morita H. Nonoperative management of hemodynamically unstable abdominal trauma patients with angioembolization and resuscitative endovascular occlusion of the aorta. J Trauma Acute Care Surg. 2015;78(1):132–5.
43. Morrison JJ, Ross JD, Rt H, Watson JD, Sokol KK, Rasmussen TE. Use of resuscitative endovascular balloon occlusion of the aorta in a highly lethal model of noncompressible torso hemorrhage. Shock. 2014;41(2):130–7.
44. Davidson AJ, Russo RM, DuBose JJ, Roberts J, Jurkovich GJ, Galante JM. Potential benefit of early operative utilization of low profile, partial resuscitative endovascular balloon occlusion of the aorta (P-REBOA) in major traumatic hemorrhage. Trauma Surgery & Acute Care Open. 2016;1(1):1–3.
45. Okumura E, Tsurukiri J, Oomura T, Tanaka Y, Oomura R. Partial resuscitative endovascular balloon occlusion of the aorta as a hemorrhagic shock adjunct for ectopic pregnancy. Am J Emerg Med. 2016;34(9):1917.e1–2.
46. Russo RM, Neff LP, Lamb CM, Cannon JW, Galante JM, Clement NF, et al. Partial resuscitative endovascular balloon occlusion of the aorta in swine model of hemorrhagic shock. J Am Coll Surg. 2016;223(2):359–68.
47. Johnson MA, Neff LP, Williams TK, DuBose JJ, Group ES. Partial resuscitative balloon occlusion of the AORTA (P-REBOA): clinical technique and rationale. J Trauma Acute Care Surg. 2016;81(5 Suppl 2):S133–7.
48. Russo RM, Williams TK, Grayson JK, Lamb CM, Cannon JW, Clement NF, et al. Extending the golden hour: partial resuscitative endovascular balloon occlusion of the aorta in a highly lethal swine liver injury model. J Trauma Acute Care Surg. 2016;80(3):372–80.
49. Saito N, Matsumoto H, Yagi T, Hara Y, Hayashida K, Motomura T, Mashiko K, Iida H, Yokota H, Wagatsuma Y. Evaluation of the safety and feasibility of resuscitative endovascular balloon occlusion of the aorta. J Trauma Acute Care Surg. 2015;78(5):897–903; discussion 904.
50. Du Bose JJ, Scalea T, Brenner M, Skiada D, Inaba K, Cannon J, Moore L, Holcomb J, Turay D, Luo-Owen X, Kirkpatrick A, Xiao J, Skarupa D, Poulin N, AAST AORTA Study Group. The AAST prospective aortic occlusion for resuscitation in trauma and acute Care Surgery (AORTA) registry: contemporary utilization and outcomes of aortic occlusion and REBOA. J Trauma Acute Care Surg. 2016;81(3):409–19.
51. Brenner ML, Moore LJ, DuBose JJ, Tyson GH, McNutt MK, Albarado RP, Holcomb JB, Scalea TM, Rasmussen TE. A clinical series of resuscitative endovascular balloon occlusion of the aorta for hemorrhage control and resuscitation. J Trauma Acute Care Surg. 2013;75(3):506–11.
52. Moore LJ, Brenner M, Kozar RA, Pasley J, Wade CE, Baraniuk MS, Scalea T, Holcomb JB. Implementation of resuscitative endovascular balloon occlusion of the aorta as an alternative to resuscitative thoracotomy for noncompressible truncal hemorrhage. J Trauma Acute Care Surg. 2015;79(4):523–30; discussion 530–2.
53. Brenner M, Hoehn M, Pasley J, Dubose J, Stein D, Scalea T. Basic endovascular skills for trauma course: bridging the gap between endovascular techniques and the acute care surgeon. J Trauma Acute Care Surg. 2014;77(2):286–91.

13 Damage Control Cardiothoracic Surgery

J. Shaw, Bradley J. Phillips, and Juan A. Asensio

13.1 Introduction

Although damage control as a surgical concept and/or technique has become part of the trauma surgeon's armamentarium for the past 25 years, it is meritorious to review its origins and indications. The concept, as described, takes its origin from Stone's [1] hallmark work describing the "bailout" approach in honor of World War II paratroopers. In his 1986 seminal paper [1], he recognized a physiological "cluster" of intraoperative signs, i.e., coagulopathy, prompting interruption of trauma surgical procedures after institution of hemorrhage containing measures and packing of the abdominal cavity. He then proposed returning patients to a critical care setting and correcting the coagulopathy of trauma to return to the operating room later for definitive surgery.

This "bailout" approach ushered the area of staged surgical procedures for trauma. With this approach Stone [1] reported a 65% versus 7% survival rate in favor of patients packed versus those undergoing definitive surgical procedures.

Subsequently Burch [2] in 1992 described the abbreviated laparotomy with planned reoperation for critically ill patients, later to be described as "damage control" by Rotondo [3] in 1993. In Rotondo's [3] study consisting of 46 patients, the authors identified a maximum injury subset of 22 patients, of which 9 underwent definitive laparotomy (DL) and 13 damage control laparotomy (DL). In this group of patients, survival rate for the damage control group was 77% versus an 11% survival rate for the definitive laparotomy (DL) group. This paper [3], based on a small number of patients, provided no statistical analysis; however, it did outline a methodology for the management of critically injured trauma patients.

In reality, damage control as a methodology emerged to deal with exsanguination, an ill-defined, easily recognized, feared entity, but not foreign to trauma surgeons. Initial attempts by Anderson [4] to define this syndrome: "Patients losing their entire blood volume" and Trunkey

J. Shaw, B.A., M.S.
Department of Surgery, Creighton University School of Medicine, Omaha, NE, USA

Department of Clinical and Translational Research, Creighton University, Omaha, NE, USA

B.J. Phillips, M.D., F.A.C.S.
Department of Surgery, Creighton University School of Medicine, Omaha, NE, USA

J.A. Asensio, F.A.C.S., F.C.C.M., F.R.C.S., (England) K.M. (✉)
Department of Surgery, Creighton University School of Medicine, Omaha, NE, USA

Department of Clinical and Translational Research, Creighton University, Omaha, NE, USA

F. Edward Hébert School of Medicine, Walter Reed National Military Medical Center, Bethesda, MD, USA
e-mail: JuanAsensio@creighton.edu

J. Duchesne et al. (eds.), *Damage Control in Trauma Care*,
https://doi.org/10.1007/978-3-319-72607-6_13

[5] who described it within the context of flow, defining outcomes for patients with severe hemorrhage and rates of blood loss exceeding 250 mL per minute launched the initial attempts at rethinking and redefining this syndrome by Asensio and Ierardi [6–8] whom described it as: "Exsanguination is the most extreme form of hemorrhage. It is usually caused by injuries to major components of the cardiovascular system, injuries to parenchymatous organs or both. It is a hemorrhage in which there is an initial loss of 40% of the patient's blood volume with an ongoing rate of blood loss, exceeding 150 mls per minute. If this hemorrhage is not controlled, the patient may lose over half of his or her entire blood volume within 10 minutes." Subsequently, Moore [9] described the "bloody vicious cycle" of acidosis hypothermia and coagulopathy, while Cosgriff [10] postulated that the ability to predict the onset of coagulopathy, perhaps the most important of the components of the "bloody vicious cycle," would impact significantly decision-making with regard to the institution of "damage control."

Asensio and colleagues [11] based on 548 patients classified as sustaining exsanguination described and statically validated by univariate and logistic regression reliable variables indicating damage control and predicting outcomes in a patient population, with very low revised trauma scores (RTS) and very high injury severity scores (ISS) consisting of thoracic, abdominal, and multiple injuries admitted in profound shock with a mean pH of 7.15 and a mean estimated blood loss of 7.3 L. Subsequently, dysthymias were added to the bloody vicious cycle and described as the "lethal tetrad" [11–14]. Although the variables and indications described by Asensio and colleagues [11] for the institution of "bailout/damage control" have been adopted and validated, yet no specific study has applied them solely for the management of cardiothoracic injuries.

Application of "bailout [1]/damage control [3]" is now considered routine for severe abdominal trauma. It is recently that this strategy has begun to find its place in the management of cardiothoracic trauma. The general principles and goals of damage control are similar to those employed for the management of abdominal trauma. Expeditious operative management of unstable patients remains the primary focus.

Severe thoracic injuries are frequently and rapidly lethal; however, there is considerably less room for the institution of staged procedures for the management of cardiac, pulmonary, or thoracic vascular injuries which demand definitive repair if the patient is to survive. Although there is limited data available on the use of damage control in cardiothoracic injuries, patients with severe thoracic trauma and subsequent physiological derangement can benefit from its implementation [15].

Several factors have limited the use of damage control in cardiothoracic surgery. First, there are valid concerns that thoracic packing may compromise cardiac filling and, thus, right and left ventricular ejection fractions, as well as restricting pulmonary expansion. It should be noted that there is a paucity of literature on this topic and most of the available literature is limited to the opinions of individual trauma surgeons. Second, a clear definition of damage control as it applies to thoracic surgery is unfortunately lacking. Abbreviated thoracotomy as a damage control technique entails rapid hemorrhage control requiring a planned return to the operating room. Additionally, some authors [15–18] include emergency department thoracotomy (EDT) as a damage control procedure, while others excluded it. Finally, the available literature describes the treatment of anatomic injuries in sufficient detail but lacks crucial physiological data and outcomes [15–18].

There are both differences and similarities in the application of "damage control" to abdominal and cardiothoracic surgeries. However, the decision to perform damage control is the same regardless of anatomic location [11, 15]. In both instances, acidosis, hypothermia, and coagulopathy are individual and valid predictors of mortality. Therefore, the severely injured patient presenting with the "lethal tetrad" should prompt the trauma surgeon to rapidly institute damage control techniques. Exsanguinating hemorrhage and physiological derangements are considered the most important selection criteria. Finally, postoperative management of the abnormal patient's physiology in the intensive care unit (ICU) is approached in a similar fashion [11, 12].

For the most part, divergence of their similarities lies in the inherent anatomic differences between cardiothoracic and abdominal surgeries. One of the most important concerns during the institution in abdominal damage control is contamination from the gastrointestinal (GI) tract due to the original injury and/or the procedures required to manage these injuries. This complication is of lesser concern in cardiothoracic damage control given that thoracic esophageal injuries are rare, thus decreasing the risk of cavitary contamination. Another important difference, meritorious to note, is that virtually all abdominal and retroperitoneal injuries are accessed via a single incision laparotomy, whereas there is a broader armamentarium of incisions required to manage cardiothoracic injuries; as the thoracic cavity is compartmentalized, thus damage control largely depends on the anatomic location of injury.

Left anterolateral thoracotomy allows rapid access to the left hemithoracic, pericardium, heart, and thoracic aorta, whereas median sternotomy provides optimal exposure to the heart and mediastinum. Extension of this incision as bilateral anterolateral thoracotomies or "clamshell thoracotomy" has also been used. Regardless of the approach, it cannot be overemphasized that the incision must provide adequate exposure of all injuries [19].

The patient most likely to require damage control for thoracic injury is the unstable patient with penetrating thoracic injuries [20]. The most common mechanisms of penetrating injury are gunshot wounds (GSWs), stab wounds (SWs), and uncommonly shotgun wounds (STWs), while motor vehicle collisions comprise the majority of blunt thoracic trauma, very rarely warranting damage control. Additional patient characteristics that predict the need to institute damage control are not unique to thoracic trauma.

13.2 Cardiothoracic Damage Control in the Trauma Center

All damage control for trauma patients begins in the trauma center. Addressing the "ABCs" of cardiothoracic trauma differs slightly from nonthoracic trauma in that both resuscitative and diagnostic techniques are performed simultaneously. Following Advanced Trauma Life Support (ATLS) principles, a definitive airway and large bore IV access for resuscitative fluids should be established. Emergency release blood should be readily available, and a blood sample should be sent promptly for typing. Activation of the massive transfusion protocol (MPT) is often required. Thoracostomy tubes can be placed for both therapeutic and diagnostic purposes along the midaxillary line at the level of the fifth intercostal space. An initial assessment of the wound should be attempted by either physical examination or radiographic imaging. Thoracostomy tube output, FAST in both pericardial and pleural views, as well as chest radiographs (CXR) should be sufficient to establish the diagnosis of injuries requiring immediate surgical intervention.

Emergency department thoracotomy (EDT) is performed under strict indications to both resuscitate and control hemorrhage as well as to repair cardiac injuries until they can be transported to the operating room. EDT also functions as a triage instrument, by ensuring that patients with lethal injuries are not routinely transported to the OR. The indications for EDT have long been a subject of intense debate. In general, the decision to perform this procedure is dictated by the presence or absence of signs of life and mechanism of injury. Survival rates following EDT in thoracic trauma are highest for patients sustaining penetrating injuries and presence signs of life either in the field or upon arrival at the trauma center.

Patients requiring EDT for blunt thoracic trauma have extremely low survival rates. Therefore, EDT in these patients is generally not indicated unless very specific criteria are met [19, 21].

The primary goals of EDT are the same in damage control: release of pericardial tamponade, control of intrathoracic hemorrhage and sources of air embolism, as well as to perform open cardiopulmonary resuscitation and cross-clamping of the descending aorta. This maneuver redistributes the remaining blood volume to perfuse both carotid and coronary arteries [19, 21, 22].

The procedure begins with a left anterolateral thoracotomy (see Figs. 13.1 and 13.2). An incision is made below the nipple in the fifth intercostal space starting at the left fifth costochondral junction in a slightly curved fashion and extends to the anterior border of the latissimus dorsi. In females, the left breast is displaced cephalad. The skin, subcutaneous tissues, and chest wall musculature are rapidly transected with a scalpel. A small incision is made through the intercostal muscles, followed by complete transection of the three layers of the intercostal musculature with Metzenbaum thoracic scissors. If extension is required for better visualization, the sternum can be divided with Bethune shears or a Lebsche knife. A Finochietto rib retractor is then placed and positioned with the handle toward the table. Upon entrance into the thoracic cavity, the trauma surgeon should note whether the blood is arterial or venous. Clots must be rapidly removed, and the pericardium must be assessed for the presence of tamponade. The lung is retracted anteromedially by placing the left hand posterior and lateral to the lung with the palm against the parenchyma. If the inflated lung significantly impairs visualization, the lung can be momentarily deflated by temporarily holding ventilation. Using Metzenbaum scissors, the mediastinal pleura is then divided immediately anterior to the aorta, avoiding injury to the esophagus. Prior placement of a nasogastric tube provides a useful landmark. The trauma surgeon then digitally develops a space between the esophagus and aorta. Subsequently, a Crafoord-DeBakey aortic clamp is placed (see Figs. 13.3, 13.4, and 13.5). If present, pericardial tamponade is released by opening the pericardium anterior to the phrenic nerve initially with a scalpel followed by complete incision with Metzenbaum scissors. Extension from the root of the aorta to the apex of the heart allows for complete delivery of the heart. Injury to the phrenic nerves, which course anterior to the pericardium, should be avoided [19–23]. The presence of an air embolus is an ominous finding and a negative predictor of outcome (see Fig. 13.6).

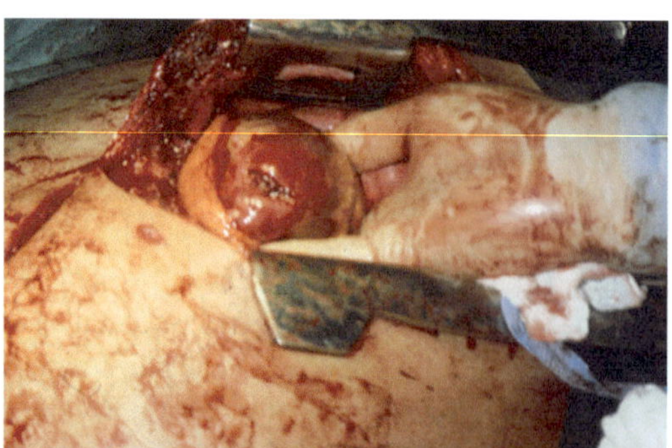

Fig. 13.1 Left anterolateral thoracotomy for gunshot wound in the left ventricle

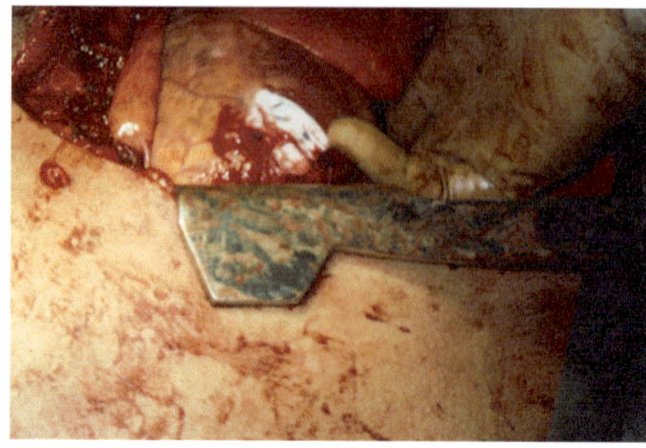

Fig. 13.2 The same patient who begun to bleed. Complex left ventricular cardiorrhaphy requiring Teflon pledgets

Once these general techniques have been implemented, additional procedures can be used based on the injury and physiological status of the patient. Hemorrhage from cardiac injuries is controlled with digital occlusion prior to performing either atrial or ventricular cardiorrhaphy with 2-0 polypropylene sutures on an MH needle [19, 23–25]. Initial management of pulmonary

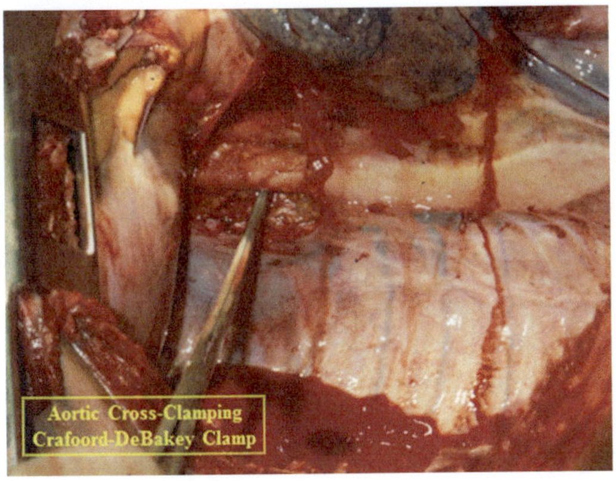

Fig. 13.3 Resuscitative thoracotomy on a patient that succumbed. Notice the left hemithoracic cavity which can harbor the entire blood volume. Thoracic aorta is dissected. Esophagus is above

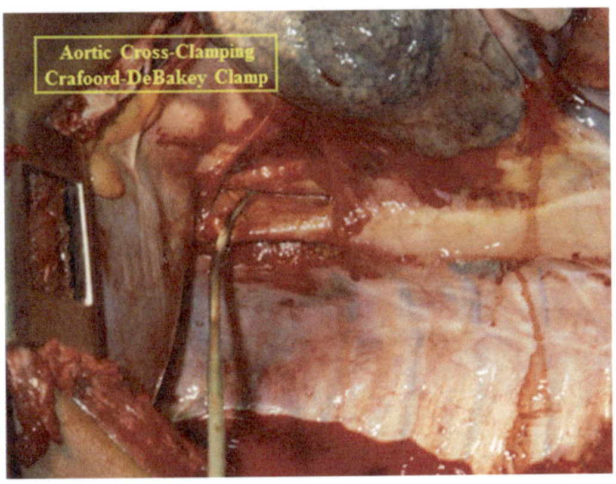

Fig. 13.4 Resuscitative thoracotomy on a patient that succumbed. Descending thoracic aorta has been clamped

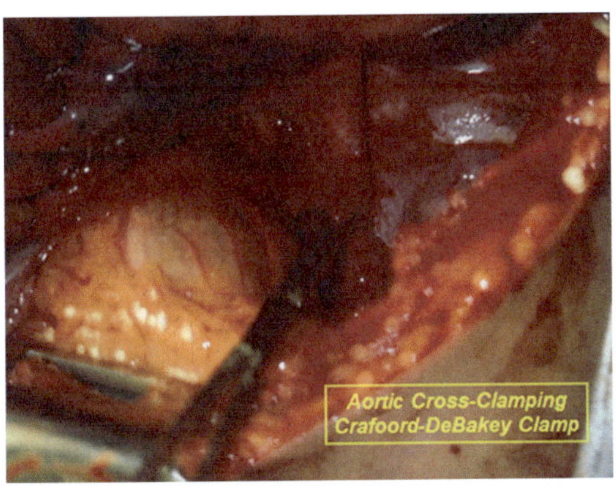

Fig. 13.5 Descending thoracic aorta cross-clamped on a live patient. Notice the decrease in size even in the largest blood vessel in the body in the presence of profound shock

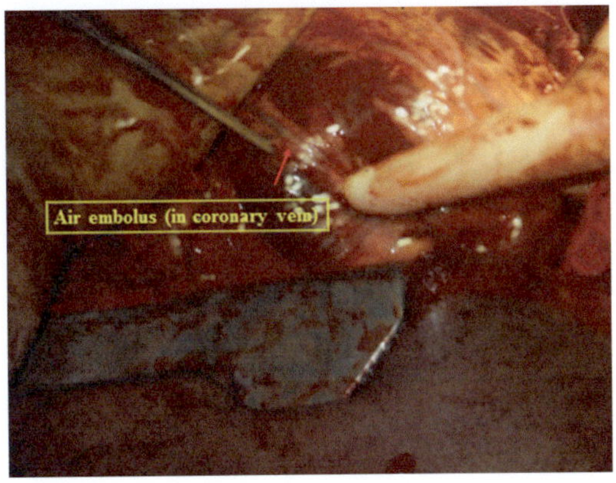

Fig. 13.6 This is an ominous finding

injuries begins with mobilization of the lung by sharply transecting and mobilizing the inferior pulmonary ligament, with the knowledge that proximity of the inferior pulmonary vein may place it at risk for iatrogenic injuries. Hemorrhage control and prevention of air embolism can be achieved by applying Duval clamps to the injured pulmonary parenchyma. Cross-clamping of the pulmonary hilum is indicated if there is an actively bleeding pulmonary hilum or if there is an expanding hilar or central hematoma. A Crafoord-DeBakey aortic clamp is also utilized [19, 23–25].

EDT is an indispensable first step in the institution of cardiothoracic damage control. Although this complex procedure is lifesaving, EDT is not without its risks or pitfalls. Overall survival rates remain low despite years of debate about the procedure and its indications. Asensio [19, 23–29] and Wall and colleagues [30] described the practice management guidelines of the American College of Surgeons Committee on Trauma (ACS-COT). In their study, a large volume of literature was reviewed, scrutinized, and stratified according to the levels of evidence. The authors reported survival rate of 7.83%. Stratified to mechanism of injury, survival rates for penetrating and blunt trauma were 11.16% and 1.6%, respectively.

EDT can also pose serious risks to the healthcare team. Rapidity of the procedure, use of sharp instruments, and suboptimal visualization make exposure to blood-borne pathogens an unequivocal risk. This risk is substantiated by reported HIV seropositivities as high as 4% in some urban trauma centers.

13.3 Cardiothoracic Damage Control in the Operating Room

13.3.1 Overall Considerations

If the patient has an organized perfusing rhythm following EDT, they are promptly transported to the operating room (OR). Upon arrival, speed is paramount and sterility a secondary concern. The patient should be placed in the supine position with both upper extremities abducted. A splash prep and draping from neck to midthighs are advisable in the event that access to the saphenous vein for an interposition reverse autogenous vein graft is required. Once the patient is properly positioned, the trauma surgeon should gown and glove immediately. Ongoing intravascular volume replacement with crystalloid, blood, and blood products should continue for the duration of the operation [23–29]. Appropriate thoracic instruments should be available (see Fig. 13.7).

Generally, the massive transfusion protocol (MPT) should be activated. Additional warming devices are used to minimize heat loss and facilitate rewarming in the hypothermic patient. Autotransfusers are viable options in thoracic injury given reduced risks of contamination. Continuous hemodynamic monitoring is achieved by placement of an arterial line. Switching to a dual-lumen endotracheal tube is usually not imperative, feasible, or recommended. If better

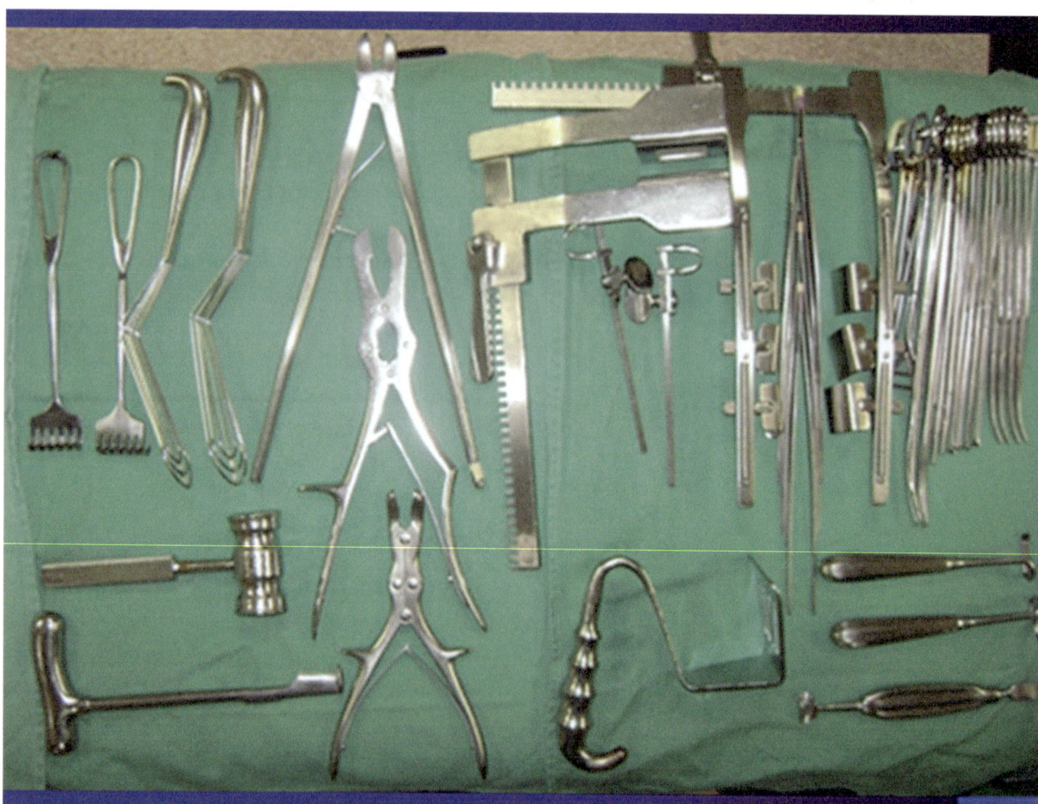

Fig. 13.7 Thoracic surgical instruments

visualization is required, the anesthesia staff may insert a bronchial blocker, or alternatively the endotracheal tube is advanced into one of the main stem bronchi to induce unilateral deflation.

13.3.2 Cardiac Injuries: Technical Aspects

For the majority of cardiac injuries, primary repair is the only option. Injuries addressed during the initial emergency department thoracotomy (EDT) should be inspected. Atrial injuries can be controlled by a Satinsky clamp and primarily repaired with 2-0 polypropylene monofilament sutures on a MH needle with horizontal mattress sutures of Halsted. Similarly, ventricular injuries are also primarily repaired in the same fashion. Occasionally, and mostly for gunshot wounds, the use of Teflon pledgets is warranted. The technical demands of suturing a functioning heart are obvious, and the difficulty of tying knots securely may be underestimated. Several techniques have been described that reduce the risk of lacerating the myocardium or exacerbating a concurrent injury [19, 23, 24, 25, 28].

Distal injuries comprise the majority of coronary vessel lacerations in those patients surviving long enough to be transported to the operating room. These injuries are often amenable to ligation with the knowledge that postoperative ischemia and intraoperative myocardial infarction are a very definite possibility. Proximal coronary artery injuries are usually fatal. Those that survive to reach the operating room will require aortocoronary artery bypass with a reverse autogenous saphenous vein graft (RSVG). In this setting, cardiopulmonary bypass is required [19, 23, 24, 25, 28]. However, one case has been described in which the LAD was repaired "off-pump" using a saphenous vein bypass graft [31]. Total inflow occlusion is indicated for injuries to the superior or inferior atriocaval junction and lateral most portion of the right atrium. This technique involves cross-clamping both the intrapericardial superior vena cava and the inferior vena

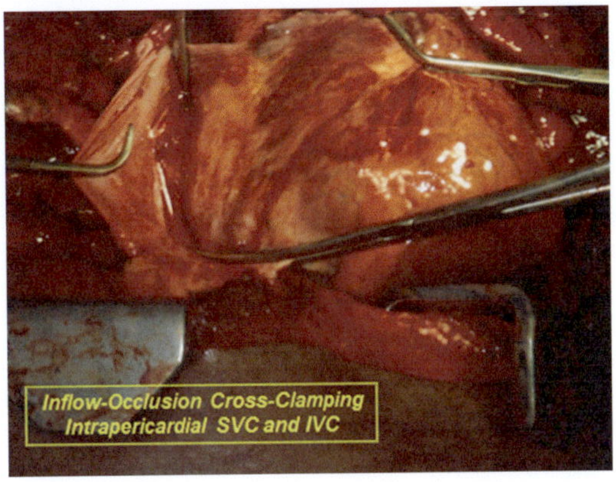

Fig. 13.8 Shumacker's maneuver

cava (IVCs), resulting in complete inflow occlusion (Shumacker's maneuver) (see Fig. 13.8) [19, 23, 24, 25, 28]. Subsequent arrest ensues along with a brief window of time to perform repairs. However, as these authors have previously warned, the safety period of this maneuver likely ranges from 1 to 3 min. If this time frame is exceeded, reestablishment of a sinus rhythm is improbable [19, 24, 25, 28].

When the repair is complete, no attempt should be made to close the pericardium. Doing so can be harmful in the event of cardiac swelling following the "stunned myocardium syndrome" and reperfusion injury. In rare instances, this may carry an increased risk of damage to the anterior cardiac surface [32].

13.3.3 Pulmonary Injuries: Technical Aspects

Management of pulmonary injuries includes pneumorraphy, non-anatomic resections, tractotomy, lobectomy, and pneumonectomy. Small peripheral injuries can be successfully managed with stapled non-anatomic resections. Most through-and-through injuries without involvement of the hilum are most amenable to pulmonary tractotomy. Clamp tractotomy, described by Wall [33], utilized aortic clamps through the wound tract which were noted to crush the pulmonary parenchyma. Asensio [34] described

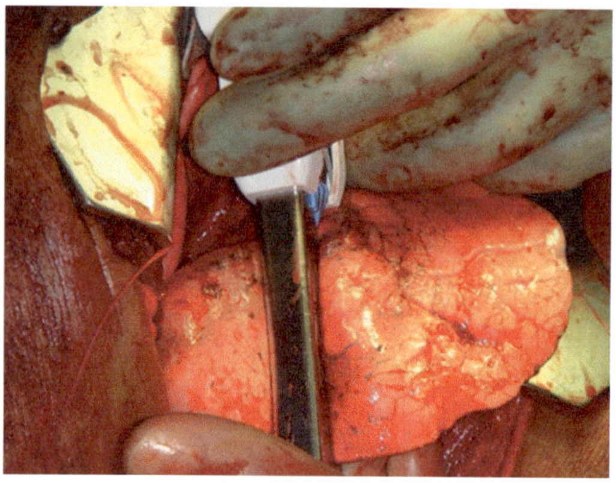

Fig. 13.9 Stapled pulmonary tractotomy

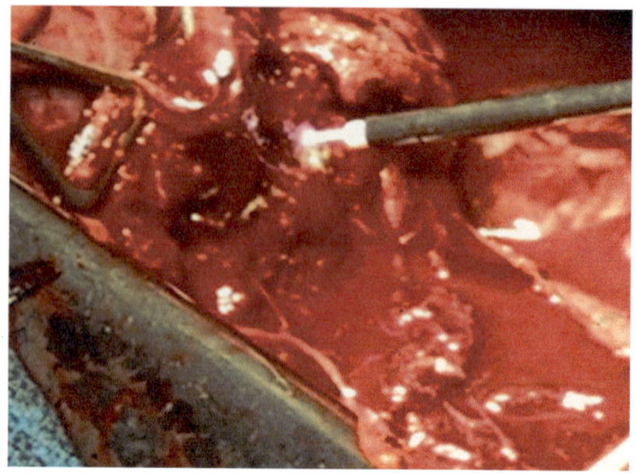

Fig. 13.11 Argon beam coagulator being utilized as an adjunct to stapled pulmonary tractotomy to control diffuse pulmonary parenchymal bleeding

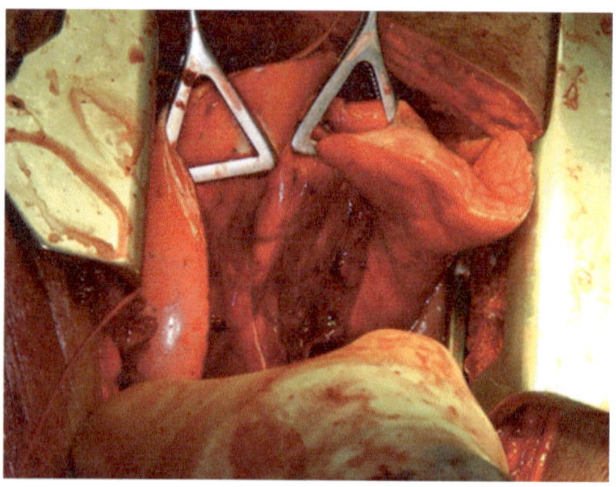

Fig. 13.10 Pulmonary parenchyma opens to identify injured blood vessels and bronchi for selective deep blood vessel ligation

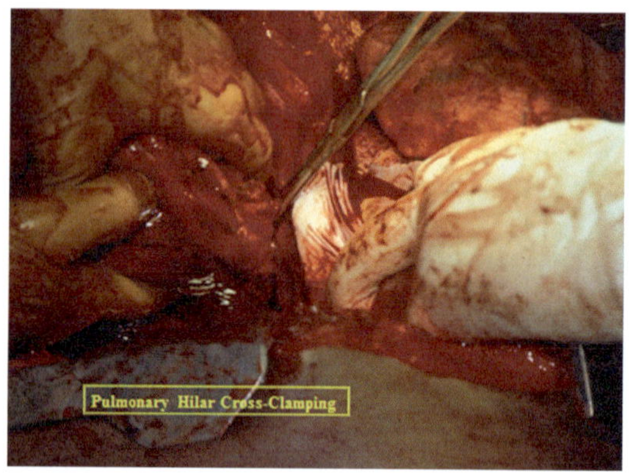

Fig. 13.12 Cross-clamping pulmonary hilum

stapled pulmonary tractotomy utilizing a GIA stapler as a tissue-sparing technique to identify and selectively ligate bleeding sources for control of hemorrhage. Once entrance and exit wounds have been identified, the stapler is placed through the wound and fired. This opens the tract, resulting in the exposure of bleeding vessels and transected bronchi [34] (see Figs. 13.9 and 13.10). Multiple studies have since shown this technique to be safe and effective [35, 36]. Similarly, Asensio and colleagues also described the use of the argon beam coagulator to control diffuse pulmonary parenchymal bleeding and as an adjunct to stapled pulmonary tractotomy [37] (see Fig. 13.11).

Pulmonary injuries that involve the hilum or hilar structures often require hilar cross-clamping and lobectomy or pneumonectomy (see Figs. 13.12 and 13.13). If time is adequate and patient physiology favorable, pulmonary vessel and bronchus isolation should be attempted (see Figs. 13.14 and 13.15). Thoracic damage control may not allow for either circumstance, in which case en bloc lobectomy or pneumonectomy using a large green load TA stapler may be required [34–36].

13.3.4 Intrathoracic Vascular Injuries: Technical Aspects

For the repair of thoracic vessels, diagnosis determines the type of incision required to gain proximal and distal control. The clear majority

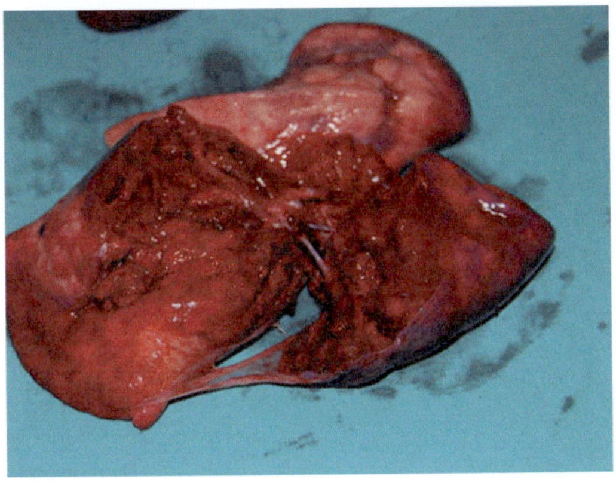

Fig. 13.13 Pneumonectomy for central hilar gunshot wound

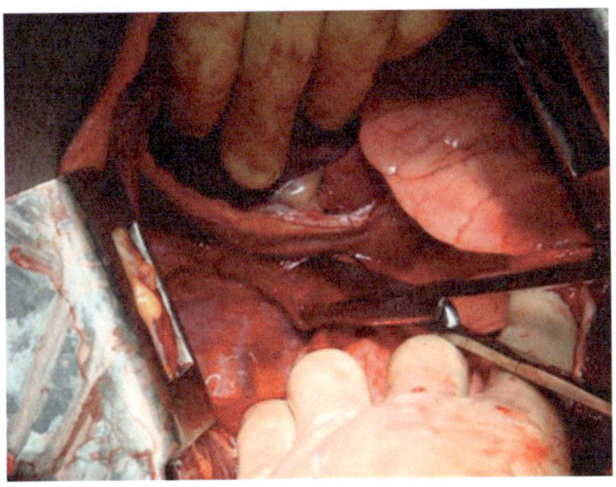

Fig. 13.14 Dissection of the extrapleural left pulmonary artery

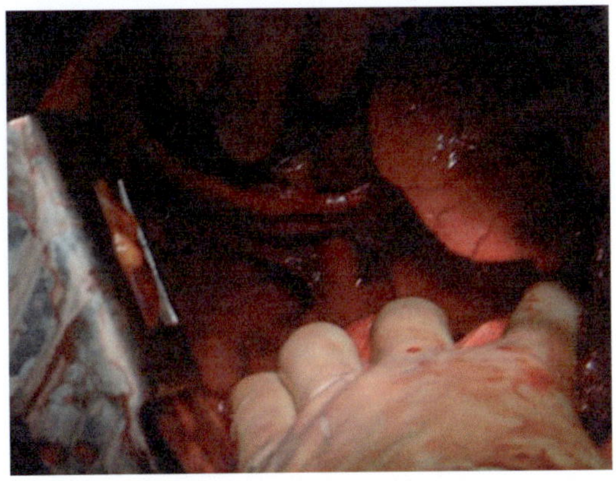

Fig. 13.15 Left main pulmonary artery

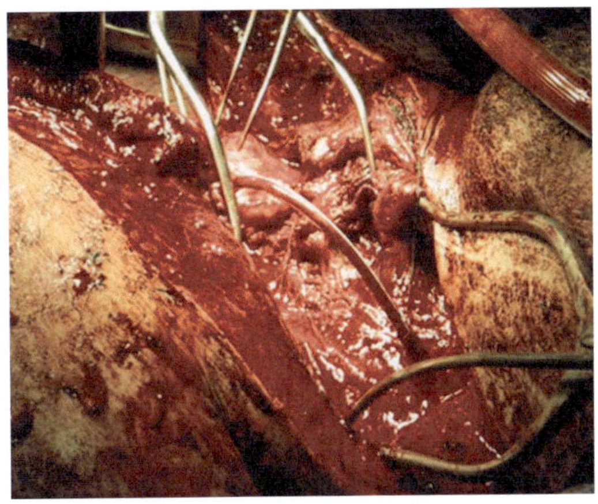

Fig. 13.16 Temporary intraluminal shunt in the left carotid artery after shotgun wound

of patients requiring damage control would have most likely undergone previous left and possibly bilateral anterolateral thoracotomies. Control of the descending thoracic aorta and proximal left subclavian artery is accessible via this incision. While an anterolateral thoracotomy provides proximal access to most other vessels, it lacks sufficient access for distal control and exposure for definitive repair [19, 38] (see Figs. 13.16 and 13.17). Injuries of the aortic arch and proximal great vessels require median sternotomy, which can be extended into the neck via the standard incision anterior to the sternocleidomastoid or as a subclavicular incision (see Figs. 13.18 and 13.19).

Injuries to the subclavian vessels are most easily accessed via a subclavicular incision with clavicle removal with or without replacement of the clavicle post-repair (see Figs. 13.20 and 13.21). If digital compression of a vessel was required at the time of EDT, the person providing digital control should be prepped in the field and digital control not removed until adequate intraoperative control is achieved. Hemorrhage originating adjacent to the clavicles can be temporarily controlled via digital pressure [19, 38, 39].

Primary repair is the preferred option in cardiothoracic damage control after satisfactory exposure and control are obtained; however, this is usually not possible given the extent of vessel damage.

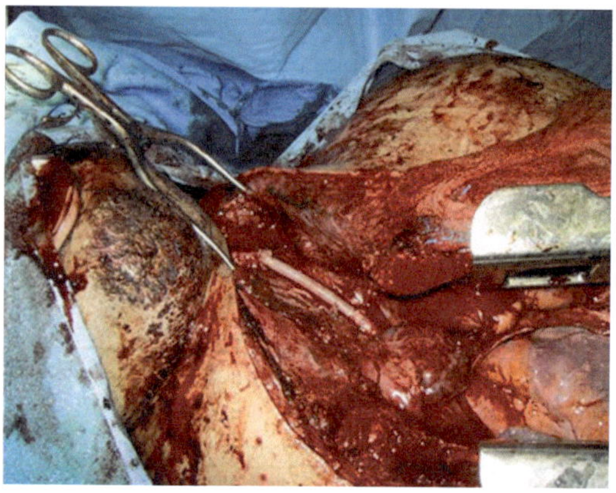

Fig. 13.17 The same patient after saphenous vein interposition graft between the proximal left carotid artery approximately 3 centimeters from its origin and the distal left common carotid artery

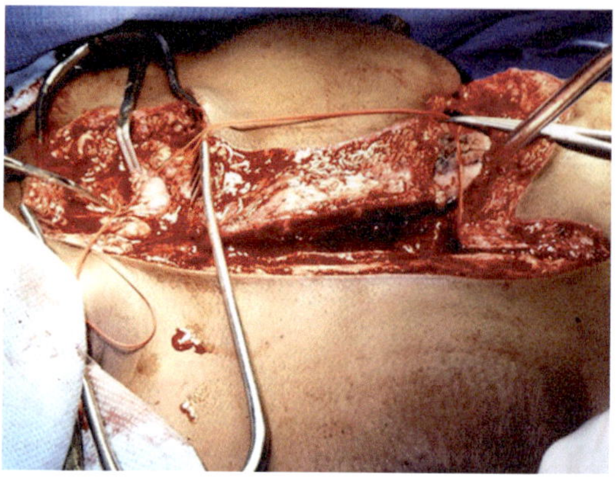

Fig. 13.20 Tangential gunshot wound. Left subclavian artery. Patient arrived in cardio pulmonary arrest. Required resuscitative thoracotomy. Transported to the OR for median sternotomy and left subclavicular incision

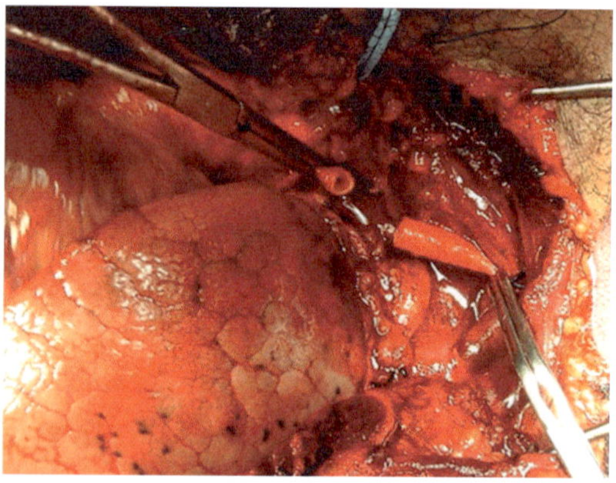

Fig. 13.18 Gunshot wound origin left common carotid artery. Proxmial and distal cross-clamping

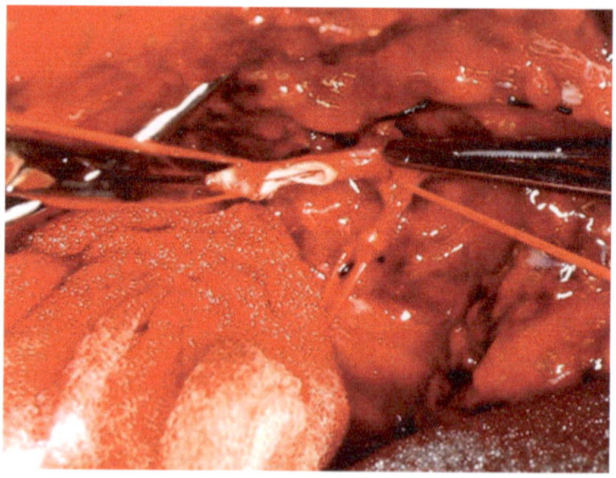

Fig. 13.21 The same patient. Left subclavian artery clamped prior to resection and PTFE interposition graft

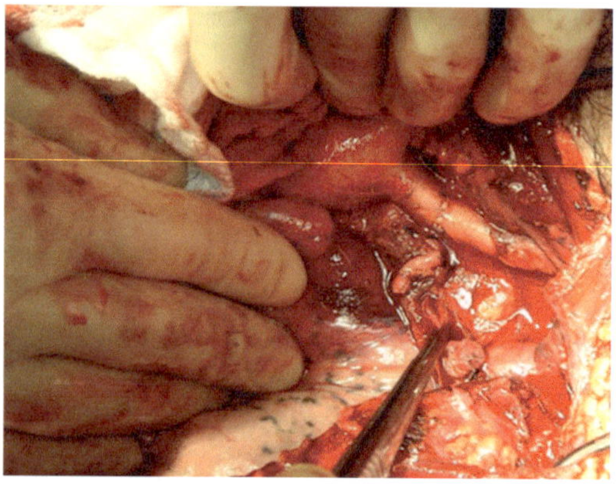

Fig. 13.19 After mobilization a primary end to and anastomosis was completed. Note arch of the aorta and transected phrenic nerve

Thus, synthetic grafts are most often used. Polytetrafluoroethylene (PTFE) or knitted Dacron grafts are the conduits of choice for vessels larger than 5 mm in diameter. Penetrating aortic injuries can usually be managed with primary repair but may require placement of a Dacron graft. In the past decade, intraluminal grafts have changed the entire spectrum of vascular injury management; however, most endografts are used for blunt thoracic aortic injuries [19, 38, 39].

Placement of intraluminal shunts to maintain blood flow in medium-sized vessels with the intention of delayed definitive repair has been rarely reported and used with some success. Shunt material and configuration are matters of personal preference, with Argyle shunts being the shunt's of choice. In areas of conflict, these authors have secured the shunts in place with 2-0 silk ties to ensure flow. Inaccessible vascular injuries can be temporized with a Fogarty catheter. In patients with rapidly deteriorating physiology, ligation is also an option. This is feasible for subclavian venous injuries but not for subclavian arterial injuries. Injuries to the subclavian, innominate, and jugular veins can be safely ligated [19, 38, 39].

13.3.5 Tracheobronchial Injuries: Technical Aspects

Penetrating injuries to the distal tracheobronchial tree are rare. In these cases, an airway should be secured prior to any specific interventions. Tracheal injuries, when suspected, can be initially managed via advancement of the endotracheal tube through the wound tract followed by wide surgical drainage. Penetrating tracheal wounds should be primarily repaired. Sutures should be applied either through or around the tracheal rings with external knot placement to reduce the risk of granuloma or stricture. These authors prefer to place sutures around the cartilaginous rings when possible and have found that to 2–3 cm defects can be approximated without tension. Bronchial injuries, although rare, should be primarily repaired if possible (see Figs. 13.22 and 13.23), or else a pneumonectomy is indicated. Postoperative suture line, dehiscence, leaks, and fistula formation are potential complications. Therefore, the intercostal muscle or other vascular pedicles can be used to buttress the repair [19, 34–36].

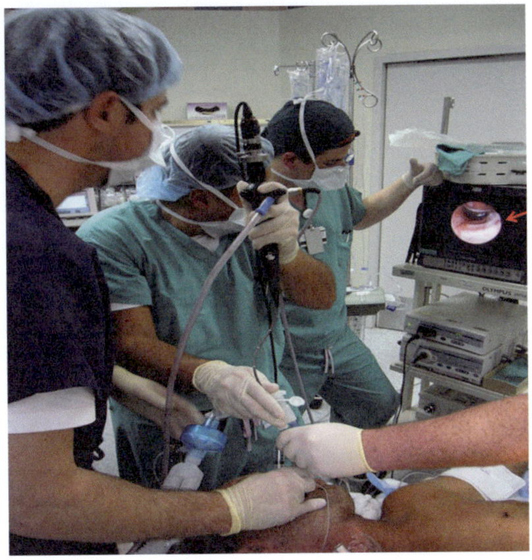

Fig. 13.22 Self-inflicted gunshot wound left chest. Massive air leak requiring multiple chest tubes. Bronchoscopy detected a left main stem bronchial laceration

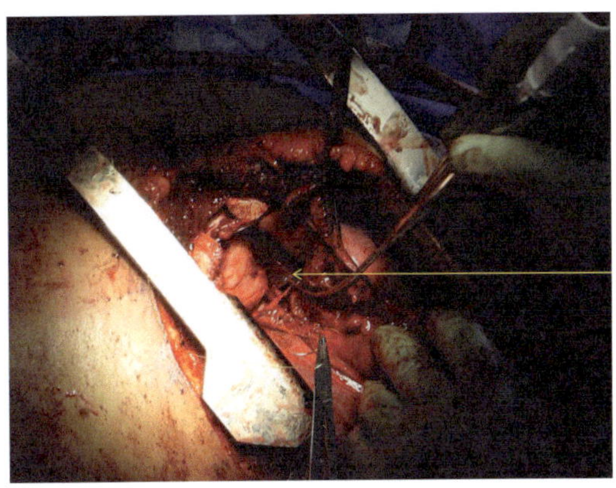

Fig. 13.23 Left mainstem bronchial laceration located after central stapled pulmonary tractotomy and primary repaired with simple interrupted 2-0 vicryl sutures

13.3.6 Esophageal Injuries: Technical Aspects

The primary goal in the management of esophageal injuries is to achieve primary repair with an excellent and functional closure without stenosis. Meticulous surgical technique will prevent suture line, dehiscence, or anastomotic failures thus avoiding risks of mediastinitis, mediastinal abscess, or empyema. Accordingly, these injuries are managed by wide drainage with two thoracostomy tubes in the setting of cardiothoracic damage control. Primary repair should be utilized and reinforced with a Grillo pleural flap or intercostal muscle [40, 41] (see Figs. 13.24 and 13.25). Non-reconstructible injuries can be temporarily managed by ligation and placement of a nasogastric tube above the level of injury with chest tubes draining the area. For complex injuries, reconstruction over a T-tube (Kehr tube) has been successfully reported [40, 41].

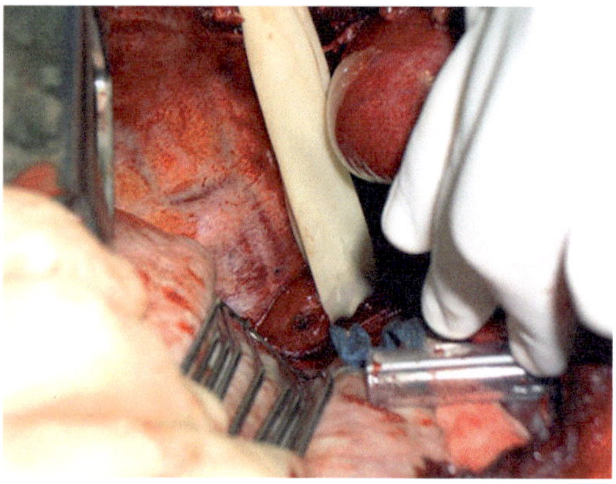

Fig. 13.24 Gunshot wound thoracic esophagus approached via right posterolateral thoracotomy esophagus mobilizes and isolated prior to double layer repair with 3-0 vicryl and 3-0 silk sutures

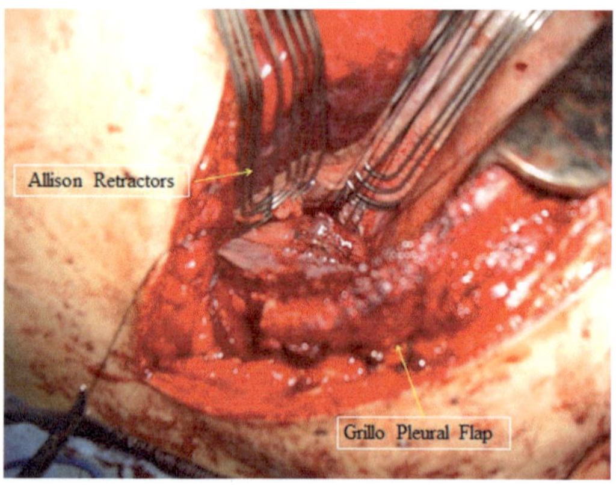

Fig. 13.25 Gunshot wound thoracic esophagus primary repaired and buttressed with grillo pleural flap

Diversion via cervical esophagostomy is a second option but adds significant time to the damage control phase and has been used infrequently. These authors prefer to wait on diversion until the second look procedure. Gastrostomy tube placement is also recommended but should be delayed until definitive repair [40, 41].

13.3.7 Thoracic Packing

Packing has long been an accepted practice for controlling hemorrhage in trauma surgery. It continues to be a useful damage control adjunct. Thoracic packing has been described as a means of controlling bleeding after cardiac surgical procedures and occasionally pulmonary resections. However, the use of packing in thoracic trauma has been less often used and at times discouraged, mainly because of concerns regarding its effects on intrathoracic pressure.

The physical space occupied by packing material combined could theoretically restrict venous return, cardiac filling, and lung expansion. This may increase the risk for the development of cardiac tamponade or inadequate ventilation [22, 38]. Specific reports substantiating these concerns are generally lacking and limited to personal experiences of trauma surgeons. Reports by Caceres [42] and Lang [43] described the application of this technique in thoracic damage control with some success. The data from these experiences seem to indicate that aforementioned concerns about possible sequelae may be unfounded. However, larger studies are needed to draw any meaningful conclusions.

Temporary packing of the chest, like the abdomen, carries an inherent risk of infection. In thoracic damage control, packing of the chest cavity is primarily used as a means of controlling bleeding, especially in the case of a massively injured chest wall. These injuries, such as those seen following close-range gunshot or shotgun wounds, often exhibit bleeding that lacks a rapid, definitive surgical solution [22]. Wall suggested the employment of chest packing as a last resort in the hypothermic, coagulopathic patient with multiple chest wall injuries and diffuse bleeding [17]. The use of gauze rolls or laparotomy pads as packing material in conjunction with the use of topical hemostatic agents may be effective in these patients. The argon beam coagulator may also be useful in this setting. Tissue debridement should only be performed if it significantly facilitates hemostasis. Otherwise, it can be delayed until the definitive operation [17, 37].

13.3.8 Temporary Chest Wall Closure

Proper closure of a thoracotomy incision requires each layer to be anatomically re-approximated. Therefore, temporary closure is a more feasible option in thoracic damage control. It allows rapid closure of the chest cavity so that the patient can be transported to the ICU where resuscitation may continue under more optimal conditions. In the setting of damage control, the thoracic cavity can be temporarily closed with towel clips, a running en masse suture, a Bogota bag, or a negative atmospheric pressure device (Wound Vac™) [24–28, 35]. For the patient in extremis, towel clips can be used as an expedient form of wound closure. However, this technique comes at the cost of reduced hemostasis and suboptimal visualization if angiography is later required. En masse closure with a single running locked suture is a second, more hemostatic option. If closure of the chest wall by either of these methods results in pulmonary or cardiac compromise, a Bogota bag can be used as a temporary closure. These authors have also used large adhesive dressings (Ioban™) to temporarily close one or both chest cavities in areas of conflict.

13.4 Cardiothoracic Damage Control in the Intensive Care Unit

The next step in the damage control sequence is continued resuscitation in the intensive care unit (ICU). Postoperative care can be just as challenging as the initial operation. Angiography, if required for vascular injuries, should be accomplished prior to arrival in the ICU [12, 16, 17, 22, 27]. Diagnostic and therapeutic bronchoscopy should also be used in patients with pulmonary injuries.

The speed with which hypothermia, acidosis, and coagulopathy are corrected is directly proportional to the likelihood of a good outcome. Hypoperfusion is the cause of acidosis in these patients. Therefore, its correction is focused on volume resuscitation and optimization of oxygen delivery. Care should be taken to address these issues while avoiding fluid overload. Many of these patients have decreased pulmonary reserve due to intraparenchymal hemorrhage, pulmonary contusions, and/or air leaks resulting from the initial injury. Excessive fluid administration can exacerbate these injuries and impair ventilation. Large intravascular volume requirements may put these patients at risk for edema. Subsequent increases in intraabdominal pressure can quickly progress to abdominal compartment syndrome, which may require decompressive laparotomy [12, 16, 17, 22, 27].

Trends in thoracostomy tube output should be monitored closely. Bleeding from thoracostomy tube drainage should decrease over the course of a few hours, as coagulopathy is addressed with blood products. Abrupt cessation of thoracostomy output should prompt suspicions of malfunction or clotting either within the drained hemithoracic cavity or the tube. If thoracostomy output remains high despite efforts to correct coagulopathy, this usually indicates that hemostasis has not been completely achieved. However, it may be difficult to know whether the cause of bleeding is surgical or because of uncorrected coagulopathy. This has long been acknowledged as one of the most difficult scenarios a trauma surgeon can encounter. The decision to return the patient to the operating room is based on clinical judgment. Unfortunately, judging incorrectly often leads to death or poor outcomes. Martin [20] advocates a threshold of six units of packed red cells transfused in 6 h without a change in hematocrit as an indication to return to the operating room. However, strict guidelines have yet to be published. These authors rely on the use of thromboelastography (TEG) and focused use of blood products to try to address the balance between a re-exploration versus continued critical care resuscitation [12, 16, 17, 22, 27].

13.5 Return to the Operating Room

Patients who have had temporizing procedures should be returned to the operating room once normal physiology and end points of resuscitation have been restored and met. The goals of reoperation are definitive organ repair and complete closure of the chest wall. At least two thoracostomy tubes should be placed at that time. These authors routinely place a 32 FR right-angled tube in the costophrenic sulcus and a 36 FR straight tube near the apex of the lung to ensure full expansion [12, 16, 17, 22, 27]. Additional tubes may be used as needed and placed in accordance with existing injuries. The thoracic cavity and incision are vigorously irrigated and hemostasis obtained prior to closing the chest wall in layers.

13.6 Complications

Complications arising from cardiothoracic damage control are common, severe, and often multiple. Those unique to this patient population are cardiac tamponade and air leak. The classical presentation of pericardial tamponade of distended neck veins, distant heart sounds, and hypotension—Beck's triad—is infrequent, even in patients presenting with cardiac injuries. In these patients findings of pericardial tamponade are often subtle, if not absent. It often presents with inadequate cardiac output and cessation of mediastinal chest tube output. Therefore, the use of noninvasive hemodynamic monitoring with a pulse wave analyzer, echocardiography, and even TEE may aid in the diagnosis [19, 23–25].

Definitive management of pericardial tamponade includes reopening of the chest and accessing the pericardium to release the tamponade. Air leaks are common following pulmonary procedures [19, 23–25]. Conservative management via thoracostomy tube drainage can initially be attempted. This often requires full expansion of the lung with adequate ventilation to be successful and avoidance if possible of high levels of positive pressure ventilation (PEEP). Persistent leaks may require reoperation to repair or resect the portion of lung parenchyma involved.

Given the condition of the patient requiring thoracic damage control, it is not surprising that mortality is very high. Mortality rates reported in the literature range from 23 to 69 %. The lowest mortality rate was reported by O'Connor [29] in the largest series to date. Variation has been attributed to differences in patient age, damage control techniques employed, and severity and mechanism of injury. In the same study, mortality rates were highest in patients requiring pneumonectomy [22].

Conclusions

Patients with severe chest trauma and marked physiological decline may benefit from cardiothoracic damage. Damage control in the chest, like in the abdomen, begins with initial management in the trauma center, followed by an abbreviated operation focused on hemorrhage and source control and temporary stabilization. This is followed by goal-directed critical care including appropriate intravascular volume replacement, normalization of end points of resuscitation, and a planned second look via re-exploration once the physiological derangements have been corrected. Cardiothoracic damage control has emphasized simple and rapid definitive procedures since there is little room for error in the management of patients "in extremis." These authors have found that the use of TTE during the initial procedure is helpful/beneficial as well as the role of TTE in the critical care unit and final chest closure. Therefore, it is imperative that the trauma surgeon be familiar with these techniques and be willing to adopt an aggressive mind-set to ensure the best opportunities for a favorable outcome. If all else fails, stop the bleeding, place thoracostomy tubes, and temporarily close the chest. Needless to say, rapid and meticulous surgical technique will influence the outcomes of these critically injured patients.

References

1. Stone HH, Storm PR, Mullins RJ. Management of the major coagulopathy with onset during laparotomy. Am Surg. 1983;197(5):532.
2. Burch JM, Oritz VB, Richardson RJ, et al. Abbreviated laparotomy and planned re-opening for critically injured patients. Am Surg. 1992;215:475–84.
3. Rotondo MF, Schwab CW, MD MG, et al. "Damage control": an approach for improved survival in exsanguinating penetrating abdominal injury. J Trauma. 1993;35:375–83.
4. Anderson KA. Pre-hospital care in traumatically induced hemorrhage and exsanguination. J Emerg Nurs. 1984;10:141.
5. Blaisdell FW, editor. Abdominal trauma: trauma management, vol. 1. Trunkey DD ed. New York: Thiemeand Straatton; 1982.

6. Asensio JA. Exsanguination from penetrating injuries. Trauma Q. 1990;6:1–25.
7. Asensio JA, Ierardi R. Exsanguination. Emerg Care Q. 1991;7(3):59–75.
8. Asensio JA, Hanpeter D, Gomez H, et al. Exsanguination. In: Shoemaker WC, Grenvik A, Ayres SM, Holbrook PR, editors. Textbook of critical care. Philadelphia: WB Saunders; 2000. p. 437–47.
9. Moore EE. Staged laparotomy for the hypothermia, acidosis, and coagulopathy syndrome. Am J Surg. 1996;172:405–10.
10. Cosgriff N, Moore EE, Sauaia A, Kenn-Moynihan M, Burch JM, Galloway B. Predicting life-threatening coagulopathy in the massively transfused trauma patient: hypothermia and acidoses revisited. J Trauma. 1997;42:857–61.
11. Asensio JA, McDuffie L, Petrone P, Roldan G, Forno W, Gambaro E, Salim A, Demetriades D, Murray J, Velmahos G, Shoemaker W, Berne TV, Ramicone E, Chan L. Reliable variables in the exsanguinated patient which indicate damage control and predict outcome. Am J Surg. 2001;182:743–51.
12. Asensio JA, Wo CJ, Li-Chien C, Lu K, Fathizadeh P, Petrone P, Kuncir E, Kimbrell B, Shoemaker WC. Non-invasive hemodynamic monitoring of patients sustaining severe penetrating thoracic, abdominal and thoracoabdominal injuries for early recognition and therapy of shock. Scand J Surg. 2006;95:152–7.
13. Asensio JA, Berne JD, Chahwan S, Hanpeter D, Demetriades D, Marengo J, Velmahos GC, Murray J, Shoemaker W, Berne TV. Traumatic injury to the superior mesenteric artery. Am J Surg. 1999;178(3):235–9.
14. Asensio JA, Britt LD, Forno W, Gambaro E, Borzotta A, Clancy KD, Peitzman A, Miller FB, Spain DA, Lukan J, Mackersie RC, Rogers S, Pasquale MD, Kurek S Jr, Patcher HL, Guth AA, Hoyt DB, Coimbra R, Kearney PA, Tsuei BJ, Ochoa JB, Boulanger BR, Wagner M, Block EFJ, Nicholas JM, Flint LM, Margulies DR, Lee SS, Fulda G, Tinkoff G, Rodriguez JL, Richardson C, Gray DK, Gracias VH, Jacobs DG, Thomason MH, Falcone R, Davis K, Durham RM, Richart CM, Anderson JT, Schenarts PJ, Diaz JJ, Coscia R, Dunham M, Indeck M, Motto C, Wargo C, Lottenberg L, Fallon WFJR, Goettler CE, Brandt MM, Taheri PA, Shah DM, Darling RCIII, Millham F, Dries DJ, McGonigal M, Ali J, Dove DB, McNeir DG, Roldan G, Salim A, Petrone P, Rowe V, Alo K, Ramicone E, Chan L. Multi-institutional experience with the management of superior mesenteric artery injuries. J Am Coll Surg. 2001;193(4):354–66.
15. Rotondo MF, Bard MR. Damage control surgery for thoracic injuries. Injury. 2004;35:649–54.
16. Vargo DJ, Battistella FD. Abbreviated thoracotomy and temporary chest closure: an application of damage control after thoracic trauma. Arch Surg. 2001;136:21–4.
17. Wall MJ Jr, Soltero E. Damage control for thoracic injuries. Surg Clin N Am. 1997;77:863–78.
18. Wilson A, Wall MJ Jr, Maxson R. The pulmonary hilum twist as a thoracic damage control procedure. Am J Surg. 2003;186:49–52.
19. Asensio JA, Stewart BM, Murray J, Fox AH, Falabella A, Gomez H, Ortega A, Fuller CB, Kerstein MD. Penetrating cardiac injuries. Surg Clin N Am. 1996;76:685–724.
20. Martin RR, Byrne M. Postoperative care and complications of damage control surgery. Sure Clin N Am. 1997;77:930–42.
21. Biffl WL, Moore EE, Harken AH. Emergency department thoracotomy. In: Mattox KL, Feliciano DV, Moore EE, editors. Trauma. New York: McGraw-Hill; 2000. p. 245–59.
22. Phelan HA, Patterson SG, Hassan MO, Gonzalez RP, Rodnig CB. Thoracic damage-control operation: principles, techniques, and definitive repair. J Am Coll Surg. 2006;203(6):933–41.
23. Asensio JA, Soto SN, Forno W, Roldan G, Petrone P, Salim A, Rowe V, Demetriades D. Penetrating cardiac injuries: a complex challenge. Injury. 2001;32(7):533–43.
24. Asensio JA, Murray J, Demetriades D, Berne J, Cornwell EE, Velmahos G, Gomez H, Berne TV. Penetrating cardiac injuries: a prospective study of variables predicting outcomes. J Am Coll Surg. 1998;186(1):24–34.
25. Asensio JA, Berne JD, Demetriades D, Chan L, Murray J, Falabella A, Gomez H, Chahwan S, Velmahos G, Cornwell EE, Belzberg H, Shoemaker W, Berne TV. One hundred five penetrating cardiac injuries: a 2-year prospective evaluation. J Trauma. 1998;44(6):1073–82.
26. Machowski MJ, Barnett RE, Harbrecht BG, Miller KR, Franklin GA, Smith JW, Richardson JD, Benns MV. Damage control for thoracic trauma. Am Surg. 2014;80(9):910–3.
27. Hunt PA, Greaves I, Owens WA. Emergency thoracotomy in thoracic trauma—a review. Injury. 2006;37(1):1–19.
28. Asensio JA, Arroyo H, Veloz W, Forno W, Gambaro E, Roldan G, Murray J, Velmahos G, Demetriades D. Penetrating thoracoabdominal injuries. The ongoing dilemma—which cavity and when? World J Surg. 2002;26(5):539–43.
29. O'Connor JV, DuBose JJ, Scalea TM. Damage-control thoracic surgery: management and outcomes. J Trauma Acute Care Surg. 2014;77(5):660–5.
30. Asensio JA, Wall M, Minei J, Demetriades D, Britt LD, Tominaga G, Weireter L, Fabian T. Practice management guidelines for emergency department thoracotomy. Am Coll Surg. 2001;193(3):303–9.
31. Fedalen PA, Bard MR, Piacentino V 3rd, Fisher CA, McCarthy JR, Schina MJ Jr, Furukawa S, Garcia JP. Intraluminal shunt placement and off-pump coronary vascularization for coronary artery stab wound. J Trauma. 2001;50(1):133–5.
32. Howells GA, Vogel LM, Krause KR, Bair HA, Chengelis DL. Temporary pericardial replacement for thoracic damage control procedures: avoidance of mechanical damage to the heart. J Trauma. 1998;45:623–5.

33. Wall MJ Jr, Villavicencio RT, Miller CC, Aucar JA, Granchi TA, Liscum KR, Shin D, Mattox KL. Pulmonary tractotomy as an abbreviated thoracotomy technique. J Trauma. 1998;45(6):1015–23.
34. Asensio JA, Demetriades D, Berne JD, Velmahos G, Cornwell EE 3rd, Murray J, Gomez H, Falabella A, Chahwan S, Shoemaker W, Berne TV. Stapled pulmonary tractotomy: a rapid way to control hemorrhage in penetrating pulmonary injuries. J Am Coll Surg. 1997;185:504–5.
35. Velmahos GC, Baker C, Demtriades D, Goodman J, Murray JA, Asensio JA. Lung-sparing surgery after penetrating trauma using tractotomy, partial lobectomy, and pneumorraphy. Arch Surg. 1999; 134:186–9.
36. Cothren C, Moore EE, Biffl WL, Franciose RJ, Offner PJ, Burch JM. Lung-sparing techniques are associated with improved outcome compared with anatomic resection for severe lung injuries. J Trauma. 2002;53:483–7.
37. Asensio JA, Mazzini FN, Gonzalo R, Iglesias E, Vu T. The Argon Beam Coagulator. An effective adjunct to stapled pulmonary tractotomy to control hemorrhage in penetrating pulmonary injuries. J Am Coll Surg. 2012;214(3):e9–e12.
38. Shapiro MB, Jenkins DH, Schwab CW, Rotondo MF. Damage control: collective review. J Trauma. 2000;49(5):969–78.
39. Aucar JA, Hirshberg A. Damage control for vascular injuries. Surg Clin N Am. 1997;77(4):853–62.
40. Asensio JA, Berne J, Demetriades D, Murray J, Gomez H, Falabella A, Fox A, Velmahos G, Shoemaker W, Berne TV. Penetrating esophageal injuries. Time interval of safety for preoperative evaluation—how long is safe. J Trauma. 1997;43(2):319–24.
41. Asensio JA, Chahwan S, Forno W, MacKersie R, Wall M, Lake J, Minard G, Kirton O, Nagy K, Karmy-Jones R, Brundage S, Hoyt D, Winchell R, Kralovich K, Shapiro M, Falcone R, McGuire E, Ivatury R, Stoner M, Yelon J, Ledgerwood A, Luchette F, Schwab CW, Frankel H, Chang B, Coscia R, Maull K, Wang D, Hirsch E, Cue J, Schmacht D, Dunn E, Miller F, Powell M, Sherck J, Enderson B, Rue L III, Warren R, Rodriquez J, West M, Weireter L, Britt LD, Dries D, Dunham CM, Malangoni M, Fallon W, Simon R, Bell R, Hanpeter D, Gambaro E, Ceballos J, Torcal J, Alo K, Ramicone E, Chan L. Penetrating esophageal injuries: multicenter study of the American Association for the Surgery of Trauma. J Trauma. 2001;50(2):289–96.
42. Caceres M, Buechter KJ, Tillou A, Shih JA, Liu D, Steeb G. Thoracic packing for uncontrolled bleeding in penetrating thoracic injuries. South Med J. 2004;97:637–41.
43. Lang JL, Gonzalez RP, Aldy KN, Carroll EA, Eastman AL, White CQ, Funk GA, Phelan HA. Does temporary chest wall closure with or without chest packing improve survival for trauma patients in shock after emergent thoracotomy? J Trauma. 2001;703:705–9.

14 Damage Control in Pediatric Patients

R. Todd Maxson

14.1 Background

The concepts of damage control surgery and resuscitation have been known for many years, as have data affirming the advantages for adult patients. There has been no doubt that the application of these damage control resuscitation principles have led to improved success of non-operative management of solid organ injury, decreased multi-system organ failure, and improved mortality [1]. As of this writing, there has been no prospective randomized trial proving the benefit of damage control resuscitation in the pediatric patient. There are several challenges with such trials; primarily, the most common injuries are traumatic brain injury, and overall mortality is low. Death from hemorrhage is rare and precludes effective trials without broad multicenter participation over an extended time frame. It should be said, however, that when a therapy or intervention is proven to have benefit in adult patients, it should be considered applicable to the pediatric population unless there is compelling reason to believe that there are differences in the pediatric anatomy or physiology that would change the efficacy of the therapy or intervention. Such is the case with damage control surgery and resuscitation. The concept of limited crystalloid resuscitation; early, balanced blood component replacement; rapid correction of physiological derangements, including coagulopathy and inflammation; and source control surgery for bleeding and contamination should all be applicable in the pediatric patient based on the developing biology of the child.

R. Todd Maxson, M.D., F.A.C.S.
Arkansas Children's Hospital, Little Rock, AR, USA

University of Arkansas for Medical Sciences, Little Rock, AR, USA
e-mail: RTMaxson@uams.edu

14.2 Differences of the Pediatric Patient

There obviously are differences in the mode of injury, the anatomical injuries sustained, and the physiological and psychological response to injury on an age-based spectrum. The infant has important differences in anatomy and physiology, while the adolescent suffers injuries and responds to them very similarly to an adult.

14.3 Mode of Injury

The young child's most common injury is fall until early adolescence where motor vehicle-related injuries dominate. Penetrating injuries are uncommon, typically unintentional and less likely to be firearm related, making the likelihood of vascular injury substantially less.

J. Duchesne et al. (eds.), *Damage Control in Trauma Care*,
https://doi.org/10.1007/978-3-319-72607-6_14

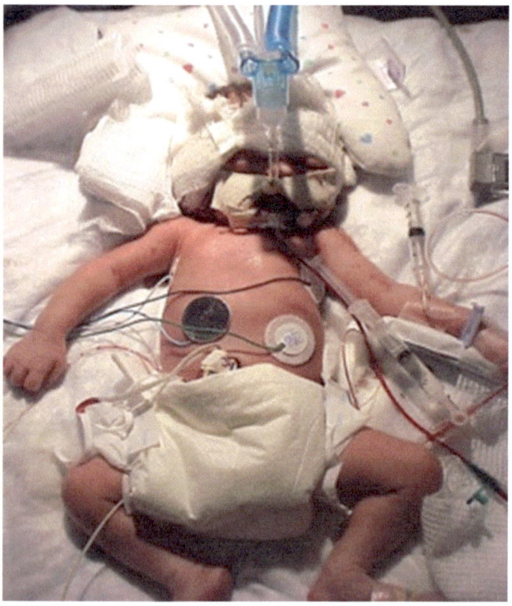

Fig. 14.1 Infant with an inflicted TBI

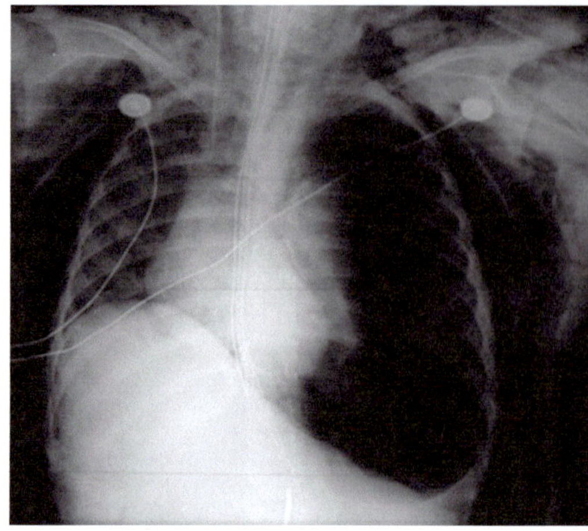

Fig. 14.2 Tension pneumothorax following blunt injury

Intentional injury is a leading cause of injury-related death in the young child when child abuse dominates the mode of injury (Fig. 14.1) [2]. Injury patterns, therefore, are primarily head injury in the young child, transitioning to more adult patterns by early adolescence.

14.4 Anatomic Differences

The young child has a relatively large head-to-body ratio and a cartilaginous skeleton, making CNS injuries and multi-system injuries common. Death is most likely from the traumatic brain injury and less likely than adults to be from hemorrhage. Specifically, the cartilaginous skeleton and lax ligaments of the pelvis make it unlikely that a young child will suffer significant pelvic injury with retroperitoneal bleeding. The growth plates are closing by the early teen years in girls and the mid-teen years in boys. This anatomic change, combined with driving motor vehicles, makes the adult pattern pelvic injuries much more common in the late teen years. These are important distinctions to make because hypotension in the younger child is less likely to be from a pelvic and retroperitoneal source. When children do suffer the rare posterior pelvic disruption from a crush mechanism, the finding is not subtle and typically easily demonstrable on physical exam in the trauma bay.

Another important difference is the mobility of the mediastinum in the young child. Small volumes of hemothorax and pneumothorax can cause significant shift, decreasing venous return (Fig. 14.2).

Therefore, early decompression of the hemithorax is prudent in the hypotensive child. Additionally, because the skeleton and specifically the ribs are cartilaginous, force may be transmitted more generally than in the adult patient, making multi-system injuries more common. The presence of a broken rib in the young child with cartilaginous ribs connotes a significant force that has been applied and is independently predictive of solid organ injury and mortality [3, 4].

14.5 Physiological Differences

Christiaans' review article in *Shock* outlines the age-dependent differences in coagulation factors. Mean values of coagulation proteins (II, V, VII, IX, X, XI, XII) are all significantly lower in the pediatric patient than the adult. There are decreased levels in the pediatric patient of tissue plasminogen, intracellular calcium, tissue plasminogen activator (t-PA), and alpha antiplasmin activity and increases in fibrinolytic activity [5–8]. These give plausible expectation that the response to injury and the induction of trauma-induced coagulopathy (TIC) may differ in the young child. The next major difference comes from the fact that the primary tissue injury is CNS. The biological differences in the mechanism of trauma-induced coagulopathy between CNS injury and hemorrhagic injury are not well delineated, but these differences may well account for much of the differences seen between pediatric and adult patients in how they manifest TIC. The third difference is in the manifestation of shock. In response to injury, the pediatric patient increases sympathetic output and increases systemic vascular resistance by increasing tone in the medium-sized arteries. This maintains mean arterial pressure and perfusion pressure to vital organs [9]. This response lessens with increasing age and is not as prevalent in the adult patient [10]. The practical point is that the child who is hypotensive from blood loss is far down the volume curve, potentially as much as 40% of total circulating blood volume has been lost.

14.6 Detection of Trauma-Induced Coagulopathy in Children

Conventional coagulation testing such as INR, aPTT, PT, and fibrinogen levels is commonly used for the evaluation of the injured pediatric patient. There are several limitations to the use of these conventional coagulation tests in the pediatric patient, including the fact that these measurements do not measure the overall coagulation system, specifically missing those components derived from injury to the endothelium and cellular components. The conventional coagulation tests also do not describe the hypercoagulable state associated with trauma. Excellent data from both Pittsburg and Houston show that trauma-induced hypercoagulable states exist more commonly in the pediatric patient than the adults [11, 12]. Tests measuring viscoelastic properties of whole blood and platelet function are available and have been used successfully in pediatric trauma patients to elucidate the hemostatic state following injury [13]. Multiple studies, both from combat and civilian practices, demonstrate a high incidence of TIC in the pediatric patient and a significant correlation to injury-related mortality [10]. Age-specific norms have been established for thromboelastography, and it has proven an extremely useful tool in characterizing the coagulation state in children. First used in the hematologic patients, its use now is common in spine, cardiac, and pediatric trauma surgery.

14.7 Treatment Options for Pediatric Patient with Trauma-Induced Coagulopathy

Little has been written to guide our approach to damage control resuscitation in the pediatric patient. A practical approach would dictate that the principles applied to the adult are a reasonable place to start a pediatric resuscitation. The challenge is that almost 80% of pediatric patients receive their initial care at a non-pediatric center and frequently receive excessive crystalloid and packed red cells prior to arrival in definitive care. Few places employ a strategy of damage control resuscitation for pediatrics prior to transfer to a pediatric trauma center.

Once in the pediatric center, a goal-directed approach for reversal of TIC is a more practical approach than an empiric method of resuscitation and blood administration [14]. Evaluation of the TIC with biological testing and replacement of specific factors to replace the deficits is a logical way to approach these transferred patients. Results following replacement of many of the specific factors are only anecdotal in the pediatric population. A replacement ratio of 0.9 (g) of fibrinogen concentrate to 1(u) pRBCs has been proposed by Schochl [10] for fibrinogen levels less than 1.5 g/dL and bleeding. Recombinant factor VIIa (90 μg/kg as a bolus and 25 μg/kg/h as a continuous infusion until bleeding has stopped) has been used successfully in children to stop bleeding but has been associated with significant thrombosis [10]. Prothrombin complexes (PCC) derived from pooled plasma have a high concentration of the proteins but significant blood exposure. Only case reports exist for the use of PCCs in pediatric care [15].

The use of the lysine analog tranexamic acid (TXA) to inhibit plasminogen activation and decrease the activity of plasmin, deceasing fibrinolysis, has been shown in the 2010 CRASH-2 trial to decrease all-cause mortality for injured patients. Anecdotal reports and Cochrane meta-analysis reviews demonstrate a benefit of the use of TXA for pediatric patients during elective cases such as craniofacial, cardiac, and scoliosis surgery. The 2014 paper from Eckert and colleagues in *The Journal of Trauma* was the first to show a decrease in injury-related mortality when TXA was used in the pediatric population in a conflict setting. Pre-teen patients with bleeding and acidosis had a reduced mortality (OR, 0.27) with the use of TXA. Further, there were no thrombotic or seizure episodes noted in the cohort in this retrospective analysis. The recommendation was, therefore, that the standard dosing protocol be utilized for pediatric patients [16].

In the United Kingdom, the Royal College of Paediatrics and Child Health and the Neonatal and Paediatric Pharmacists Group issued evidence-based statements recommending dosing TXA for injured children at 15 mg/kg loading (max 1 g) over 10 min and 2 mg/kg/h until bleeding stops [17]. Trauma care providers have three choices when considering TXA administration: (1) provide it for all patients with potential significant bleeding, (2) provide it for patients known to have significant bleeding and confirmed acidosis, and (3) provide it for patients known to have hyperfibrinolysis based on biological testing. While definitive data is lacking, at our institution, we begin TXA if there is significant bleeding prior to thromboelastography confirmation of hyperfibrinolysis [18].

14.8 Massive Transfusion in Children

The use of a massive transfusion protocol (MTP) is rare in the young child because of the infrequent incidence of hemorrhagic shock. The use of MTP in pediatric trauma centers is variable and historically has been based on practitioner preference rather than evidence. Neff retrospectively looked at the threshold of blood products given in a combat setting and determined that one-half of a pediatric patient's circulating blood volume or 40 cm^3/kg of all products given over 24 h defined a patient at risk for mortality from bleeding with TIC [19]. Others have used proven coagulopathy by conventional coagulation testing methods along with bleeding and acidosis to define the need for a MTP [20]. There have been no studies that have definitively defined those patients who need an MTP prospectively, and little evidence guides our decision to initiate the MTP in the trauma bay [21].

The physiological difference in children where they maintain mean arterial pressure would suggest that the child who is already hypotensive is significantly volume depleted and may benefit from earlier institution of an MTP. The American College of Surgeons Committee on Trauma's Resources for the Optimal Care of the Injured Patient (2014) requires a weight-based MTP in pediatric trauma centers [22]. Most centers divide the MTP protocol into distinct weight groups. Table 14.1 is an example of a weight-based transfusion threshold for initiation of MTP. Table 14.2 is an example of the weight-based transfusion protocol.

Table 14.1 Example of a weight-based transfusion threshold for initiation of MTP

Patient weight (kg)	Patient meets MTP criteria when RBCs transfused within 3 h equals	Patient meets MTP criteria when RBCs transfused within 24 h equals
<20 g	>1 unit or 40cc/kg	>3 units or 75 cm^3/kg
20–35	3 units	5 units
36–50	4 units	6 units
>50	6 units	10 units

Table 14.2 Example of a weight-based transfusion protocol

Blood/blood component	Initial pack # of adult units	Second pack # of adult units	Third pack # of adult units	Fourth pack # of adult units	Fifth pack # of adult units
For patients weighing ≤20 kg					
RBC	1	1	1	1	1
FFP	1	1	1	1	1
PLT	0.5	0.5	0.5	0.5	0.5
Cryo	Order as needed	2 units	Order as needed	2 units	Order as needed
Alternatively the small child would receive 20 cm^3/kg of PRBCs and FFP and 10 cm^3/kg platelets in each pack					
For patients weighing 21–50 kg					
RBC	2	2	2	2	2
FFP	2	2	2	2	2
PLT	1	1	1	1	1
Cryo	Order as needed	4 units	Order as needed	4 units	Order as needed
For patients weighing >50 kg					
RBC	4	4	4	4	4
FFP	4	4	4	4	4
PLT	1	1	1	1	1
Cryo	Order as needed	10 units	Order as needed	10 units	Order as needed

14.9 Summary of Damage Control Resuscitation

While little evidence exists that a damage control resuscitation (DCR) strategy decreases mortality in the pediatric trauma population, there are enough circumstantial evidence and evidence of success of the various components to recommend its use. An "expert opinion" recommendation would be:

(1) Minimize crystalloid use to maintain minimally acceptable, age-specific, systolic pressures in the prehospital and ED setting.
(2) Initiate TXA for confirmed hypotension from hemorrhage.
(3) Initiate a weight-based MTP for confirmed hypotension from hemorrhage.
(4) Initiate viscoelastic biological testing as soon as feasible in the resuscitation.
(5) Transition to a goal-directed replacement strategy based on the results from testing.

14.10 Damage Control in the Neonatal Period

The neonatal patient suffers from few surgical catastrophes, but among them are those resulting from congenital anomalies such as malrotation with midgut volvulus. In these cases, the rapid laparotomy, reduction of the volvulus, and rapid resection, if required, of frankly dead intestine, followed by resuscitation and reoperation, are the preferred methods (Fig. 14.3). If a second look operation is planned, then temporary closure with a silo of material from Gore-Tex to Silastic is an option (Figs. 14.4 and 14.5).

Another catastrophe that benefits from a damage control procedure is fulminant necrotizing enterocolitis in the premature infant under 1 kg. Such infants often benefit from a temporizing abdominal drainage with or without lavage, further resuscitation, and later definitive operation if necessary (Fig. 14.6). Frequently, however, the temporizing drainage procedure is the only intervention

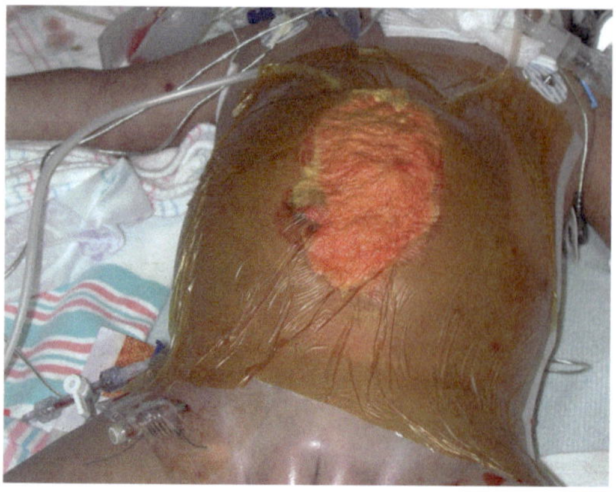

Fig. 14.3 Laparotomy

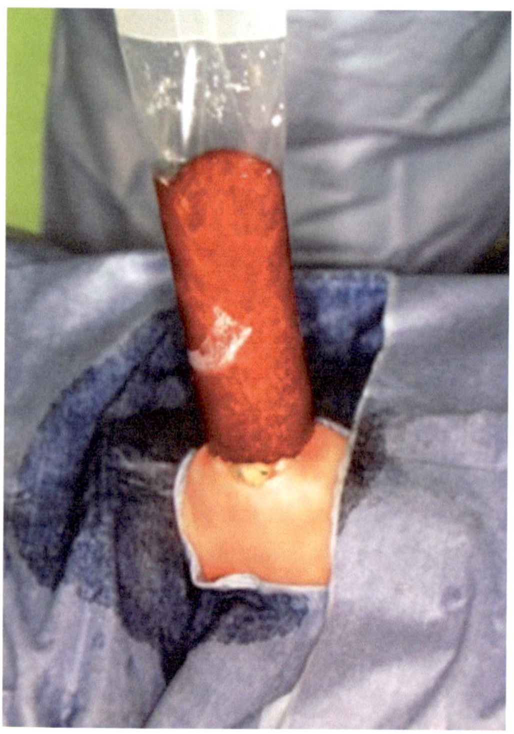

Fig. 14.4 Silastic silo

required as the perforation will, at times, seal spontaneously or the baby will progress to a more fulminant total intestinal involvement for which operation is not curative.

The use of umbilical catheters in the neonatal intensive care unit has become ubiquitous. The use of these catheters is not without risk, including vascular and liver injuries. Rapid fluid bolus,

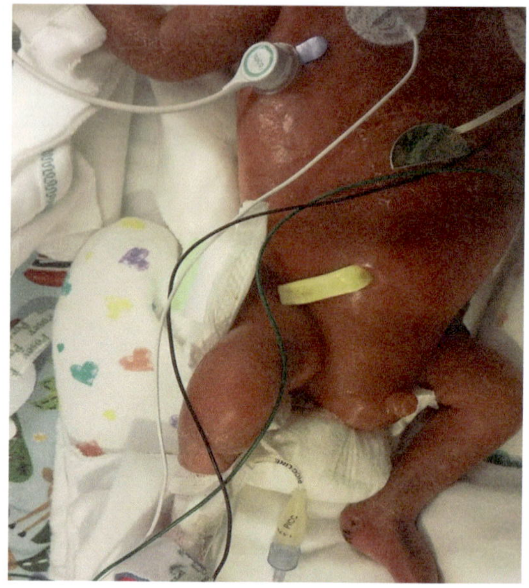

Fig. 14.5 Penrose drainage of an extremely premature infant

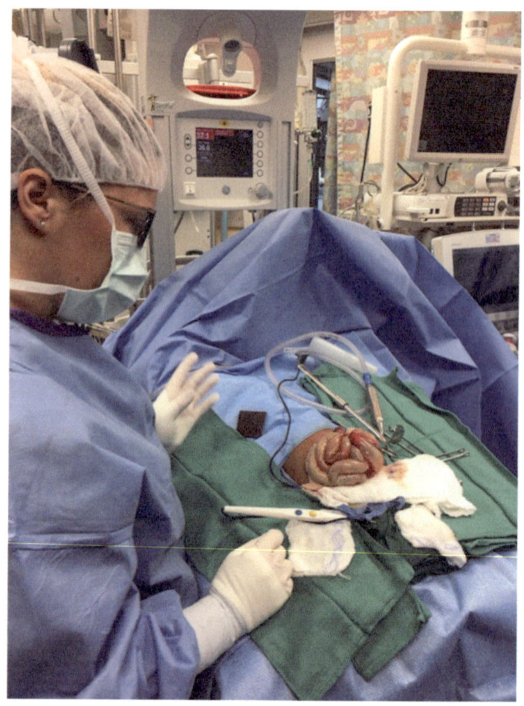

Fig. 14.6 Bedside operation in the ICU for necrotizing enterocolitis

particularly through an umbilical venous catheter, can have serious consequences, including opening of previously closed ductus arteriosus and rapid liver expansion with capsular rupture, the latter being a catastrophic consequence. Expanding liver capsular bleeding can occur intraoperatively with minimal contact with the neonatal liver and similarly can be catastrophic [23]. Packing the neonatal liver injury can be lifesaving and is often accomplished with hemostatic gauze alone [24]. The same principles apply, as they do in the adult patient—rapid control of the hemorrhage, correction of the acidosis and coagulopathy, and then reassessment of the hemorrhage.

One benefit of resuscitation of the neonatal patient is the availability of whole blood, which is often used in neonatal cardiac surgery and in many neonatal ICUs. Units that do not have whole blood still likely benefit from packed cells that have had a much shorter shelf life than those sent to non-neonatal units.

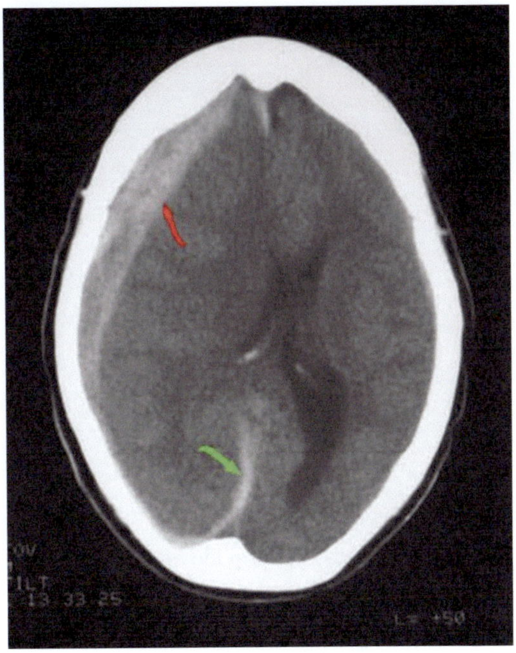

Fig. 14.7 Subdural hematoma with midline shift

14.11 Damage Control for Neurological Injury

The incidence of coagulopathy in children suffering isolated traumatic brain injury is high and, in a paper from USC-LA County, was over 40% in the pediatric population. The release of tissue factor associated with parenchymal brain injury is frequently the inciting factor for the coagulopathy. Researchers have shown that this coagulopathy occurs later than the coagulopathy induced from bleeding but is still significantly associated with mortality [25, 26]. The term "damage control neurosurgery" was coined by JV Rosenfeld (Injury 2004) and referred to abbreviated operation to control bleeding, debride devitalized tissue, and replace dura with a temporary closure (Figs. 14.7 and 14.8) [27]. The Brain Trauma Foundation guidelines endorse early decompressive craniectomy for pediatric patients with intracranial hypertension [28, 29]. While there is no compelling data proving a benefit from this approach, it remains the expert opinion of the foundation and the modern standard of care.

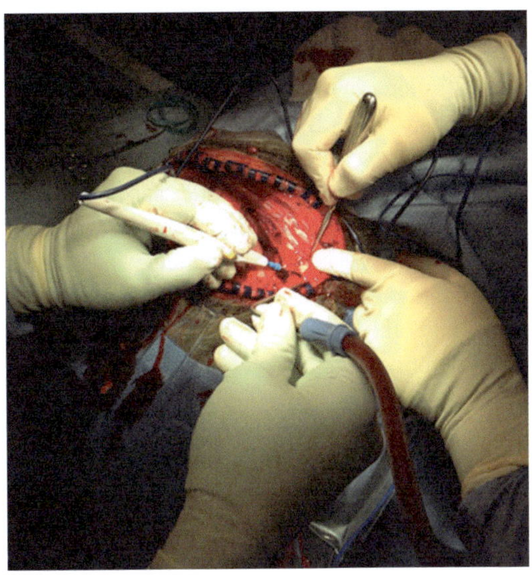

Fig. 14.8 Craniotomy

14.12 Damage Control Orthopedic Surgery

The concept of damage control orthopedics was described initially by Scalea et al. in 2000 [30]. The concept involved temporarily stabilizing a fracture

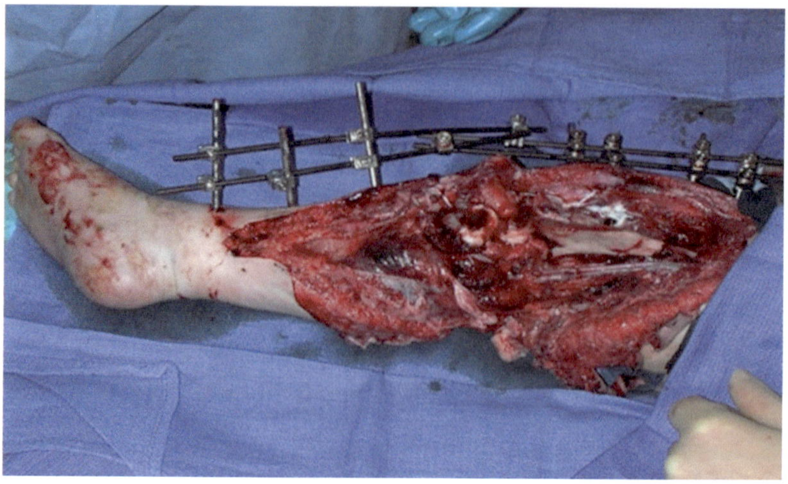

Fig. 14.9 Damage control in severe orthopedic injuries with early bleeding control followed by bony stabilization

with external fixation to provide time for resuscitation and correction of coagulopathy and acidosis before proceeding to a definitive repair (Fig. 14.9). Since the early reports describing its use in adults, there has been very little written regarding children. External fixation was originally felt to be the temporizing method of choice but carried a higher complication rate than internal fixation. Complications, in both adults and children include non-union, joint stiffness, and pin site infections. More recent case series and reports are of submuscular bridge plating and antibiotic spacers that have been described with fewer complications.

The triage of patients to a damage control procedure is often predicated on the resuscitation status and other injuries present [31]. Adult literature demonstrates that the use of serum lactate levels or other biological markers of adequacy of resuscitation is valuable in determining the need for a damage control procedure versus an early definitive operation. Adult patients with high injury severity scores and preoperative lactate levels >3.7 had need for longer ventilation postoperatively than did those with lower lactate levels [32]. Other publications have demonstrated that preoperative lactate levels above 2.5 mmol/L had increased complication rates [33]. There are no such studies in the pediatric population, but there is no reason to believe that if the child is under-resuscitated, as determined by any valid method, delaying definitive repair would not be prudent. In such cases, a temporizing damage control procedure may be warranted.

The optimal timing of long bone fractures in the pediatric patient is also unknown. Again, adult data demonstrates a clear benefit in fixation of femur fractures within 24 h of injury. The primary benefit seems to be a decrease in pulmonary complications, particularly ARDS. The physiological differences in children make the overall incidence of ARDS much less; therefore, if studied, the outcomes may not be similar in children. The one injury pattern that is most bothersome in children is the concomitant long bone and traumatic brain injury because fixation should be accomplished as soon as possible before the cerebral edema precludes.

14.13 Vascular Injuries

Vascular injuries in civilian trauma are not common and even more infrequent in the pediatric population. It is estimated that less than 1% of all injuries are vascular in nature. As more trauma care is delivered in freestanding children's hospitals, the experience of surgeons in dealing with significant and complex vascular injuries is diminishing. Most pediatric vascular injuries are due to an accidental penetrating mechanism (Fig. 14.10), occur in males, and are in the extremities. Many are not isolated and are seen concurrently with other significant injuries. There are physiological differences in the child that must be considered when planning a reconstruction. Pediatric vessels are prone to vasospasm. This fact can be protective

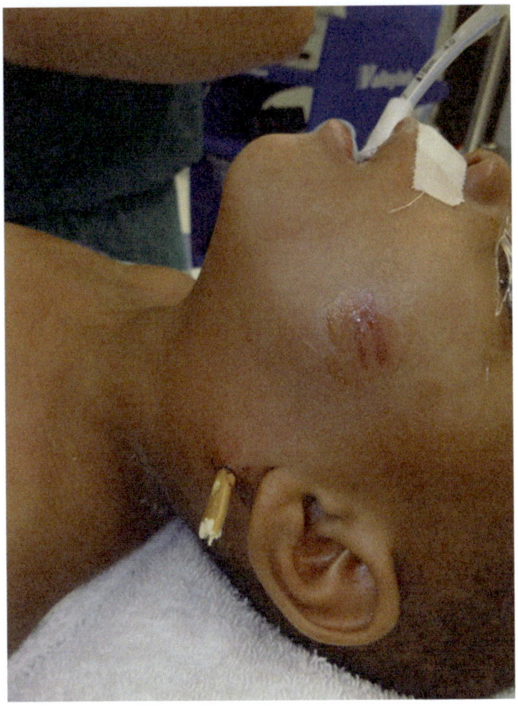

Fig. 14.10 Penetrating injury

preoperatively but can be clinically confusing intraoperatively. The use of a vasodilator around the repair is often necessary. There is also the consideration of growth in the pediatric limb and the need for growth in the vessel. Because of this concern, interrupted sutures are often used instead of a "running" suture. The benefit of this, however, has never been proven.

The last consideration is that of the use of synthetic graft material in the reconstruction [34]. The recommendation is that vascular reconstructions utilize native vessels as a conduit rather than synthetic graft material. The recommendation is based on the belief that autologous material will have a longer patency rate than a synthetic material. This however, must be balanced against the additional time that may be needed to obtain autologous conduit in a damage control situation.

Given the lack of pediatric-specific vascular expertise, the need for autologous conduit, and the likelihood of concomitant injuries, damage control for pediatric vascular injuries with temporary vascular shunts is an attractive tool to have in the armamentarium, since definitive repair of the pediatric vascular injury may not be feasible [35]. The use of such shunts is well-documented in the military and urban civilian trauma literature but is limited to anecdotal reports in the pediatric patient population.

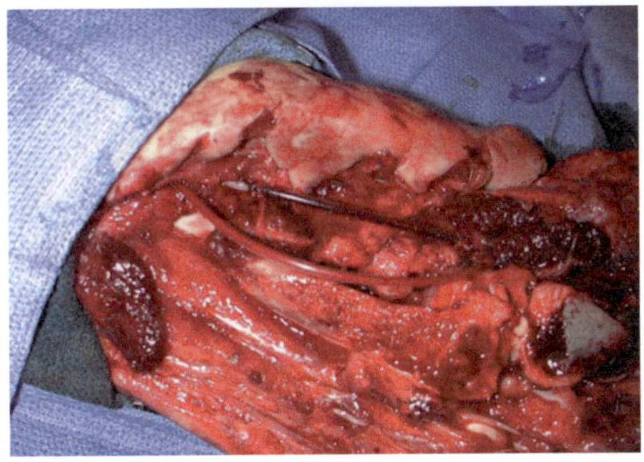

Fig. 14.11 The use of temporary shunts to restore flow in a complex pediatric injury

Argyle™ carotid shunts are ideal conduits for temporary vascular shunts in children. They range in size from 8 to 14 French. The straight shunts are 6 in. long and the looped shunts are 11 in. (Fig. 14.11). The ends are rounded and less likely to cause intimal injury for dissection with passage, and they are sufficiently stiff to tie in place with a suture to prevent dislodgement. The shunts can be used for both arterial and high flow venous injuries as a temporizing means to definitive repair.

Systemic heparinization is often used when temporizing shunts are deployed, but there are case reports of long-term use in the arterial position without heparinization with no untoward consequence.

14.14 Other Adjuncts

Blunt tracheobronchial injuries are rare in the pediatric population, but in the adolescent population, when motorized vehicles are involved, the force and complexity increase significantly. Injuries seen are typically managed with gentle ventilation and chest drainage, but the occasional high force injury sheers the bronchus at or near the carina creating a bronchopleural fistula, where hypoxia precludes successful thoracotomy and repair. The mortality reported in the adult literature is between 8 and 16%. There are no case series large enough to define a reliable mortality rate in children. In these rare incidences, extracorporeal membrane oxygenation (ECMO) has been used successfully with differential lung ventilation to manage these children through resuscitation and even into the OR for repair [36]. ECMO is a valuable tool for the stabilization of patients with respiratory or cardiac compromise; its use is limited to situations where systemic anticoagulation is feasible [37].

14.15 Summary

The changes in anatomy and physiology that occur as a child matures to adulthood influence the pattern and response to injury. While the specific response to damage control resuscitation may vary in an age-dependent way, the principles appear to be applicable to the pediatric patient. The use of damage control surgery has broad applicability in both trauma and non-trauma settings. Rapidly controlling the source of bleeding or infection, relief of intracranial pressure, and stabilization of the bony skeleton followed by continued, targeted resuscitation are undoubtedly equally beneficial in the child as it is in the adult. The opportunities presently facing us in the care of injured children are to adapt technology to aid in the damage control procedures and to elucidate further the changing physiologic response to injury and resuscitation. Only through this understanding will we take full advantage of these concepts.

References

1. Shrestha B, Holcomb JB, Camp EA, Del Junco DJ, Cotton BA, Albarado R, Gill BS, Kozar RA, Kao LS, McNutt MK, Moore LJ, Love JD, Tyson GH 3rd, Adams PR, Khan S, Wade CE. Damage-control resuscitation increases successful nonoperative management rates and survival after severe blunt liver injury. J Trauma Acute Care Surg. 2015;78(2):336–41.
2. Centers for Disease Control. Web-based Injury Statistics Query and Reporting System (WISQARS). Atlanta, GA: US Department of Health and Human Services, 10 Leading Causes of Nonfatal Injury, United States; 2014. https://www.cdc.gov/injury/wisqars. Accessed 1 Dec 2016.
3. Al-Hassani A, Abdulrahaman H, Afifi I, Almadani A, Al-Den A, Al-Kuwari A, Recicar J, Nabir S, Maull KI. Rib fracture patterns predict thoracic chest wall and abdominal solid organ injury. Am Surg. 2010; 76(8):888–91.
4. Rosenberg G, Bryant AK, Davis KA, Schuster KM. No breakpoint for mortality in pediatric rib fractures. J Trauma Acute Care Surg. 2016;80(3):427–32.
5. Andrew M, Paes B, Johnston M. Development of the hemostatic system in the neonate and young infant. Am J Pediatr Hematol Oncol. 1990;12(1):95–104.
6. Andrew M, Milner R, Johnston M, Mitchell L, Tollefsen DM, Castle V, Powers P. Development of the human coagulation system in the healthy premature infant. Blood. 1988;72(5):1651–7.
7. Andrew M, Paes B, Milner R, Johnston M, Mitchell L, Tollefsen DM, Powers P. Development of the human coagulation system in the full-term infant. Blood. 1987;70(1):165–72.
8. Andrew M, Vegh P, Johnston M, Bowker J, Ofosu F, Mitchell L. Maturation of the hemostatic system during childhood. Blood. 1992;80(8):1998–2005.
9. Advanced Trauma Life Support (ATLS). American College of Surgeons' Committee on Trauma, and International ATLS Working Group. 9th ed. Chicago, IL: The ATLS Subcommittee. 2012.
10. Christiaans SC, Duhachek-Stapelman AL, Russell RT, Lisco SJ, Kerby JD, Pittet JF. Coagulopathy after severe pediatric trauma. Shock. 2014;41(6):476–90.
11. Liras IN, Cotton BA, Cardenas JC, Harting MT. Prevalence and impact of admission hyperfibrinolysis in severely injured pediatric patients. Surgery. 2015; 158(3):812–8.
12. Leeper CM, Neal MD, McKenna C, Sperry J, Gaines BA. Abnormalities in fibrinolysis at the time of admission are associated with DVT, mortality and disability in a pediatric trauma population. J Trauma Acute Care Surg. 2017;82(1):27–34.
13. Vogel AM, Radwanss ZA, Cox CS Jr, Cotton BA. Admission rapid thromboelastography delivers real-time "actionable" data in pediatric trauma. J Pediatr Surg. 2013;48(6):1371–6.
14. Hendrickson JE, Shaz BH, Pereira G, Atkins E, Johnson KK, Bao G, Easley KA, Josephson CD. Coagulopathy is prevalent and associated with adverse outcomes in transfused pediatric trauma patients. J Pediatr. 2012;160(2):204–9.
15. Navaratnam M, Ng A, Williams GD, Maeda K, Mendoza JM, Concepcion W, Hollander SA, Ramamoorthy C. Perioperative management of pediatric en-bloc combined heart-liver transplants: a case series review. Paediatr Anaesth. 2016;26(10):976–86.
16. Eckert MJ, Wertin TM, Tyner SD, Nelson DW, Izenberg S, Martin MJ. Tranexamic acid administration to pediatric trauma patients in a combat setting: the pediatric trauma and tranexamic acid study (PED-TRAX). J Trauma Acute Care Surg. 2014;77(6): 852–8.

17. Nishijima DK, Monuteaux MC, Faraoni D, Goobie SM, Lee L, Galante J, Holmes JF, Kuppermann N. Tranexamic acid use in United States Children's Hospitals. J Emerg Med. 2016;50(6):868–74.
18. Arkansas Children's Hospital Clinical Laboratory: Massive Transfusions. ACH Policy and Procedures, November 2016.
19. Neff LP, Cannon JW, Morrison JJ, Edwards MJ, Spinella PC, Borgman MA. Clearly defining pediatric massive transfusion: cutting through the fog and friction with combat data. J Trauma Acute Care Surg. 2015;78(1):22–8.
20. Chidester SJ, Williams N, Wang W, Groner JI. A pediatric massive transfusion protocol. J Trauma Acute Care Surg. 2012;73(5):1273–7.
21. Nosanov L, Inaba K, Okoye O, Resnick S, Upperman J, Shulman I, Rhee P, Demetriades D. The impact of blood product ratios in massively transfused pediatric trauma patients. Am J Surg. 2013;206(5):655–60.
22. Resources for Optimal Care of the Injured Patient. Chicago, IL: American College of Surgeons, Committee on Trauma. 2014. Print.
23. Pumberger W, Kohlhauser C, Mayr M, Pomberger G. Severe liver haemorrhage during laparotomy in very low birthweight infants. Acta Paediatr. 2002;91(11): 1260–2.
24. Villalona GA, Mckee MA, Diefenbach KA. Damage control surgery in a <1 kg neonate: a brief report. Yale J Biol Med. 2013;86(3):385–7.
25. Talving P, Lustenberger T, Lam L, Inaba K, Mohseni S, Plurad D, Green DJ, Demetriades D. Coagulopathy after isolated severe traumatic brain injury in children. J Trauma. 2011;71(5):1205–10.
26. Harhangi BS, Kompanje EJ, Leebeek FW, Maas AI. Coagulation disorders after traumatic brain injury. Acta Neurochir. 2008;150(2):165–75. discussion 175
27. Rosenfeld JV. Damage control neurosurgery. Injury. 2004;35(7):655–0.
28. The 4th Edition of Guidelines for Management of Severe Traumatic Brain Injury. Campbell, CA: Brain Trauma Foundation; 2016.
29. Kochanek PM, Carney N, Adelson PD, Ashwal S, Bell MJ, Bratton S, Carson S, Chesnut RM, Ghajar J, Goldstein B, Grant GA, Kissoon N, Peterson K, Selden NR, Tasker RC, Tong KA, Vavilala MS, Wainwright MS, Warden CR. Guidelines for the acute medical management of severe traumatic brain injury in infants, children, and adolescents—second edition. Pediatr Crit Care Med. 2012;13(Suppl 1):S1–82, Erratum in: Pediatr Crit Care Med. 2012 Mar;13(2):252.
30. Mooney JF. The use of 'damage control orthopedics' techniques in children with segmental open fractures. J Pediatr Orthop B. 2012;21(5):400–3.
31. Flynn JM, Schwend RM. Management of pediatric femoral shaft fractures. J Am Acad Orthop Surg. 2004;12(5):347–59.
32. Richards JE, Matuszewski PE, Grififin SM, Koehler DM, Guillamondegui OD, O'Toole RV, Bosse MJ, Obremskey WT, Evans JM. The role of elevated lactate as a risk factor for pulmonary mortality after early fixation of femoral shaft fractures. J Orthop Trauma. 2016;30(6):312–8.
33. Crowl AC, Young JS, Kahler DM, Claridge JA, Chrzanowski DS, Pomphrey M. Occult hypoperfusion is associated with increased morbidity in patients undergoing early femur fracture fixation. J Trauma. 2000;48(2):260–7.
34. Kirkilas M, Notrica DM, Langlais CS, Muenzer JT, Zoldos J, Graziano K. Outcomes of arterial vascular extremity trauma in pediatric patients. J Pediatr Surg. 2016;51(11):1885–90.
35. Inaba K, Aksoy H, Seamon MJ, Marks JA, Duchesne J, Schroll R, Fox CJ, Pieracci FM, Moore EE, Joseph B, Haider AA, Harvin JA, Lawless RA, Cannon J, Holland SR, Demetriades D, Multicenter Shunt Study Group. Multicenter evaluation of temporary intravascular shunt use in vascular trauma. J Trauma Acute Care Surg. 2016;80(3):359–64; discussion 364–5.
36. Garlick J, Maxson T, Imamura M, Green J, Prodhan P. Differential lung ventilation and venovenous extracorporeal membrane oxygenation for traumatic bronchopleural fistula. Ann Thorac Surg. 2013;96(5): 1859–60.
37. Cornfield DN. Acute respiratory distress syndrome in children: physiology and management. Curr Opin Pediatr. 2013;25(3):338–43.

Damage Control Resuscitation in Surgical Critical Care

15

Asanthi Ratnasekera, Patrick Reilly, and Paula Ferrada

15.1 Introduction

Damage control surgery was born out of the need to adapt surgical procedures to fit the physiological state of the patient. Although today leaving an open abdomen and performing a trauma procedure in stages are widely practiced, this was not the case decades ago [1]. Other procedures beyond laparotomy have also been employed, prioritizing trauma patient survival by using a damage control philosophy [2].

Damage control resuscitation (DCR) combines multiple principles that support the surgical approach described above. These include early resuscitation of the multi-injured patient with blood products; avoiding hypothermia, acidosis, and coagulopathy; prioritizing the control of hemorrhage in (and outside of) the operating room; and avoiding massive crystalloid resuscitation. The DCR approach begins in the trauma bay, continues in the operating room, and extends to the intensive care unit as well as other areas of the hospital (e.g., interventional radiology) where the multi-injured patient may require care. In the rural setting where prehospital times may be prolonged, DCR combined with permissive hypotension may also be employed.

15.2 Blood Product Resuscitation

Early initiation of blood product resuscitation is the hallmark of DCR for the bleeding multi-injured patient. Crystalloid resuscitation is extensively limited as red cell, plasma, and platelet transfusion are administered to resuscitate, while concomitant attempts at bleeding control are undertaken. Attempts to limit trauma-induced coagulopathy are of paramount importance as its development increases the mortality rate in a critically ill trauma patient.

Electronic supplementary material The online version of this chapter (https://doi.org/10.1007/978-3-319-72607-6_15) contains supplementary material, which is available to authorized users.

A. Ratnasekera, D.O.
Department of Surgery, Virginia Commonwealth University, Richmond, VA, USA

P. Reilly, M.D.
Department of Surgery, University of Pennsylvania, Philadelphia, PA, USA

P. Ferrada, M.D., F.A.C.S. (✉)
Department of Surgery, Virginia Commonwealth University, Richmond, VA, USA

West Hospital, Richmond, VA, USA
e-mail: pferrada@mcvh-vcu.edu

J. Duchesne et al. (eds.), *Damage Control in Trauma Care*,
https://doi.org/10.1007/978-3-319-72607-6_15

The pathogenesis of trauma-induced coagulopathy is complex and however is important to understand. The prospective, observational, multicenter, major trauma transfusion (PROMMTT) study by Cohen et al., which enrolled 1245 bleeding trauma patients from ten major trauma centers, analyzed blood samples from a subset of 165 patients who had coagulation factor levels obtained [3]. The investigators found that the combination of increased injury severity and increased hypoperfusion was significantly associated with increased activated protein C (APC) activity, prolonged PT and PTT, increased fibrinolysis, and depletion of factors I, II, V, VII, VIII, IX, and X. The decreases in factor levels and increased activated protein C levels correlate with hypoperfusion and injury severity [4–6].

APC cannot be held the single culprit for coagulopathy of trauma. In the setting of trauma, multiple factors are associated. Endothelial injury from trauma has been recognized to upregulate both procoagulant and anticoagulant mechanisms. Endothelial injury can lead to microthrombosis to maintain perfusion to end organs but can also cause an anticoagulant effect to counterbalance the procoagulant effects [7, 8].

Injury to the endothelial glycocalyx by trauma, hypoxemia, or hypoperfusion leads to extravasation of protein and fluid leading to edema. Components of endothelial glycocalyx such as chondroitin sulfate and heparin sulfate can lead to anticoagulation pathways. Transfused plasma is known to repair endothelial glycocalyx compared to crystalloids. In the setting of an injured endothelial glycocalyx, crystalloid use can aggravate peripheral and bowel edema [8].

Platelet dysfunction is known to contribute to coagulopathy of trauma; however, the exact mechanism is unknown. In hemorrhagic shock, the mass activation of platelets to achieve hemostasis may exhaust platelet function and thereby cause coagulopathy. Platelet dysfunction in the setting of hemorrhagic shock, acidosis, and hypothermia may cause inactivation of the platelet. Platelet transfusion along with other blood products may improve survival. The pragmatic, randomized optimal platelet and plasma ratios (PROPPR) study randomized 680 bleeding trauma patients to receive high or low ratios of plasma and platelets to packed red blood cells (1:1:1 vs. 1:1:2). The high plasma and platelet ratio (1:1:1) group had reduced risk of exsanguination (9% vs. 15%) and improved achievement of clinical hemostasis (86% vs. 78%) compared with the 1:1:2 group [4].

The breakdown of fibrinogen to fibrin is an important part of the coagulation pathway in forming a stable clot to maintain hemostasis. Lower clot strength was found in trauma patients which can increase coagulopathy and mortality. Trauma patients with low levels of fibrinogen may benefit replacement with cryoprecipitate. Fibrinolysis which is the degradation of the fibrin matrix by plasmin is also an important part of the coagulation pathway. Plasmin is created by cleavage of plasminogen by tissue plasminogen activators (TPA). TPAs are secreted in response to injury and catecholamines by the endothelium. Hyperfibrinolysis can also lead to hemorrhagic shock. The clinical randomization of an antifibrinolytic in significant hemorrhage 2 (CRASH-2) trial was performed to analyze the effect of empiric antifibrinolytic treatment. The trial randomized over 20,000 trauma patients at risk for hemorrhage to receive placebo or tranexamic acid (TXA), which binds to plasminogen and inhibits its activation by TPA. TXA reduced death due to bleeding. The largest reduction of exsanguination was seen when TXA was given within 1 hour of injury (RR, 0.68; 95% CI, 0.57–0.82), with a lesser benefit observed when given between 1 and 3 hours (RR, 0.79; 95% CI, 0.64–0.97), whereas exsanguination was increased when TXA was given after 3 hours (RR, 1.44; 95% CI, 1.12–1.84). For patients receiving TXA within 3 h of injury, the absolute risk reduction for exsanguination was 1.9% [9, 10].

Shock itself is a cause of coagulopathy of trauma. Shock can lead to acidemia and hypoperfusion of tissues which leads to inactivation of coagulation factors and proteins. A base deficit greater than six was also shown to have an effect of acidemia and hypoperfusion which in turn will lead to coagulopathy. Hemodilution with crystalloid solution resuscitation has been studied to decrease clot function and stability. Acidemia can also result from excessive crystalloid use which can lead to an unstable clot formation [5, 11].

Although coagulopathy of trauma is multifactorial and can resemble disseminated intravascular coagulopathy, the management may be different. Prolonged PT, PTT, and INR are commonly seen in cases of DIC and however may not be evident in coagulopathy of trauma. The use of thromboelastography (TEG) may provide more information regarding the phase of coagulation pathway that may be affected in the multi-injured trauma patient (see Fig. 15.1). TEG is a method to analyze the capacity to clot. The test determines four values that represent clot formation: reaction time *R*, *K* value, the angle, and the maximum amplitude (MA).

The *R* value is the time that takes to produce a clot. The *K* value represents the speed of clot formation. The angle is the tangent of the curve made as the *K* is reached and offers similar information to *K*. The MA is an indicator of clot strength.

The identification of the deficiency in the clot forming pathway is important in the patient with coagulopathy of trauma. This will guide blood product transfusion and resuscitation [5, 9, 10].

15.2.1 Summary

- Coagulopathy of trauma is multifactorial and can lead to hemorrhagic shock and increase mortality.
- Shock itself can cause coagulopathy of trauma with destruction of glycocalyx and platelet dysfunction.

15.3 Resuscitation to Euvolemia

Resuscitation to normovolemia is one of the most important aspects of DCR [12–14]. A multimodality approach to goals of resuscitation should be utilized. Goal-directed therapy and resuscitation to normovolemia are important to avoid over-resuscitation with blood products and crystalloids. An analysis of the National Trauma Data Bank in 2011 demonstrated that intravenous fluid (IVF) administration was associated with higher mortality in trauma patients, including a significant increase in mortality in patients with penetrating

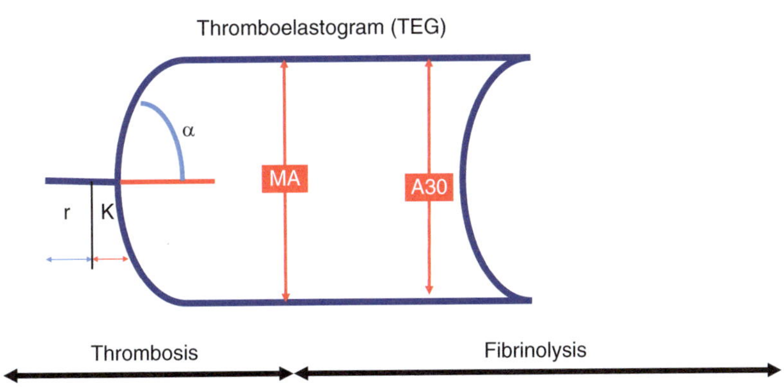

Fig. 15.1 Thromboelastography (TEG): R = the reaction; it represents the time until the first evidence of a clot is detected. K = value of time from the end of R until the clot reaches 20 mm, and this represents the speed of clot formation. α: The angle is the tangent of the curve made as the K is reached and offers similar information to K. MA = maximum amplitude. It is a reflection of clot strength

mechanism. While coagulopathy of trauma is a major concern, over-resuscitation with blood products also carries rates of increased hypocalcemia and coagulopathy of massive transfusion [7].

Volume status evaluation continues to be a complex issue to obtain. While in the intensive care unit, advanced hemodynamic monitoring can be utilized, and in austere circumstances, less advanced methods need to be considered to help the patient in need [15]. It is important to recognize that we are trying to achieve perfusion and that all the tools we use for hemodynamic monitoring add to the picture to help us guide therapy. There are no perfect tools for hemodynamic monitoring, and none of them replaces clinical judgment.

Basic goals of resuscitation including urine output of >0.5 cm^3/kg/h and MAP goals >65 are accepted but by no means perfect when addressing volume status. Other clinical indicators may include tachycardia, tachypnea, prolonged capillary refill, and diaphoresis. These clinical parameters are subjective and require the clinical acumen of the provider to be recognized as a sign of lack of perfusion [7].

The primary resuscitation question is whether the patient will increase their cardiac output in response to intravascular volume infusion. This will depend on the physiological state of the patient as well as potential comorbidities. One way to address this is with the response to passive leg rising. Other noninvasive modalities include use of stroke volume variation and/or continuous cardiac output monitors. It is important to understand the limitation of these devices in patients with arrhythmias and spontaneously breathing.

Central venous pressure can be used as trend; however the values in patients with high ventilator pressures this parameter is very limited. Pulmonary artery catheters may still be indicated in some clinical scenarios. However, the operator must infer volume status secondary to a pressure reading. It places patients at risk for complications such as pulmonary emboli and other risks inherent to the placement. These and other methods to evaluate volume status are examined below.

15.4 Cardiac Ultrasound

Cardiac ultrasound has been demonstrated to be simple to undertake, reproducible, and accurate to guide therapy. It has limitations, most of them linked to operator expertise. Ultrasound-guided resuscitation is a dynamic and noninvasive method of goal-directed resuscitation in a multi-injured patient. Basic understanding of ultrasound physics is necessary since ultrasonography is operator dependent. Use of ultrasonography can provide the critical care surgeon with accurate hemodynamic information rapidly. It is essential to understand the components of the ultrasound system. The transmitter controls electrical signals sent to the transducer. The receiver processes the electrical signal. The transducer or probe contains piezoelectric crystals to convert electric and acoustic energy. The monitor displays the image transmitted. A diagnostic ultrasound uses transducer frequencies ranging from 2.5 to 10 MHz. High-frequency ultrasound shows excellent resolution in superficial structures such as soft tissue abscesses and is used in breast imaging. Lower-frequency transducers can emit waves deep into the tissues and can visualize organs. Increasing frequency of an image can also increase resolution. Speed at which sonography is propagated through is dependent on the medium. Ultrasound waves travel better through solids and liquids. They do not travel well through structures with air. A good ultrasound image is generated by the medium the waves travel through and the amount of waves reflected once it hits a target organ. Amplitude which is the height of the wave is reduced as waves travel through tissue. The higher the frequency, the less the transducers can visualize deep structures. Increasing gain can increase the amplitude of the returning ultrasound waves [15–18].

Use of ultrasound to ensure resuscitation to normovolemia is a rapid and dynamic modality. Assessment of normovolemia can be facilitated by a few ultrasound views. A subcostal view or a right midaxillary posterior view of the IVC in long axis approximately 2 cm from the atriocaval junction can be useful. The measurement of IVC and the variability in respirations can be used in a hypovolemic patient with positive pressure ventilation. IVC size variability with respirations >50% collapse or a flat IVC is indicative of a hypovolemic patient. However, a full IVC does not rule out hypovolemia. The IVC variability must be assessed in a full respiratory cycle [4].

The parasternal long axis view can be obtained by placing the probe left of the sternum with the arrow of the probe pointing to the right shoulder between the second and third intercostal space. This will show the contractility of the left and right ventricles as well as the left ventricular outflow tract.

The apical view can be obtained by placing the probe at the point of maximal impulse or below the nipple with the probe in a horizontal manner. This view is excellent to view all the chambers and the pericardium.

These views can demonstrate the contractility of the heart, the collapsibility of the IVC, and the right ventricle demonstrating volume status. The use of ultrasound to guide resuscitation is a quick method that can aid the clinician obtain information regarding the patient's hemodynamic and volume status [12, 16, 19]. Figures 15.2 and 15.3 show an empty and full IVC. Videos 15.1 and 15.2 are the dynamic view of these parameters.

Advantages

- Gives dynamic images and information of the current volume status of the patient
- Able to obtain critical information in an efficient manner
- Noninvasive modality of assessing normovolemia

Pitfalls

- User training is required to obtain clinically significant images.
- User dependency on obtaining accurate information.

15.5 Stroke Volume Variation

There are several devices available that measure stroke volume variation (SVV). The FloTrac/Vigileo monitor (Edwards Lifesciences, Irvine, CA) measures pulse pressure-derived cardiac output (CO) without external calibration. It is a noninvasive method of obtaining CO and SVV measurements. It also provides calculations in stroke volume (SV) and cardiac index (CI). The Vigileo monitor requires the presence of an arterial catheter. The third-generation and fourth-generation software has provided the above information calculated every 20 s to 1 min. The software analyzes arterial waveform with a frequency of a 100 Hz. The Vigileo system can provide dynamic information on the patient's

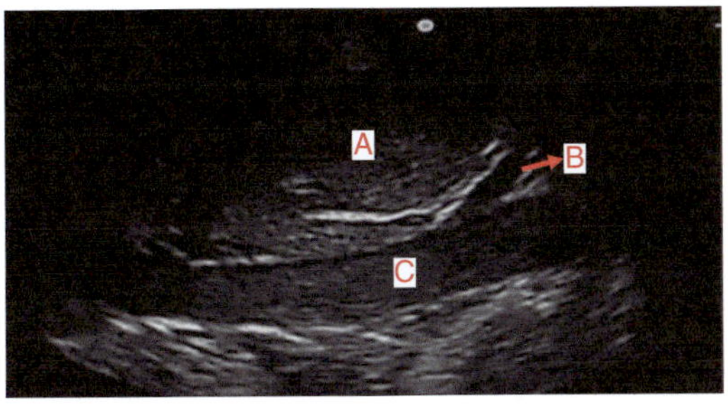

Fig. 15.2 Full inferior vena cava. Picture of a full Inferior Vena Cava with minimal variation. *A*: Liver, *B*: hepatic veins. *C*: IVC

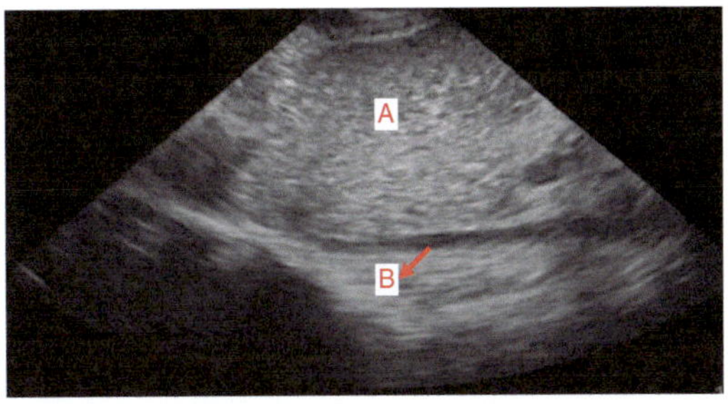

Fig. 15.3 Empty IVC. Picture of a flat inferior vena cava. *A*: Liver, *B*: IVC. Hepatic veins not visible

hemodynamic status with ease. However, it carries its own disadvantages. Studies have shown that Vigileo information is not accurate in patients with arrhythmias and hyperdynamic cardiac output and patients with low SVRs. The patient should also ideally have no spontaneous breathing efforts [20].

Advantages

- The clinician can easily access information from the Vigileo monitor which can easily be set up.
- Provides access to information in a real-time setting.
- Mostly minimally invasive for the patient.

Pitfalls

- Requires an arterial catheter
- Information inaccurate in patients with arrhythmias and spontaneously breathing

15.6 Swan-Ganz Catheter

The Swan-Ganz catheter or pulmonary arterial catheter (PAC) has long been used in the ICU setting. It was first introduced in 1970 by HJ Swan and W Ganz. It has recently been trending out of favor in the ICU setting due to the advent of other noninvasive modalities for hemodynamic monitoring. The PAC is still used in the ICU setting in a variety of clinical situations. The PAC requires placement of a large-bore central line such as a Cordis® catheter through the internal jugular or subclavian vein. Then the PAC is passed through the right atrium and right ventricle and "floated" into the pulmonary artery. Waveform monitoring is used during the procedure to establish placement of the PAC into the pulmonary artery.

Once the catheter is "floated," a pulmonary artery wedge pressure can be obtained. The wedge pressure can provide an estimate of the left ventricular preload. With the PAC, pulmonary artery pressure, central venous pressure (CVP), CO, pulmonary artery saturation, mixed venous oxygen saturation, and core temperatures can be measured. The SVR, SV, oxygen delivery, oxygen consumption, pulmonary vascular resistance, and ventricular pressures are calculated. Real-time monitoring of these parameters is useful in resuscitation to normovolemia in the critically ill patient.

User technical training is required to "float" the PAC. While the PAC assists in the management of the critically ill patient, literature has proven no benefit or improvement in mortality with the use of PAC. The PAC is still used in many settings such as intraoperative and postoperative management of liver transplant patients, open cardiac bypass patients, and patients with severe pulmonary hypertension. There are several complications that arise from the PAC. Those that are related to central venous access are air embolus, pneumothorax, and inadvertent arterial puncture. The complications related to the catheterization itself are dysrhythmias and heart block. Finally, complications related to catheter presence are pulmonary artery rupture and pulmonary vein thrombus [21].

Advantages

- Real-time monitoring of CO, SVR, CI, and intracardiac pressures which may guide resuscitation to normovolemia
- Can be effectively used in certain surgical patient population such as open cardiac surgery and liver transplant surgery patients

Pitfalls

- No proven benefit in mortality or length of stay in critically ill patients
- Requires central venous access and catheter "floating" and placement in the pulmonary artery for accurate information
- Has intrinsic complications related to central venous access, catheterization, and catheter presence

15.7 Esophageal Doppler

Transcutaneous Doppler ultrasound (Cardio Q™, Deltex, UK) has been in use to measure pulse velocity in peripheral and central vessels for a long time. The use of Doppler ultrasound via a probe in the esophagus has been used to measure the blood velocity in the descending aorta. The blood velocity measurement in the descending aorta can be used to calculate cardiac output and stroke volume. A flexible probe is inserted through the mouth into the esophagus to 40 cm length. The probe has piezoelectric crystals that produces ultrasound images. The probe tip lies along the descending aorta. The velocity of the red blood cells is obtained and is converted to flow using an algorithm. Factors such as age, gender, weight, and height are considered. This relatively noninvasive method can provide real-time cardiac output and stroke volume measurements beat by beat. The distribution of cardiac output in the setting of varying sympathetic tone in the critically ill patients may provide inaccurate measurements. Also, the diameter of the descending aorta is calculated based on patient characteristics. If the patient is not thoroughly sedated, movement of the Doppler may occur and loss of signal may result [22].

Advantages

- Provides real-time information on CO and SV
- Relatively noninvasive

Pitfalls

- May represent inaccurate information based on patients requiring vasopressors.
- Diameter of the descending aorta is not measured but calculated using patient characteristics.
- Requires patient sedation.

15.7.1 Summary

- Many noninvasive and invasive modalities are used in the ICU setting for hemodynamic monitoring.
- One modality may not be sufficient to obtain the whole picture on volume status.
- Resuscitation to normovolemia should be the goal for every surgical critical care patient using these modalities.
- Each modality carries its own advantages and pitfalls.

15.8 Fluid Overload

Avoiding massive crystalloid resuscitation is one of the mainstays of DCR. Resuscitation to fluid overload status can cause congestive heart failure, compartment syndromes, and coagulopathy. Therefore, resuscitation to normovolemia is important in the multi-injured trauma patient in the ICU.

Assessing fluid overload in the critically ill trauma patient is also a multimodality method. Signs of fluid overload can be visualized in physical exam by increasing daily weights, peripheral edema, and pulmonary vascular congestion seen on chest X-ray. Signs of cephalization and curly B lines are commonly seen on chest X-ray in patients with fluid overload [7, 8, 11, 13, 14, 23–26].

Another method of assessing fluid overload is with ultrasound. The IVC may appear "full" and does not change with fluid challenges. During respiratory cycle, the IVC may not have any variation in size. Visualizing ultrasound lung comets can also indicate pulmonary congestion due to fluid overload. Ultrasound comet tails originate from water-thickened interlobular septa and fan out from the lung surface. The technique requires ultrasound scanning of the anterior right and left chest, from the second to the fifth intercostal space [16, 19, 27].

Compartment syndrome is a complication from over-resuscitation. Compartment syndrome can occur from severe injuries, burns, and sepsis. Literature describes the detrimental effect on the glycocalyx from over-resuscitation. The destruction of the glycocalyx can lead to capillary leak and extravasation of fluid from the intravascular space to the interstitial space. The fluid in the interstitial space can lead to bowel edema, increased intracranial pressures, and pulmonary edema. It may also manifest as extremity and abdominal compartment syndrome. Compartment syndrome is defined as organ failure or dysfunction due to decreased perfusion pressures or blood flow to the organ and may occur with over-resuscitation with fluid or blood products. A normal intra-abdominal pressure in a supine, relaxed patient is below 10 mmHg. A pressure of greater than 12 mmHg is intra-abdominal hypertension. In the surgical intensive care unit, a catheter can be placed into the stomach or the bladder for measurement of abdominal pressures. The most commonly used method is a catheter placed into the bladder with the patient supine and relaxed. 25 cm^3 of saline is injected into the empty bladder and is connected to a pressure transducer or manometer. This is a reliable method of trending abdominal pressures. Peak airway pressures if the patient is mechanically ventilated can also be useful. Peak pressures greater than 45 and difficulty in ventilation can be indicative of abdominal compartment syndrome.

Treatment varies with grade of abdominal hypertension. Use of diuretics such as mannitol may be helpful to excrete excess fluid. In the presence of ascites, abdominal paracentesis or laparoscopic-guided drainage of ascites will be helpful. However, decompressive laparotomy is required to relieve abdominal compartment syndrome and reestablish abdominal perfusion pressures.

15.9 Overstretching of the Heart

With over-resuscitation and increasing preload, an increase in CVP and atrial stretching can be noted. Arial stretching can cause release of atrial natriuretic peptide (ANP) and brain natriuretic peptide (BNP). These peptides released by the atrial myocytes in response to atrial distension from hypervolemic states inhibit the renin–angiotensin–aldosterone system causing natriuresis and diuresis. These peptides also increase glomerular filtration rate causing increased diuresis as well. This effect decreases plasma volume and preload. ANP and BNP directly vasodilate arteries and decrease SVR. They can also venodilate and decrease preload in turn. This may cause decreased perfusion to the end organs and cause ischemia of the organs as well [28].

15.9.1 Summary

- Resuscitation to normovolemia is key in critically ill patients in the ICU.
- Resuscitation causing volume overload has many adverse effects including coagulopathy, pulmonary edema, bowel edema, and abdominal compartment syndrome.
- Resuscitation causing volume overload can also increase ANP and BNP levels causing reflex hypovolemia, hypotension, and decreased perfusion to end organs.

15.10 Recurrent Hypovolemia

Hypovolemia and hypovolemic shock are most commonly caused by hemorrhage in trauma or surgery and intestinal losses from GI-related diseases. Hypovolemia causes decreased preload and therefore decreased cardiac output and can decrease perfusion to end organs causing ischemia. End organ ischemia can result in lactic acidosis and oxygen deficiency and dysfunction in tissue. In the presence of oxygen, a glucose molecule can create 38 ATP molecules which can provide energy for cellular function. In the absence of oxygen, glucose cannot be taken into cells due to insufficient pyruvate. Pyruvate is converted into lactate: lactate ratio is increased in oxygen absent states. In states of hypovolemia, systemic oxygen delivery is decreased, and in turn tissue oxygen extraction is increased. This can be demonstrated by decreased percentage of mixed central venous oxygen saturations (SVO2 or SCVO2). When levels of oxygen needed for tissues are not maintained, anaerobic metabolism ensues with increasing lactate production.

Under resuscitation can lead to tissue ischemia, decreased organ perfusion, and lactic acidosis. Under resuscitation with hypotension can lead to a state of shock and organ dysfunction. End organ dysfunction can be manifested in many signs of symptoms. Neurologically patients may present with altered mental status or state of anxiety. In cardiovascular setting, patient may present with tachycardia and hypotension. Bowel edema and ischemia may present with decreased perfusion to bowel. Acute kidney injury may occur in the event of decreased perfusion to the kidneys with decreased urine output [7, 12, 13].

15.10.1 Summary

- Hypovolemia from hemorrhagic shock or septic shock can lead to tissue ischemia with decreased oxygen delivery.
- 1:1:1 resuscitation in hemorrhagic shock with early blood product use is a new paradigm.
- Permissive hypotension has shown to decrease mortality in patients with hemorrhagic shock.

Figure 15.4 represents recommendations when revaluating a hypotensive ICU patient for resuscitation to normovolemia.

15.11 The ICU as a State of Mind Not a Physical Location

Resuscitation to normovolemia should be accepted as paradigm not only in the ICU but also in the trauma bay, the operating room, and wherever the injured patient requires care. In trauma, most patients' hypotension will be associated with hypovolemia. However, there are other causes of hypotension to consider such as pump failure (either secondary to cardiac contusion or a cardiac event prior to the trauma), neurogenic shock, and in late stages of severe traumatic brain injury. Furthermore, once the patient is resuscitated and the bleeding has been stopped, care must be taken not to swing the pendulum to the other extreme. Elderly patients are at a high risk for deleterious effects form over-resuscitation.

Resuscitation to normovolemia can be accomplished in the trauma bay using ultrasound and the use of other end points of resuscitation.

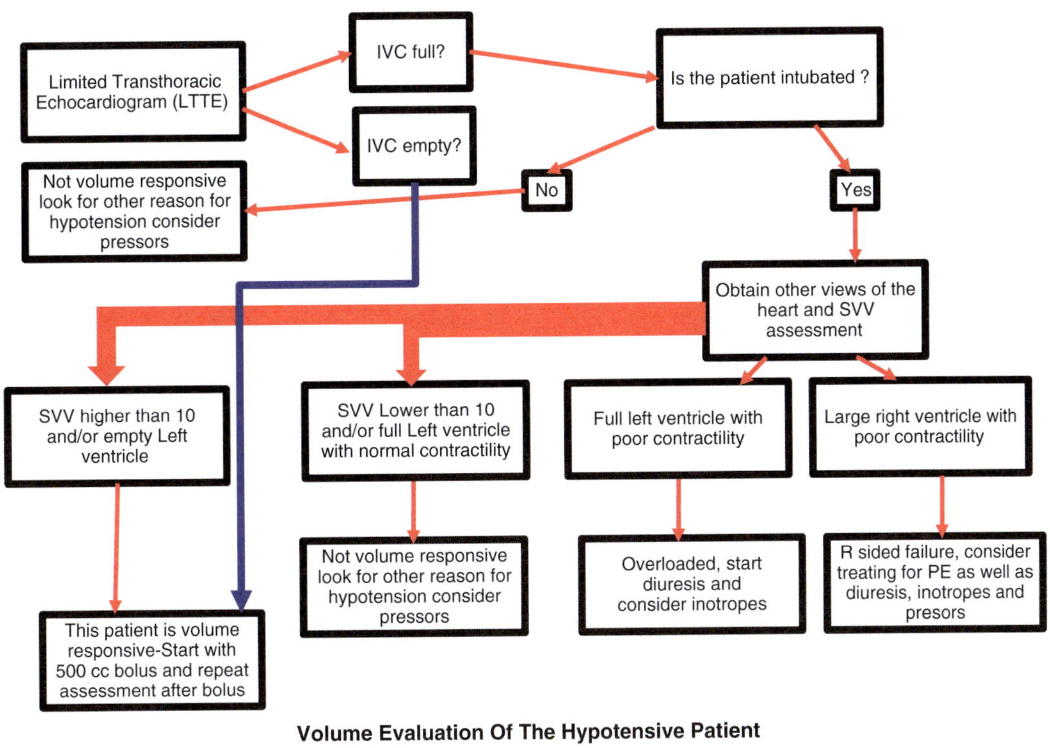

Fig. 15.4 How to evaluate a hypotensive patient

Communication with anesthesia during damage control surgery and goal to achieve hemostasis and normovolemia are important concepts in the operating room. The use of esophageal Doppler intraoperatively would be helpful in maintaining normovolemia during damage control surgery.

In rural or underserved trauma communities, access to advanced hemodynamic monitoring and specialized testing may be limited. However, damage control resuscitation can be achieved in rural and underserved communities. Use of ultrasound for assessment of normovolemia can be used in these communities with ease. The ownership and education of surgeons regarding ultrasound modalities for damage control resuscitation can easily be achieved. The American College of Surgeons offers basic and advanced ultrasound courses that may be completed with easy access. The use of ultrasound can be extended for bedside procedures and in diagnosing deep vein thrombosis as well. The use of ultrasound can also be extended to mid-level providers who aid in the care of the critically ill trauma patient.

Damage control resuscitation and resuscitation to normovolemia are concepts that should be utilized in all trauma patients and should be a vital part of management of the trauma patient and not an adjunct.

15.11.1 Summary

- Damage control resuscitation can be used in the trauma bay, OR, and ICU.
- Multimodality approach can be used to resuscitate to normovolemia in these places.
- DCR can be extended to rural and underserved trauma communities.

References

1. Rotondo MF, Schwab CW, McGonigal MD, Phillips GR 3rd, Fruchterman TM, Kauder DR, et al. 'Damage control': an approach for improved survival in exsanguinating penetrating abdominal injury. J Trauma. 1993;35(3):375–82; discussion 2–3.
2. Waibel BH, Rotondo MM. Damage control surgery: it's evolution over the last 20 years. Rev Col Bras Cir. 2012;39(4):314–21.
3. Holcomb JB, del Junco DJ, Fox EE, Wade CE, Cohen MJ, Schreiber MA, et al. The prospective, observational, multicenter, major trauma transfusion (PROMMTT) study: comparative effectiveness of a time-varying treatment with competing risks. JAMA Surg. 2013;148(2):127–36.
4. Baraniuk S, Tilley BC, del Junco DJ, Fox EE, van Belle G, Wade CE, et al. Pragmatic Randomized Optimal Platelet and Plasma Ratios (PROPPR) Trial: design, rationale and implementation. Injury. 2014; 45(9):1287–95.
5. Chang R, Cardenas JC, Wade CE, Holcomb JB. Advances in the understanding of trauma-induced coagulopathy. Blood. 2016;128(8):1043–9.
6. Engels PT, Rezende-Neto JB, Al Mahroos M, Scarpelini S, Rizoli SB, Tien HC. The natural history of trauma-related coagulopathy: implications for treatment. J Trauma. 2011;71(5 Suppl 1):S448–55.
7. Edwards MR, Mythen MG. Fluid therapy in critical illness. Extreme Physiol Med. 2014;3:16.
8. Funk D, Bohn J, Mutch W, Hayakawa T, Buchel EW. Goal-directed fluid therapy for microvascular free flap reconstruction following mastectomy: a pilot study. Plastic Surg. 2015;23(4):231–4.
9. Dente CJ, Shaz BH, Nicholas JM, Harris RS, Wyrzykowski AD, Patel S, et al. Improvements in early mortality and coagulopathy are sustained better in patients with blunt trauma after institution of a massive transfusion protocol in a civilian level I trauma center. J Trauma. 2009;66(6):1616–24.
10. Teixeira PG, Inaba K, Shulman I, Salim A, Demetriades D, Brown C, et al. Impact of plasma transfusion in massively transfused trauma patients. J Trauma. 2009;66(3):693–7.
11. Cantle PM, Cotton BA. Prediction of massive transfusion in trauma. Crit Care Clin. 2017;33(1):71–84.
12. Lee CW, Kory PD, Arntfield RT. Development of a fluid resuscitation protocol using inferior vena cava and lung ultrasound. J Crit Care. 2016;31(1):96–100.
13. Duchesne JC, Heaney J, Guidry C, McSwain N Jr, Meade P, Cohen M, et al. Diluting the benefits of hemostatic resuscitation: a multi-institutional analysis. J Trauma Acute Care Surg. 2013;75(1):76–82.
14. Carrico CJ, Coln CD, Lightfoot SA, Allsman A, Shires GT. Extracellular fluid volume replacement in hemorrhagic shock. Surg Forum. 1963;14:10–2.
15. Ferrada P. Image-based resuscitation of the hypotensive patient with cardiac ultrasound: an evidence-based review. J Trauma Acute Care Surg. 2016;80(3): 511–8.
16. Ferrada P, Anand RJ, Whelan J, Aboutanos MA, Duane T, Malhotra A, et al. Qualitative assessment of the inferior vena cava: useful tool for the evaluation of fluid status in critically ill patients. Am Surg. 2012;78(4):468–70.
17. Ferrada P, Wolfe L, Anand RJ, Whelan J, Vanguri P, Malhotra A, et al. Use of limited transthoracic echocardiography in patients with traumatic cardiac arrest decreases the rate of nontherapeutic thoracotomy and hospital costs. J Ultrasound Med. 2014;33(10):1829–32.

18. Wesson HK, Khan S, Ferrada P. Ultrasound as a tool for fluid status assessment in the trauma and critically ill patient. Int J Surg. 2016;33(Pt B):190–5.
19. Ferrada P, Murthi S, Anand RJ, Bochicchio GV, Scalea T. Transthoracic focused rapid echocardiographic examination: real-time evaluation of fluid status in critically ill trauma patients. J Trauma. 2011;70(1):56–62; discussion 4
20. Krige A, Bland M, Fanshawe T. Fluid responsiveness prediction using Vigileo FloTrac measured cardiac output changes during passive leg raise test. J Intensive Care. 2016;4:63.
21. Rajaram SS, Desai NK, Kalra A, Gajera M, Cavanaugh SK, Brampton W, et al. Pulmonary artery catheters for adult patients in intensive care. Cochrane Database Syst Rev. 2013;2:CD003408.
22. Warnakulasuriya SR, Davies SJ, Wilson RJ, Yates DR. Comparison of esophageal Doppler and plethysmographic variability index to guide intraoperative fluid therapy for low-risk patients undergoing colorectal surgery. J Clin Anesth. 2016;34: 600–8.
23. Bickell WH, Wall MJ Jr, Pepe PE, Martin RR, Ginger VF, Allen MK, et al. Immediate versus delayed fluid resuscitation for hypotensive patients with penetrating torso injuries. N Engl J Med. 1994;331(17):1105–9.
24. Cosnett JE. The origins of intravenous fluid therapy. Lancet. 1989;1(8641):768–71.
25. Duchesne JC, Guidry C, Hoffman JR, Park TS, Bock J, Lawson S, et al. Low-volume resuscitation for severe intraoperative hemorrhage: a step in the right direction. Am Surg. 2012;78(9):936–41.
26. Dutton RP, Mackenzie CF, Scalea TM. Hypotensive resuscitation during active hemorrhage: impact on in-hospital mortality. J Trauma. 2002;52(6):1141–6.
27. Ferrada P, Evans D, Wolfe L, Anand RJ, Vanguri P, Mayglothling J, et al. Findings of a randomized controlled trial using limited transthoracic echocardiogram (LTTE) as a hemodynamic monitoring tool in the trauma bay. J Trauma Acute Care Surg. 2014;76(1):31–7; discussion 7–8
28. Mitchell JR, Wang JJ. Expanding application of the Wiggers diagram to teach cardiovascular physiology. Adv Physiol Educ. 2014;38(2):170–5.

16 Damage Control Anesthesia

Shihab Sugeir, Itamar Grunstein, and Joshua M. Tobin

Abstract

The role of the anesthesiologist in damage control trauma care is that of resuscitation consultant. Damage control anesthesia must occur in concert with damage control resuscitation and surgery to optimize the physiology of the shocked patient, while ensuring adequate surgical conditions for the operative team. Damage control anesthesia encompasses a variety of procedural skills, from the induction of anesthesia to advanced airway management techniques and to the full spectrum of vascular access options. Beyond providing only procedural assistance in the resuscitation, the anesthesiologist offers the unique perspective of a physician who spends each day monitoring and correcting deranged physiology in the operating room.

Participation in the initial phases of trauma care ensures seamless transition from the trauma bay to the operating room and into the intensive care unit. A consideration for resuscitation end points and their impact on multiple organ systems is vital to the successful conduct of damage control anesthesia. The following chapter will review the anesthesiologist's role in the induction of anesthesia, airway management, and hemodynamic monitoring of the trauma patient, as well as resuscitation end points, neurotrauma concerns, renal protection issues, and pulmonary management.

S. Sugeir, M.D. • I. Grunstein, M.D.
J.M. Tobin, M.D. (✉)
Division of Trauma Anesthesiology, Keck School of Medicine at USC, Los Angeles, CA, USA
e-mail: Shihab.Sugeir@med.usc.edu; Itamar.Grunstein@med.usc.edu; joshua.tobin@med.usc.edu

16.1 Induction of Anesthesia in Damage Control Trauma Care

Prior to the induction of the trauma patient, two large bore IVs should be secured, and a fluid bolus should be ongoing. Even with this precaution in place, the induction of the trauma patient is extremely challenging, as trauma patients are commonly in a shocked state. Regardless of the etiology of the shock (e.g., hypovolemic, neurogenic, etc.), the patient will almost certainly require less medication than what is commonly used for the induction of sedation in more routine cases. The exact medication choice is complex, as the immediate and long-term effects of the pharmacokinetics and pharmacodynamics of medications used in the shocked patient must be considered. The anesthesiologist is uniquely qualified to make these decisions and will be responsible for management of the resuscitation of the patient over the ensuing hours in the operating room.

J. Duchesne et al. (eds.), *Damage Control in Trauma Care*,
https://doi.org/10.1007/978-3-319-72607-6_16

All patients should be treated as full stomach, and a rapid sequence induction should be followed. The head of the bed should be elevated if possible to ensure that passive reflux is hindered by gravity. The induction agent should be immediately followed by the neuromuscular blocking (NMB) agent.

While etomidate (0.3 mg/kg) is likely to be the most hemodynamically stable medication to choose, the long-term effects of adrenal suppression after even a single dose are concerning [1, 2]. Etomidate at 0.3 mg/kg will often cause a sudden drop in blood pressure as the sympathetic nervous system activation is lost with the analgesia from induction. Propofol (1.5 mg/kg) can cause drops in blood pressure that may result in significant drops in cardiac output and possible cardiac arrest. Ketamine (1.5 mg/kg) is a centrally acting sympathomimetic but can directly cause cardiac depression. This dose may result in a dangerous drop in blood pressure and therefore should be used with caution. A choice that is gaining popularity is using both ketamine and propofol; however, in this patient population, severe hypotension remains a possibility [3, 4].

Fentanyl and midazolam are two other medications that can be used in the trauma patient either individually or in combination to help prepare the patient for intubation. These medications are not used traditionally to provide amnesia and analgesia alone for intubation, but in the trauma patient in extremis, both medications may be sufficient for anesthesia prior to intubation. Fentanyl may cause a drop in blood pressure with the blunting of the sympathetic stimulation due to analgesia. Midazolam will cause anterograde amnesia, with little impact on the blood pressure. There is no specific dose that can be recommended for fentanyl or midazolam as these medications are not used for induction outside of the trauma bay. Any medication used to induce amnesia and analgesia at recommended doses will cause significant drops in blood pressure that may be unrecoverable. Medications used in damage control anesthesia must be titrated to effect, and pharmacologic agents to address drops in cardiac output must be readily available.

The choice of NMBs is simpler but is still fraught with potential complications. Succinylcholine (1 mg/kg) will cause ideal intubating conditions in 60–90 s. However, succinylcholine may also cause hyperkalemia in certain patient populations and has a duration of action of 3–5 min. In a trauma situation, rocuronium (1.2 mg/kg) can be given to achieve full paralysis in about 90 s, with a duration of action of at least 20 min. Once the patient is anesthetized and paralyzed, the airway can be secured.

16.2 Airway Management in Damage Control Anesthesia

Airway management of the trauma patient can present special challenges; however, it is important to understand that all airway management can be temporized with good basic airway maneuvers. In the appropriate patient, a simple jaw thrust with placement of an oropharyngeal airway can open the airway and facilitate oxygenation sufficiently to allow the anesthesiologist to quickly evaluate the patient and formulate a plan for intubation. In the case of an awake patient, placement of supplemental oxygen can provide a depot of oxygen that can last for several minutes of apneic oxygenation. Leaving a nasal cannula in situ set at a high flow rate (i.e., 15 L/min) during intubation has been postulated to extend the period of apneic oxygenation [5]. A promising trend in the intensive care unit that may be useful in the trauma bay is the use of high flow nasal cannula for both supplemental oxygenation and apneic oxygenation while intubating the trauma patient [6].

An investigation of 6088 patients intubated by experienced trauma anesthesiologists at a Level I trauma center over a 10-year period found that 6008 (98.7%) were intubated successfully via the orotracheal route [7]. Roughly 0.3% of patients required a surgical airway. Another study evaluated prehospital intubation on a Scandinavian prehospital team [8]. A total of 240 endotracheal intubation attempts resulted in 238 successes (99.2%). The small number of unsuccessful attempts involved complex cases with distorted facial/airway anatomy.

16.3 Cervical Spine Considerations

If a cervical spine injury is suspected, careful attention must be paid during intubation to ensure that any injury is not worsened. Shatney and colleagues examined 81 patients with cervical vertebral body fractures of whom 26 required intubation [9]. Twenty-two of these patients were intubated via the oral tracheal route with no resulting neurological deficit. In 69 patients with high spinal cord injuries, 29 required endotracheal intubation, of which 26 were intubated via oral tracheal intubation. No further neurological deficit resulted. It is reassuring to know that in trauma, even with spinal fractures or spinal cord injuries, oral tracheal intubation does not result in higher rates of neurological injury.

Part of a careful plan for intubation in the trauma patient in whom cervical spine injury may be suspected is the use of manual in-line stabilization (MILS). This involves simply holding gentle support on both sides of the head during laryngoscopy. The objective is to prevent excessive extension of the neck during intubation. The efficacy of MILS however, remains debated. Investigations using similar methodology have found conflicting results on the use of MILS. In one investigation, a cadaver model was evaluated under fluoroscopy and found that MILS did not affect measured subluxation, angulation, or distraction of the cervical spine [10]. Other work using a similar cadaver model, however, found that MILS offered significantly less anterior-posterior subluxation of the cervical spine than a cervical collar [11]. While it is an interesting exercise to debate the merits and limitations of MILS, a practical clinical approach to the topic may be found in simply applying MILS in cases in which cervical spine injury is suspected. If MILS somehow diminishes the view that the person intubating has, then it can be relaxed somewhat.

16.4 Video Laryngoscopy

Video laryngoscopy (VL) offers a tool that can improve visualization of the vocal cords. It is uncertain, however, if this confers an advantage in securing the airway. In a meta-analysis of 17 trials including 2000 patients, Griesdale and colleagues found that VL improved glottic visualization but did not impact success of first attempt intubation or time to intubation [12]. In another analysis of VL, 623 trauma patients were randomized to either VL or direct laryngoscopy [13]. No difference in mortality was noted, but time to intubation was longer in the VL group. Subgroup analysis of patients who had suffered traumatic brain injury (TBI) found higher mortality with VL; however, this analysis was not identified a priori, and the results should be taken with caution.

Non-expert experience with VL has been more positive. When medical students, paramedic students, and nurses who had previously only intubated manikins used VL, they had greater overall success and faster time to intubation [14]. Subjects intubated five patients with either VL or direct laryngoscopy. Although first attempt success and time to intubation were improved in the first four patients, by the fifth patient, there was no significant difference between VL and direct laryngoscopy.

A retrospective review of 2004 cases found that VL was successful in securing the airway in 98% of cases when used as a primary technique and in 94% of cases when used as a rescue technique after direct laryngoscopy [15]. While useful, the authors caution against over reliance on VL at the expense of direct laryngoscopy and flexible bronchoscopy skill sets. If the trauma bay does not have an anesthesiologist available for intubation, the use of VL may be a helpful adjunct to providers who do not intubate as often.

16.5 Other Airway Adjuncts

If one is unable to intubate the trauma patient, other airway alternatives must be considered. The laryngeal mask airway (LMA) is one option. When used as a rescue device in a case series of 15 patients, the LMA was able to facilitate oxygenation and ventilation in patients who were entrapped or otherwise not able to be intubated [16]. There are many different variations of LMAs, but familiarity with at least one is helpful for the trauma patient that cannot be intubated successfully.

It is important to appreciate that laryngeal airways do not secure the airway and that a risk of aspiration remains after placement. It can be difficult to ventilate non-compliant lungs with positive pressure ventilation via a supraglottic airway. One case report of a drowning patient noted an inability to achieve peak pressure necessary for lung inflation with a supraglottic airway and subsequent insufflation of air into the stomach [17].

The intubating LMA uses a stylet to advance an endotracheal tube through the vocal cords via an acutely angled supraglottic airway. While this technique can secure the airway with a cuffed endotracheal tube, it is a multi-step process that can be a challenge to perform in an emergency. A case report documented successful intubation of a morbidly obese patient with chest trauma with an intubating LMA [18]. Other modest case series have also documented the successful use of the intubating LMA in out-of-operating room emergency intubations [19].

Another alternative is the laryngeal tube suction, another supraglottic airway, which was successfully placed in 57 trauma patients either as a primary or rescue technique [20]. Most laryngeal tube suctions were placed by providers who had used the technique ten or fewer times, suggesting relative ease of use during an emergency. Supraglottic airways use a high-volume balloon to seat the device in the posterior oropharynx and direct gas from the tube toward the glottic opening. Again, this does not secure the airway but can be helpful in cannot intubate–cannot ventilate emergencies, as may be found with the trauma patient in extremis. When used in 351 out-of-hospital nontrauma cardiac arrests, basic life support crews using a laryngeal tube suctions were more successful in achieving first attempt success than paramedics using endotracheal intubation [21].

16.6 Awake Intubation

In certain cases, the trauma patient may require awake airway management. Cases in which this may be considered include cervical spine injury or hemodynamically stable patients in whom induction of anesthesia could result in airway compromise (e.g., extensive facial trauma). Awake intubation is a safe but rarely performed procedure [22]. Out of 146,252 general anesthetics, awake intubation was performed 1544 times (1%) with a failed intubation rate of 31 (2%).

In a retrospective analysis of 1055 awake flexible intubations, complications (e.g., mucus plug, cuff leak, inadvertent extubation) occurred in 1.6% of cases, and failed intubation occurred in 1% of cases [23]. Propensity matching of awake intubation to intubation post-induction found that awake intubation took longer (16 min vs. 4 min).

During awake fiber-optic intubation, it is important to explain the need for the procedure to the patient, surgeon, and support staff to avoid a loud distracting environment that may alarm an already anxious patient. Remember that the patient just suffered a traumatic injury, is having difficulty breathing, and now has several people around him/her saying that they are going to put a tube down his/her throat while he/she is awake! Taking the time to explain to the patient and team what is being done and why will help alleviate any anxiety.

Application of standard monitoring can occur as one speaks to the patient. An infusion of dexmedetomidine (1 mcg/kg over 10 min) provides sedation while maintaining the patient's normal minute ventilation, but hypotension may occur and should be anticipated. Nebulized viscous lidocaine provides anesthesia to the airway, to include the area below the vocal cords. Additional topicalization of the airway can be achieved with atomized viscous lidocaine "painted" across the posterior oropharynx. The pharynx is innervated by the glossopharyngeal nerve (IX), and the hypopharynx is innervated by the glossopharyngeal and hypoglossal (XII) nerves. Both the pharynx and hypopharynx can be anesthetized with atomized viscous lidocaine or nebulized lidocaine. The total amount of lidocaine given should not exceed 3 mg/kg to help prevent local anesthetic toxicity.

The larynx is innervated by the vagus (X) nerve, with the internal branch of the superior laryngeal nerve providing innervation from the epiglottis to the vocal cords. A nerve block at the cornu of the hyoid bone can be undertaken with two milliliters (mL) 2% lidocaine to effectively decrease sensation in this nerve distribution. The recurrent laryngeal nerve (RLN) branch of the vagus nerve provides sensation below the vocal cords. The RLN can be blocked with 3–5 mL of transtracheal local anesthetic applied via a trans-cricothyroid membrane approach. This technique almost always results in coughing which can serve to aerosolize the local anesthetic. If rigorous coughing is a concern (i.e., unstable cervical spine fracture), then the transtracheal block merits careful consideration. Using the regional blocks should not be done when anatomy has been significantly changed with trauma. The regional blocks can be used in place of nebulized lidocaine, but the two techniques should not be used in combination unless careful attention is paid to the total dose of lidocaine given.

After the patient has had sufficient topicalization of the airway, an "intubating oropharyngeal airway" can be gently placed in the airway. If the patient does not tolerate the airway, then a small bolus of ketamine may augment the sedative profile while maintaining airway reflexes. Consider using glycopyrrolate if hypersalivation from the use of ketamine is a concern.

Once the intubating oropharyngeal airway is in place, pass a well-lubricated and focused flexible bronchoscope through the airway's central aperture. Slow, deliberate movements will bring the vocal cords into view. Pass the vocal cords and visualize the carina. An assistant can pass the preloaded endotracheal tube over the flexible bronchoscope and into the trachea. Withdraw the bronchoscope and attach the ventilator circuit. Ensure end-tidal carbon dioxide is present and proceed with securing the endotracheal tube.

16.7 Cricothyroidotomy

Surgical airway management is the final option in a "cannot intubate–cannot ventilate" situation. Cricothyroidotomy is perhaps the most common emergency surgical airway technique and is rarely needed. Rather than being the heroic lifesaving procedure that is often portrayed in the media, it may more appropriately be regarded as a failure of all other techniques. With that said, when a patient needs a surgical airway, they need one in seconds. When the decision has been made to proceed with a surgical airway, one must move quickly and efficiently.

In a prospective observational study of airway management among 282 patients in a combat setting, 17 cricothyroidotomies were performed with four failures [24]. Other investigations have found a similarly high rate of complication with cricothyroidotomy [25]. Among patients who received cricothyroidotomies, 82% had suffered a gunshot wound to the face, neck, or head; and 66% died. Prehospital cricothyroidotomy failed to cannulate the trachea in 26% of cases. Physicians and physician assistants had lower failure rates than medics (15% vs. 33%). Given the high rate of failure and relatively infrequent performance of the procedure, it is important to train for this potentially lifesaving technique with simulation or other techniques. Many difficult airway workshops allow hands on training of this technique, and online resources provide excellent review of this rare but critical procedure.

16.8 Awake Tracheostomy

In some cases of massive trauma to the upper airway, the patient may not be willing to undergo awake or asleep intubation (or even to consider lying down!) If that is the case, then let the patient adopt a comfortable posture and consider awake tracheostomy. This must be undertaken with careful coordination with the surgeon and patient. Topicalization of the airway as noted above can provide adequate anesthesia, along with infiltration of local anesthetic in the anterior neck. Mild sedation can offer the patient some anxiolysis without compromising the airway. With sedation and local anesthetic being used, airway reflexes will be decreased, and the risk of aspiration will be much higher. Monitoring must be in place, and vascular access must anticipate the surgical procedure that will immediately follow the placement of the tracheostomy. Formal tracheostomy (versus cricothyroidotomy) can be safely undertaken in the emergent, awake patient but requires excellent communication between the surgical and anesthetic teams.

16.9 Resuscitation End Points in Damage Control Anesthesia

The goal of a damage control anesthetic is to ensure adequate resuscitation while maintaining a depth of anesthesia appropriate for the procedure being undertaken. It can be challenging to quantify the effectiveness of the resuscitation in a critically ill trauma patient. Traditional normal values may need to be significantly reevaluated and other resuscitation end points considered.

16.10 Blood Pressure

Noninvasive blood pressure (NIBP) devices occlude blood flow by compressing an artery against a proximate bone. As pressure is decreased and pulsatile flow returns, the NIBP cuff measures oscillations in pressure. The point of maximum oscillation is defined as the mean arterial pressure (MAP), and the systolic and diastolic pressures are calculated from that value.

An arterial line waveform is a processed signal that serves as a proxy for the arterial blood pressure. A catheter in the artery transmits the arterial pressure via a fluid column to a Wheatstone bridge. This electrical device converts the mechanical pulsation to an electrical signal via a diaphragm. The pulsatile diaphragm results in differences in resistance in the arms of the Wheatstone bridge. These differences are processed via a Fourier analysis that reduces the signal to smaller characteristic waveforms and then integrates the area under those curves to derive a MAP. This electronic signal is sent to the monitor as a function (i.e., $y = f(x)$), which is then represented as the familiar arterial line waveform.

In a pairwise comparison of 27,022 NIBP measurements and arterial line measurements, it was found that NIBP overestimates systolic blood pressure in hypotensive patients [26]. This raises the question of whether NIBP systolic blood pressure measurements fail to recognize end organ hypoperfusion. The authors found that the mean arterial pressure of NIBP and arterial line measurements correlated reasonably well and suggested that MAP be used as the "preferred metric" in critical care.

Differences in blood pressure measurement from NIBP and arterial lines continue to inspire controversy. In one prospective observational study of patients in the intensive care unit who were on norepinephrine infusions with a goal MAP greater than 70 mmHg, NIBP measurements were found to be 6.6 mmHg higher than arterial line MAP [27]. The difference was unrelated to the age of the catheter or the dose of norepinephrine. This serves to underscore the need to evaluate a range of resuscitation metrics when treating a critically ill patient in extremis.

A benefit of having an arterial line is the ability to monitor stroke volume variability. Stroke volume variability (SVV) offers a unique perspective on the interpretation of blood pressure. SVV is defined as the difference between the maximum and minimum stroke volumes divided by the average of the minimum and maximum over a floating 30-second period (i.e., SVV = (Max − Min)/Mean). In one investigation, SVV greater than 9.5% predicted a 5% increase in stroke volume with a 100 mL fluid bolus [28]. Fluid responsiveness correlated well with SVV (area under the receiver operating curve (ROC) = 0.87) but not with heart rate (ROC = 0.59) or central venous pressure (ROC = 0.49). To date, there are few studies in trauma patients looking at SVV and its utility in identifying hypovolemia. While most hypotensive trauma patients will benefit from fluid resuscitation, end points for that resuscitation remain a challenging and exciting area for future research.

16.11 Base Deficit

Base deficit is the amount of base required to bring 1 L of whole blood at body temperature and a partial pressure of carbon dioxide of 40 to a pH of 7.4. This methodology attempts to isolate the metabolic contribution to the acid-base status. In 209 trauma patients, a deranged base deficit correlated with a decreased MAP and higher volume requirements [29]. In patients with a deranged base deficit (i.e., less than 10), administration of bicarbonate resulted in greater fluid and blood requirements, as well as a more deranged base deficit at 1 h and 24 h (with no difference in base deficit at 2 and 4 h). The same group found that worsened base deficit at admission in 2954 trauma patients predicted the need for transfusion as well as complications (e.g., ARDS, multi-organ failure, renal failure) [30].

When used as a resuscitation end point during damage control anesthesia, base deficit is reliable, rapidly obtainable, and well validated [31]. A four-stage classification system for base deficit (I = BD < 2 mmol/L, II = BD 2–6 mmol/L, III = BD 6–10 mmol/L, IV = BD >10 mmol/L) has compared favorably to more traditional shock classifications [32]. In an investigation of 16,305 patients, the base deficit classification system correlated well with the need for massive transfusion (class I = 5% vs. class IV = 52%), as well as mortality (class I = 7.4% vs. class IV = 51.5%). The authors found that the base deficit system predicted the need for massive transfusion and mortality better than the more traditional ATLS classification system for hypovolemic shock.

16.12 End-Tidal Carbon Dioxide

End-tidal carbon dioxide ($ETCO_2$) can serve as a surrogate for the measurement of dead space ventilation, such as occurs during low-flow peri-arrest states seen in damage control anesthesia. A return of spontaneous circulation (ROSC) following cardiac arrest has been correlated with a higher peak $ETCO_2$, larger area under the $ETCO_2$ curve, and a rising $ETCO_2$ slope [33]. In an investigation of 30 patients who underwent cardiopulmonary resuscitation (CPR) in a hospital setting, an $ETCO_2$ greater than 20 mmHg between 5 and 10 min post intubation was associated with ROSC, as was a maximum $ETCO_2$ of 25 mmHg between 5 and 10 min or an $ETCO_2$ slope greater than zero between 0 and 8 min.

End-tidal carbon dioxide provides some prognostic ability for trauma patients. In 106 trauma patients, $ETCO_2$ was evaluated in the context of mortality [34]. The authors found that an $ETCO_2$ of 27 or higher was associated with 5% mortality, whereas an $ETCO_2$ of less than 24 was associated with 68% mortality. It may be that a rapidly decreasing $ETCO_2$ suggests the need for more aggressive damage control resuscitation. If a trauma patient has loss of spontaneous circulation during resuscitation, it is important to refer to the $ETCO_2$ to ensure adequate compressions and note the ROSC.

16.13 Hypocalcemia

While not a resuscitation end point per se, serum calcium levels are decreased during massive transfusion. This is related to the chelating effect that the preservative, citrate, included in blood products has on serum calcium concentration. The effect of hypocalcemia in resuscitation can be devastating. In one investigation of 352 critically ill bleeding patients who required massive transfusion, hypocalcemia was associated with increased mortality with an odds ratio of 1.25 [35]. Hypocalcemia is even present in trauma patients at the time of initial evaluation (i.e., before blood transfusion) [36]. Two hundred and twelve trauma patients with a mean injury severity score (ISS) of 34 were stratified by serum ionized calcium (iCa) concentration. Three-quarters of trauma patients at the time of emergency department admission were either hypocalcemic (iCa < 1.15 mmol/L; 64%) or severely hypocalcemic (iCa < 0.9 mmol/L; 10%). It was noted that hypocalcemia is correlated with colloid but not crystalloid administration.

Indeed, admission hypocalcemia in trauma was associated with worsened mortality in 591 trauma patients [37]. Admission iCa < 1 was associated with 15.5% mortality, whereas iCa ≥ 1 had significantly lower mortality (8.7%). Ionized calcium <1 was further found to be an independent predictor of the need for massive transfusion (OR 2.2, 95% CI 1.053–4.996). Given the frequency of hypocalcemia on admission and after transfusion, it is reasonable to include administration of exogenous calcium as part of any damage control anesthetic.

The use of these variables throughout the trauma activation, the operating room, and into the intensive care unit will be helpful in guiding resuscitation and ensuring that hypocalcemia is not missed.

16.14 Neurotrauma and Damage Control Anesthesia

The polytrauma patient may have significant neurological injury involving either the brain or the spinal cord. These injuries certainly make anesthetic management more challenging as some of the goals for neuroprotection may be in direct conflict with other resuscitative goals. The anesthesiologist must balance these sometimes competing interests to ensure that the patient is given the best opportunity to make a full and meaningful recovery.

The trauma patient who has sustained a spinal cord injury must be managed carefully throughout the trauma activation and treatment in the operating room. Per the updated 2013 guidelines, the use of methylprednisolone or other steroids is contraindicated, as the harm that steroids cause outweighs any benefit that they may provide [38]. While this is typically well understood by all team members, it sometimes bears reinforcement from the anesthesiologist during the operation.

A mean arterial pressure goal of 85–90 mmHg in traumatic brain injury (TBI) can be challenging to achieve in a hypotensive trauma patient. This goal will certainly be challenging to achieve intraoperatively and may go against the desire to assist the surgeon with decrease blood loss until the vascular injury has been identified and repaired. The use of vasopressors to increase the MAP to 85–90 mmHg can worsen outcomes in trauma patients, despite being recommended for some spinal cord injury patients.

Trauma patients with concomitant TBI have other challenges that must be addressed. The most recent recommendations advise against using mannitol until intracranial pressure (ICP) monitoring has been established unless the patient shows signs of progressive neurologic deterioration [39]. Hyperventilation should be avoided during the first 24 h and then should only be used as a temporizing measure to treat acute neurologic decline. Steroids have not been shown to improve outcome or decrease ICP. Blood pressure recommendations are based on age, and the goal is to maintain adequate cerebral perfusion pressure (CPP). The goal CPP is between 60 and 70 mmHg. Without ICP monitoring, the best estimate will be from the systolic blood pressure (SBP) and central venous pressure. The goal SBP for 50–69 year olds is ≥100 mmHg and for 15–49 or >70 years old is ≥110. Both SBP ranges are more easily obtainable during damage control resuscitation.

The current recommendations for neuroprotection highlight what is likely to be a growing problem, the conflict of interest between different organ systems. The SBP goals in TBI patients are more reasonable and obtainable than the MAP goals in spinal cord injury patients. Patients should not receive steroids, and the use of hyperosmotic solutions and hyperventilation should be used as part of rescue therapy.

16.15 Renal Protection in Damage Control Anesthesia

When discussing renal protective management strategies and acute kidney injury (AKI) in the trauma patient, it is useful to refer to the RIFLE criteria or the AKIN classification. The RIFLE criteria were formulated in 2004 by the Acute Dialysis Quality Initiative (ADQI) to promote an objective and uniform definition of AKI [40]. The RIFLE criteria divide AKI into two groups. The risk, injury, and failure groups are considered mild and reversible forms of AKI, while the loss and end-stage group are severe and irreversible forms of AKI. The AKIN classification was formulated in 2007 by the Acute Kidney Injury Network. It simplified the classification further by discarding the latter, irreversible group, broadening the "risk" category (stage 1), and defining the "failure" category (stage 3) as the need for the renal replacement therapy [41]. Both classifications are in common use in the medical literature.

Acute kidney injury is common among trauma patients. A recent study using the RIFLE criteria found that half of all intensive care unit trauma admissions had AKI. Among these patients, class R, I, and F were most common and comprised 47%, 36%, and 17% of AKI, respectively [41]. These milder forms of AKI are likely related to the initial trauma and surgery. Persistent or irreversible AKI with need for RRT is rare (0.1–8.4% in one study) among trauma patients in the ICU and is related to the sequelae of severe trauma with subsequent multi-organ failure [42].

All degrees of AKI are associated with worse key outcome measures including increased length of stay and increased duration of mechanical ventilation in the ICU. While all forms of AKI are associated with increased mortality, this association is greater for AKI requiring RRT (40–70% increase in mortality) [43]. In trauma patients, for whom the majority will have normal renal function prior to their traumatic injuries, preoperative and intraoperative renal protective management are of great importance in minimizing the incidence and severity of AKI.

The pathophysiology of AKI has traditionally been divided into prerenal, intrinsic renal, and post renal etiologies. When considering renal protective measures in the trauma patient, it is useful to think about causes of AKI in this manner. The most common etiologies of AKI encountered in the trauma patient are listed in Table 16.1.

Considering the etiologies of AKI in this manner is helpful in structuring a comprehensive approach to diagnosing and treating infrequent but easily reversible causes of AKI. In reality, AKI is a complex and multifactorial process that can blur these distinctions. ATN is traditionally considered as an intrinsic renal pathology, for example. It is the most common cause of post-traumatic AKI and is the result of multiple insults that may occur in the early management of the trauma patient (e.g., contrast-induced nephropathy (CIN), renal hypoperfusion from hemorrhage and/or "third-space" fluid shifts, and direct trauma to the kidney and renal vasculature). Myoglobin and fibrin complex deposition resulting from injury and DIC, respectively, can also cause or exacerbate ATN.

Table 16.1 Etiologies of acute kidney injury

Prerenal	Intrinsic (ATN)	Post renal
Hemorrhage	Ischemia	Obstructed Foley
Trauma and surgery	Myoglobin	Blood clots
Burns	DIC	Inadvertent ureter ligation
Abdominal compartment Syndrome	Contrast	Retroperitoneal hematoma

ATN acute tubular necrosis

The AKI continuum of renal insults is a "multiple hit model." The importance of sequential renal protective measures that begin early in the resuscitation in the emergency department and are carried through the intraoperative management and into the ICU can be readily appreciated. Contrast-induced nephropathy is an iatrogenic contributor to AKI that can be modified early in the trauma patients' hospital course. Computer tomography with contrast is an important diagnostic tool that helps identify injuries and informs surgical planning. However, most commercial contrasts contain agents that are nephrotoxic and may contribute significantly to ATN. When time allows, contrast protective strategies are often employed to decrease the risk of CIN. Developing a risk stratification tool to identify patients at increased risk for CIN, as well as alternative imaging strategies and iso-osmolar contrast agents may be important measures to mitigate the risk of ATN.

Most of the studies regarding preoperative AKI were performed in patients after cardiac surgery, and the risk stratification tools for AKI after cardiac surgery have been tested and validated [44]. Risk factors for AKI in trauma patients are less well studied; however, some of the accepted risk factors for AKI in this population are summarized in Table 16.2.

Optimization of hemodynamic status and intravascular volume is the single most beneficial measure in ensuring adequate renal perfusion. Maintaining adequate renal perfusion is a cornerstone of renal protective management; however, this can often be challenging during the intraoperative phase of care. The traditional marker of renal perfusion (i.e., urine output) is an inaccurate marker of intravascular volume and renal perfusion in the trauma patient undergoing general anesthesia. Anesthesia and the stress of trauma and surgery can decrease the glomerular filtration rate (GFR) through indirect sympathetic and humoral responses. Many commonly used parenteral agents (e.g., benzodiazepines, opioids) also reduce GFR and urine output. An approach that incorporates multiple indices of renal perfusion, in addition to urine output, to assess the adequacy of renal perfusion during the resuscitation may offer benefit and is reviewed in Table 16.3.

Table 16.2 Risk factors for acute kidney injury

Patient-related factors	Procedure-related risk factors	Contrasts-related risk factors
Age >60	Intraoperative hypotension	Volume of contrast
Diabetes	Suprarenal aortic cross clamping	Low-osmolar contrast Medium > iso-osmolar
Hypertension	Massive blood transfusion	Nonionic > ionic
CHF	Vasopressors and inotropes	Arterial > venous
CKD	Diuretic use (mannitol and loop diuretics)	
Renal transplant		
Hypotension		

Table 16.3 Indices of renal perfusion

Hemodynamics	MAP > 65 mmHg
Urine output	>0.5 mL/kg/h
Lactate and lactate clearance	Lactate <2.5 mmol/L, clearance >20%/h
Base deficit	>−4
Stroke volume variation	8–12%

AKI secondary to rhabdomyolysis is a distinct form of ATN in which myoglobin is thought to result in direct nephrotoxicity, renal vasoconstriction, and renal tubular obstruction. Crush injuries, vascular injuries, and compartment syndromes lead to muscle necrosis with the release of myocyte contents into the circulation. Creatine kinase (CK) is a useful biomarker for tracking the severity and resolution of rhabdomyolysis. The risk and severity of AKI generally correlate with the degree of CK elevation. Traditionally, management of this condition has advocated the use of bicarbonate solution to alkalinize the urine and favor a soluble form of myoglobin. Volume expansion and administration of mannitol promote urine output of 2–3 mL/kg/h in an effort to "flush" the renal tubules of insoluble myoglobin precipitates [45].

It is important to understand that mannitol and bicarbonate administration are controversial therapies for the prevention and treatment of rhabdomyolysis-induced AKI. The literature on this topic does not demonstrate conclusive benefit, and these treatments may be harmful in the under-resuscitated trauma patient by further exacerbating intravascular volume loss and masking worsening acidemia [45]. These therapies may be selectively applied if goal urine output is not achieved despite adequate volume expansion.

Other alternative practices include the use of loop diuretics, typically furosemide, to promote diuresis in oliguric patients under general anesthesia. As mentioned, urine output is not an accurate intraoperative indicator of intravascular volume and renal perfusion in severe trauma patients, and the benefit of inducing diuresis with loop diuretics is unknown. Studies in critical ill patients with AKI have demonstrated that non-oliguric AKI has lower rates of progression to RRT and is associated with lower mortality than oliguric renal failure. Of note, however, is that the use of loop diuretics in this population has never been shown to reduce progression of renal failure or reduce intensive care unit length of stay or mortality. A meta-analysis on this topic demonstrated no benefit to the use of loop diuretics either in reducing progression to RRT or in reducing all-cause mortality and suggested a tendency toward harm [46].

In the operative setting, loop diuretics increase urine output but do not increase GFR or creatinine clearance. In addition, furosemide induces aciduria that may favor precipitation of urinary proteins and promotes free radical formation by radiocontrast dyes. For this reason, furosemide may promote AKI in patients with rhabdomyolysis and in patients who have had recent contrast-enhanced CT imaging. While the use of loop diuretics to reduce volume overload as part of a conservative fluid management strategy in patients with ARDS has demonstrated benefit in decreasing intensive care unit ventilator days and length of stay, there is no date to suggest that this strategy is renal protective [47].

Mild reversible AKI is a frequent sequela of severe trauma and an important contributor to the need for prolonged intensive care unit stay. Early renal protective measures should focus on identifying patients at increased risk for AKI secondary to nephrotoxic agents (radiocontrast dyes) and prevention of exposure if possible. Hemodynamic resuscitation with volume expansion and blood products is the cornerstone of renal protective management and should begin as early as possible and continue intraoperatively. Multiple indices of adequate hemodynamic and renal perfusion should be utilized intraoperatively as urine output by itself is not an accurate intraoperative marker of renal perfusion and GFR in the trauma patient. The use of bicarbonate solutions and mannitol after adequate volume expansion in the prevention of AKI secondary to rhabdomyolysis is controversial. The routine use of loop diuretics to promote urine output is without benefit and may be harmful.

16.16 Pulmonary Protection in Damage Control Anesthesia

The continuum of care for damage control anesthesia must anticipate the physiologic needs of the patient as they depart the operating room (OR)/interventional radiology (IR) suite. One must consider the next 12–24 h of the patient's hospital course as care is handed from the anesthesiologist to the intensivist. For example, has the resuscitation team avoided transfusion associated circulatory overload (TACO)? Has the resuscitation team set the critical care team up for success? Have they avoided the acute respiratory distress syndrome (ARDS) and is the patient oxygenating and ventilating well?

TACO is a genuine concern in the patient who has received a massive transfusion/damage control anesthetic. TACO is associated with hemorrhagic shock, the number of blood products transfused, as well as with premorbid renal failure and congestive heart failure [48]. Patients who develop TACO are at an increased risk of inhospital mortality, as well as longer hospital and ICU lengths of stay.

The acute respiratory distress syndrome (ARDS) has been historically described in healthy trauma patients following resuscitation, sometimes called "Da Nang Lung" in the Vietnam War. The ARDS Net investigation was an impactful publication in the care of the critically ill ventilated patient [49]. Low lung compliance and elevated peak pressures seen in ARDS were treated with lower tidal volumes. Permissive hypercarbia and escalating fractions of inspired oxygen (FiO_2) paired with increasing positive end-expiratory pressure (PEEP) improved oxygenation in this critically ill patient population.

Neuromuscular blockade (NMB) was evaluated in the context of ARDS and found to improve 90-day mortality [50]. Three hundred and forty patients with ARDS were randomized to receive cisatracurium or placebo for 48 h. Mortality was improved in the NMB group with no increase in ICU-acquired paresis; however, off-label use of NMB, varied positioning techniques (e.g., prone), and uses of other modalities (e.g., nitric oxide) make these data difficult to interpret on a broader scale.

Given the limited options for treating ARDS in the ICU, one wonders if there is a way to preemptively mitigate the development of ARDS. A meta-analysis looked at initiation of low lung volume ventilation in the operating room [51]. In 20 articles including over 2000 patients, lower tidal volume used in the OR resulted in decreased development of lung injury and mortality. Additionally, there was a lower incidence of pulmonary infection and shorter hospital length of stay (LOS).

Protective and conventional ventilation during surgery were further evaluated in an analysis of 15 randomized control trials including 2127 patients [52]. Postoperative lung injury, infection, and barotrauma were tracked in patients who received low volume ventilation/protective versus conventional ventilation. The protective ventilation group had a lower incidence of pulmonary complications (PC). Elevated levels of PEEP, however, did not result in a decreased incidence of PC. Interestingly, a protocol for protective lung ventilatory strategies in the noninjured lung has been developed for use in the operating room [53].

Alternative therapies of treatment of ARDS/lung injury have been proposed. In the CESAR trial, extracorporeal membrane oxygenation (ECMO) evaluation was compared to conventional therapy for treatment of ARDS. Patients with a Murray score >3 and a pH <7.2 were randomized to conventional therapy or referral to an EMCO capable center. Of those patients who were evaluated for ECMO 75% (68/90) actually received ECMO. Disability-free survival at 6 months was 63% in the ECMO group versus 47% in the conventional therapy group. This study needs to be replicated as those patients transferred to the ECMO capable center may have also received better, non-ECMO, ARDS care.

In trauma, heparin-free ECMO has been used in limited number of patients [54]. A total of ten patients were treated with ECMO (seven with veno-venous ECMO and three with veno-arterial ECMO). Improved gas exchange and correction of cardiopulmonary failure were noted, with six of the ten patients recovering without handicap.

The objective of damage control anesthesia is to carry the resuscitation seamlessly from one phase of care to the next. Initiation of low lung volume ventilation in the OR/IR suite can help mitigate the risk of ARDS and TACO in the critical care setting. Experimental modalities like NMB and ECMO have yet to demonstrate a proven benefit in pulmonary management of damage control resuscitation but offer exciting opportunities for future research.

16.17 Transfer to the Intensive Care Unit in Damage Control Anesthesia

At the end of the operation, it is imperative that the surgical team and the anesthetic team continue to have good communication. The intensive care unit bed should be brought into the operating room, and the transport monitor should be connected to the patient while they remain on the operating table. Once all monitors have been attached and a review of the vital signs has confirmed the patient is stable, then the anesthesiologist should lead the team in safely transferring the patient to the intensive care unit bed. The head of the bed should be raised unless concern for spinal fractures prevents the team from doing so.

A member from the surgical team should accompany the anesthesia team to the intensive care unit, and the patient should be constantly monitored. Transport should occur with emergency drugs and back up airway supplies in case something changes acutely during transport. Once the patient has arrived to the intensive care unit, everyone should work in unison to apply the intensive care unit monitors onto the patient. Assuming the patient is stable, a formal handoff should occur. McElroy showed that unorganized handoffs with ambiguous roles increase the risk of patient harm [55].

The handoff should include the bedside nurse, the intensive care unit team, the surgical team, and the anesthesia team. A standardized handoff should be used with a consistency and concerns from each group being highlighted. Salzwedel showed that a standardized checklist for patient handoffs increased both the quantity and quality of the information relayed [56]. Before leaving the patient's bedside, the nurse and intensive care unit team should "read back" what they understood to ensure that all concerns have been understood and the next goals of care are appropriately prioritized. Implementation of a handoff checklist can help make the transition of care more complete and safer for the patient.

Conclusion

The anesthesiologist plays an integral role in the care of the trauma patient from the trauma bay to the intensive care unit. Their understanding of cardiopulmonary physiology and resuscitation pharmacology, as well as an appreciation for the priorities of care for the trauma patient, makes them a valuable resuscitation consultant. Damage control anesthesia encompasses anesthetic induction, airway management, hemodynamic monitoring, and resuscitation coordination, as well as consideration of neuro, renal, and pulmonary protection. The damage control approach with "all hands" contributing their expertise offers potential for successful care of the critically ill trauma patient.

References

1. Bruder EA, Ball IM, Ridi S, Pickett W, Hohl C. Single induction dose of etomidate versus other induction agents for endotracheal intubation in critically ill patients. Cochrane Database Syst Rev. 2015;1:CD010225.
2. Coursin DB, Fish JT, Joffe AM. Etomidate-trusted alternative or time to trust alternatives? Crit Care Med. 2013;41(3):917–9.
3. Jabre P, Combes X, Lapostolle F, Dhaouadi M, Ricard-Hibon A, Vivien B, Bertrand L, Beltramini A, Gamand P, Albizzati S, et al. Etomidate vs ketamine for rapid sequence intubation in acutely ill patients: a multicentre randomized controlled trial. The KETASED trial. Lancet. 2009;374:293–300.
4. Ray DC, McKeown DW. Effect of induction agent on vasopressor and steroid use, and outcome in patients with septic shock. Crit Care. 2007;11(3):1–8.
5. Weingart SD, Levitan RM. Preoxygenation and prevention of desaturation during emergency airway management. Ann Emerg Med. 2012;59:165–75. e1
6. Miguel-Montanes R, Hajage D, Messika J, Bertrand F, Gaudry S, Rafat C, Labbe V, Dufour N, Jean-Baptiste S, Bedet A, Dreyfuss D, Richard JD. Use of high-flow nasal cannula oxygen therapy to prevent desaturation during tracheal intubation of intensive care patients with mild-to-moderate hypoxemia. Crit Care Med. 2015;43:574–83.
7. Stephens CT, Kahntroff S, Dutton RP. The success of emergency endotracheal intubation in trauma patients: a 10-year experience at a major adult trauma referral center. Anesth Analg. 2009;109:866–72.
8. Sollid SJ, Lossius HM, Soreide E. Pre-hospital intubation by anaesthesiologists in patients with severe trauma: an audit of a Norwegian helicopter emergency medical service. Scand J Trauma Resusc Emerg Med. 2010;18:30.
9. Shatney CH, Brunner RD, Nguyen TQ. The safety of orotracheal intubation in patients with unstable cervical spine fracture or high spinal cord injury. Am J Surg. 1995;170:676–9; discussion 9–80.
10. Turner CR, Block J, Shanks A, Morris M, Lodhia KR, Gujar SK. Motion of a cadaver model of cervical injury during endotracheal intubation with a Bullard laryngoscope or a Macintosh blade with and without in-line stabilization. J Trauma. 2009;67:61–6.
11. Gerling MC, Davis DP, Hamilton RS, et al. Effects of cervical spine immobilization technique and laryngoscope blade selection on an unstable cervical spine in a cadaver model of intubation. Ann Emerg Med. 2000;36:293–300.

12. Griesdale DE, Liu D, McKinney J, Choi PT. Glidescope((R)) video-laryngoscopy versus direct laryngoscopy for endotracheal intubation: a systematic review and meta-analysis. Can J Anaesth. 2012; 59(1):41–52.
13. Yeatts DJ, Dutton RP, Hu PF, et al. Effect of video laryngoscopy on trauma patient survival: a randomized controlled trial. J Trauma Acute Care Surg. 2013;75:212–9.
14. Nouruzi-Sedeh P, Schumann M, Groeben H. Laryngoscopy via Macintosh blade versus GlideScope: success rate and time for endotracheal intubation in untrained medical personnel. Anesthesiology. 2009; 110:32–7.
15. Aziz MF, Healy D, Kheterpal S, Fu RF, Dillman D, Brambrink AM. Routine clinical practice effectiveness of the Glidescope in difficult airway management: an analysis of 2,004 Glidescope intubations, complications, and failures from two institutions. Anesthesiology. 2011;114:34–41.
16. Hulme J, Perkins GD. Critically injured patients, inaccessible airways, and laryngeal mask airways. Emerg Med J. 2005;22:742–4.
17. Baker PA, Webber JB. Failure to ventilate with supraglottic airways after drowning. Anaesth Intensive Care. 2011;39:675–7.
18. Bindra T, Nihalani SK, Bhadoria P, Wadhawan S. Use of intubating laryngeal mask airway in a morbidly obese patient with chest trauma in an emergency setting. J Anaesthesiol Clin Pharmacol. 2011;27:544–6.
19. Tobin JM. Usage and efficacy of airway adjuncts in an emergency intubation kit. Emerg Med Australas. 2011;23:514–5.
20. Schalk R, Meininger D, Ruesseler M, et al. Emergency airway management in trauma patients using laryngeal tube suction. Prehosp Emerg Care. 2011; 15:347–50.
21. Gahan K, Studnek JR, Vandeventer S. King LT-D use by urban basic life support first responders as the primary airway device for out-of-hospital cardiac arrest. Resuscitation. 2011;82:1525–8.
22. Law JA, Morris IR, Brousseau PA, de la Ronde S, Milne AD. The incidence, success rate, and complications of awake tracheal intubation in 1,554 patients over 12 years: an historical cohort study. Can J Anaesth. 2015;62:736–44.
23. Joseph TT, Gal JS, DeMaria S Jr, Lin HM, Levine AI, Hyman JB. A retrospective study of success, failure, and time needed to perform awake intubation. Anesthesiology. 2016;125:105–14.
24. Adams BD, Cuniowski PA, Muck A, De Lorenzo RA. Registry of emergency airways arriving at combat hospitals. J Trauma. 2008;64:1548–54.
25. Mabry RL. An analysis of battlefield cricothyrotomy in Iraq and Afghanistan. J Spec Oper Med. 2012;12:17–23.
26. Lehman LW, Saeed M, Talmor D, Mark R, Malhotra A. Methods of blood pressure measurement in the ICU. Crit Care Med. 2013;41:34–40.
27. Pytte M, Dybwik K, Sexton J, Straume B, Nielsen EW. Oscillometric brachial mean artery pressures are higher than intra-radial mean artery pressures in intensive care unit patients receiving norepinephrine. Acta Anaesthesiol Scand. 2006;50:718–21.
28. Berkenstadt H, Margalit N, Hadani M, et al. Stroke volume variation as a predictor of fluid responsiveness in patients undergoing brain surgery. Anesth Analg. 2001;92:984–9.
29. Davis JW, Shackford SR, Mackersie RC, Hoyt DB. Base deficit as a guide to volume resuscitation. J Trauma. 1988;28:1464–7.
30. Davis JW, Parks SN, Kaups KL, Gladen HE, O'Donnell-Nicol S. Admission base deficit predicts transfusion requirements and risk of complications. J Trauma. 1996;41:769–74.
31. Connelly CR, Schreiber MA. Endpoints in resuscitation. Curr Opin Crit Care. 2015;21:512–9.
32. Mutschler M, Nienaber U, Brockamp T, et al. Renaissance of base deficit for the initial assessment of trauma patients: a base deficit-based classification for hypovolemic shock developed on data from 16,305 patients derived from the TraumaRegister DGU(R). Crit Care. 2013;17:R42.
33. Einav S, Bromiker R, Weiniger CF, Matot I. Mathematical modeling for prediction of survival from resuscitation based on computerized continuous capnography: proof of concept. Acad Emerg Med. 2011;18:468–75.
34. Tyburski JG, Collinge JD, Wilson RF, Carlin AM, Albaran RG, Steffes CP. End-tidal CO_2-derived values during emergency trauma surgery correlated with outcome: a prospective study. J Trauma. 2002;53:738–43.
35. Ho KM, Leonard AD. Concentration-dependent effect of hypocalcaemia on mortality of patients with critical bleeding requiring massive transfusion: a cohort study. Anaesth Intensive Care. 2011;39:46–54.
36. Vivien B, Langeron O, Morell E, et al. Early hypocalcemia in severe trauma. Crit Care Med. 2005;33:1946–52.
37. Magnotti LJ, Bradburn EH, Webb DL, et al. Admission ionized calcium levels predict the need for multiple transfusions: a prospective study of 591 critically ill trauma patients. J Trauma. 2011;70:391–5; discussion 5–7.
38. Walters BC, Hadley MN, Hurlbert RJ, Aarabi B, Dhall SS, Gelb DE, Harrigan MR, Rozelle CJ, Ryken TC, Theodore N. Guidelines for the management of acute cervical spine and spinal cord injuries: 2013 update. Clin Neurosurg. 2013;60:82–91.
39. Carney N, Totten AM, O'Reilly C, Ullman JS, GWJ H, Bell MJ, Bratton SL, Chesnut R, Harris OA, Kissoon N, Rubiano AM, Shutter L, Tasker RC, Vavilala MS, Wilberger J, Wright DW, Ghajar J. Guidelines for the management of severe traumatic brain injury, fourth edition. Neurosurgery. 2017;80(1):6–15.
40. Gomes E, Antunes R, Dias C, Araujo R, Costa-Pereira A. Acute kidney injury in severe trauma assessed by RIFLE criteria: a common feature without implications on mortality? Scand J Trauma Resusc Emerg Med. 2010;18:1.

41. Bellomo R, Ronco C, Kellum JA, Mehta RL, Palevsky P. Acute dialysis quality initiative workgroup. Acute renal failure—definition, outcome measures, animal models, fluid therapy and information technology needs: the Second International Consensus Conference of the Acute Dialysis Quality Initiative (ADQI) group. Crit Care. 2004;B(4):R204–12.
42. Liaño F, Junco E, Pascual J, Madero R, Verde E. The spectrum of acute renal failure in the intensive care unit compared with that seen in other settings. The Madrid Acute Renal Failure Study Group. Kidney Int. 1998;53:S16–24.
43. Cosentino F, Chaff C, Piedmonte M. Risk factors influencing survival in ICU acute renal failure. Nephrol Dial Transplant. 1994;9:179–82.
44. Huen SC, Parikh CR. Predicting acute kidney injury after cardiac surgery: a systematic review. Ann Thorac Surg. 2012;93(1):337–47.
45. Brown C, Rhee P, Chan L, Evans K, Demetriades D, Velmahos D. Preventing renal failure in patients with rhabdomyolysis: do bicarbonate and mannitol make a difference? J Trauma Inj Infect Crit Care. 2004;56(6):1191–6.
46. Ho KM, Power BM. Benefits and risks of furosemide in acute kidney injury. Anesthesia. 2010;65(3):283–93.
47. Comparison of two fluid-management strategies and acute lung injury. The National Heart, Lung, and Blood Institute Acute Respiratory Distress Syndrome (ARDS) clinical trials network. N Engl J Med. 2006;354:2564–75.
48. Murphy EL, Kwaan N, Looney MR, et al. Risk factors and outcomes in transfusion-associated circulatory overload. Am J Med. 2013;126:357.e29–38.
49. The Acute Respiratory Distress Syndrome Network. Ventilation with lower tidal volumes as compared with traditional tidal volumes for acute lung injury and the acute respiratory distress syndrome. N Engl J Med. 2000;342:1301–8.
50. Papazian L, Forel JM, Gacouin A, et al. Neuromuscular blockers in early acute respiratory distress syndrome. N Engl J Med. 2010;363:1107–16.
51. Serpa Neto A, Cardoso SO, Manetta JA, et al. Association between use of lung-protective ventilation with lower tidal volumes and clinical outcomes among patients without acute respiratory distress syndrome: a meta-analysis. JAMA. 2012;308:1651–9.
52. Serpa Neto A, Hemmes SN, Barbas CS, et al. Protective versus conventional ventilation for surgery: a systematic review and individual patient data meta-analysis. Anesthesiology. 2015;123:66–78.
53. Guldner A, Kiss T, Serpa Neto A, et al. Intraoperative protective mechanical ventilation for prevention of postoperative pulmonary complications: a comprehensive review of the role of tidal volume, positive end-expiratory pressure, and lung recruitment maneuvers. Anesthesiology. 2015;123:692–713.
54. Arlt M, Philipp A, Voelkel S, et al. Extracorporeal membrane oxygenation in severe trauma patients with bleeding shock. Resuscitation. 2010;81:804–9.
55. McElroy LM, Macapagal KR, Collins KM, Abecassis MM, Holl JL, Ladner DP, Gordon EJ. Clinician perceptions of operating room to intensive care unit handoffs and implications for patient safety: a qualitative study. Am J Surg. 2015;210(4):629–35.
56. Salzwedel C, Mai V, Punke MA, Kluge S, Reuter DA. The effect of a checklist on the quality of patient handover from the operating room to the intensive care unit: a randomized controlled trial. J Crit Care. 2016;32:170–4.

Are We Doing Too Much Damage Control?

17

John A. Harvin

Abstract

Unfortunately, a large proportion of care delivered to trauma patients is not based upon high-quality evidence. Poor external funding of research, difficulty studying emergent interventions, and regulatory burdens create a high burden to overcome to successfully design, implement, and interpret emergent clinical trials. The lack of high-quality evidence for interventions results in variations of practice and outcomes across trauma centers. Damage control techniques have certainly saved lives since their introduction into modern trauma care. However, some of these techniques lack rigorous evidence. Other techniques have high-quality evidence but suffer from a lack of generalizability as resuscitation has dramatically evolved over the last 15 years.

17.1 Introduction

Are we doing too much damage control? The short answer—probably. Too much or too little of any intervention is highly subject to the local environment in which these decisions are made. The same goes for damage control. There is significant heterogeneity in the types of patients trauma centers treat, and this heterogeneity leads to dissimilar utilization of damage control surgery. In this chapter, we will review the evidence for damage control surgery, discuss the difficulties in interpreting the evidence, and make the argument that high-quality studies of damage control interventions are both feasible and necessary.

J.A. Harvin, M.D., F.A.C.S.
McGovern Medical School at UT Health, Houston, TX, USA
e-mail: John.Harvin@uth.tmc.edu

17.2 The Evidence

17.2.1 Damage Control Laparotomy

The initial indications described for damage control laparotomy were the onset of coagulopathy during emergency laparotomy and an intra-abdominal vascular injury combined with two or more visceral injuries in a massively transfused, penetrating trauma patient [1, 2]. This concept was innovative at the time and led to the application of this technique to other situations, such as hepatic packing, second-look trauma laparotomy, need for a time-consuming operation in a marginally resuscitated patient, and abdominal compartment syndrome prophylaxis and treatment [3]. Improvements in patient care were seen immediately leading to an even more liberal application of damage control laparotomy with rates reaching in the 30–40% range at some institutions [4, 5].

J. Duchesne et al. (eds.), *Damage Control in Trauma Care*,
https://doi.org/10.1007/978-3-319-72607-6_17

While clinical experience with damage control laparotomy is now quite robust, there continues to be a dearth of level 1 evidence to support its use. Even decades after its first implementation and widespread dissemination, appropriateness of indication is still based upon expert opinion and experience [6, 7]. A major impediment to studying damage control laparotomy is surgeon equipoise. Quite simply, surgeons disagree on appropriate and inappropriate indications for damage control (Fig. 17.1).

This variability, however, is proof that *group* equipoise exists. This group equipoise should be the basis for future clinical trials of damage control laparotomy. While it may be uncontroversial to perform a damage control laparotomy in a coagulopathic patient with severe hepatic injury requiring packing, certainly some indications are debatable, such as second-look laparotomies. It is these indications in which controversy exists that we should study this intervention.

17.2.2 Damage Control Orthopedics

Unlike damage control laparotomy, there are multiple randomized clinical trials evaluating damage control orthopedics [8–10]. In general, early fracture fixation has not been associated with increased rates of acute respiratory distress syndrome or mortality. There may be a subgroup of severely injured patients ("borderline" patients), in whom damage control orthopedics is helpful; however no adequately powered study exists to support this concept [11]. So, again, there is limited high-quality data to guide surgeon decision-making.

An additional concern about previous clinical trials evaluating early total care versus damage control orthopedics is generalizability. Most studies on the subject were performed in an era where crystalloid was a large component of massive resuscitations [12, 13]. The harms of crystalloid and their association with acute respiratory

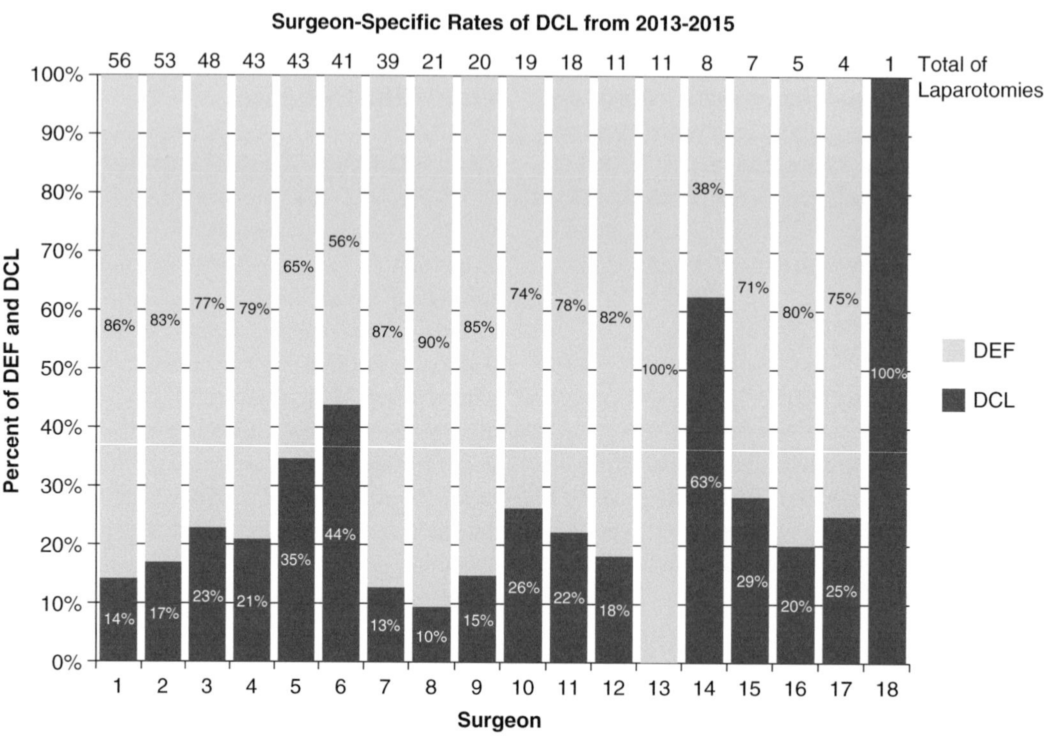

Fig. 17.1 Surgeon-specific rates of damage control laparotomy at the Red Duke Trauma Institute at Memorial Hermann Hospital—Texas Medical Center in Houston, Texas (unpublished data)

distress syndrome and mortality are becoming clear as the benefits of balanced resuscitation have become evident [14]. As in damage control laparotomy, where minimization of crystalloid and high ratios of plasma, platelets, and red blood cells have helped prevent and reverse coagulopathy and acidosis allowing surgeons to stay in the operating room longer, improved resuscitation may also better optimize patients for early total care as opposed to damage control orthopedics.

17.3 Difficulties Interpreting the Evidence

There are several difficulties in interpreting the data available on all forms of damage control surgery. First, there is a dearth of clinical trials on the subject, leaving mostly retrospective studies available to interpret and apply to current clinical situations. Because most available studies are retrospective, selection bias and the presence of known and unknown confounders limits the ability to accurately determine the effect of damage control surgery. That is, patients who were treated with a damage control intervention were more severely injured or more physiologically deranged than those treated with definitive interventions. No amount of matching or regression can account for all the confounding factors that go along with being more severely injured. Thus, morbidity associated with damage control interventions is likely to be higher than present. This helps to limit the prospective study of damage control interventions because disproportionate and unrealistic harm is associated with the damage control intervention.

Second, more often than not, studies detailing damage control interventions—especially damage control laparotomy—fail to report the rate of and indications for those interventions. Any surgeon evaluating their own institution might find it difficult to evaluate the question "Are we doing too much damage control?" without baseline rates of these interventions and commonly accepted indications being published. Indeed, a standard requirement for any publication on a damage control intervention should be the overall rate of use and a breakdown of the indications for that intervention.

Lastly, the generalizability of studies to one's own institution and patient population can be difficult. There are two methods by which generalizability can be improved. First, studies should describe the context in which they are performed. Examples of this include overall trauma volume per year, number of laparotomies per year, level of trauma center designation, and a description of the patient population (rural, urban, mixed). Second, multicenter studies can provide more generalizable knowledge to apply to local practices.

17.4 The Future

At this point, no damage control intervention has sufficient high-quality evidence to make strong recommendations to support its use [15]. The vast majority of interventions only have biased treatment effects to guide decision-making. The Institute of Medicine lists aim to improve healthcare quality, including that care be safe, effective, patient-centered, timely, efficient, and equitable. If our goal is to provide quality trauma care to our patients, the available literature is simply not capable of directing us. Unfortunately, this statement is true for most interventions we provide to patients, not simply damage control interventions.

It is difficult to perform prospective clinical trials in trauma and acute care surgery. Individual informed consent often cannot realistically be obtained. The simple act of opening an envelope to randomize a patient can be challenging in the middle of a hectic resuscitation. Nevertheless, many recent clinical trials have shown that it is possible to overcome these obstacles [16, 17]. The use of exception from informed consent appears to be increasing in trauma research. This tool provided by the US Department of Health and Human Services allows for enrollment of patients into clinical trials and delayed consent once the patient has stabilized [18]. The process of obtaining an exception from informed consent has been improved and facilitated by the use of social media [19, 20].

Surgeon equipoise can also limit the ability to perform clinical trials in trauma. Many experienced surgeons can either feel strongly in favor of or against any intervention that has low-quality evidence. This decisiveness is necessary for them to provide timely care to injured patients. This decisiveness also may limit the ability of those surgeons to feel ethically justified to enroll patients into clinical trials evaluating the effect of those interventions. The focus of equipoise should not be on surgeon equipoise, but group or clinical equipoise [21]. If there is controversy among the experienced surgeons in the trauma community about any particular intervention, then clinical equipoise likely exists and surgeons should feel ethically justified to participate in such a clinical trial. This requires the transparent acknowledgment that the best treatment is currently unknown.

Conclusion

Are we doing too much damage control? Probably. A recent quality improvement study at the Red Duke Trauma Institute at Memorial Hermann Hospital—Texas Medical Center resulted in a reduction in damage control laparotomy from 39 to 23% [22]. The rate continued to decrease ultimately averaging 18% over the most recent 8 months. Despite this decrease, no change in morbidity or mortality was observed. This brings into question the morbidity typically associated with damage control laparotomy. Other centers have also reported similar successful efforts to decrease the rate of damage control surgery [5].

Despite using damage control techniques for decades, there is still too little high-quality data to definitively answer that question. The trauma community should acknowledge that clinical equipoise exists for many of the interventions being performed daily in the United States. Clinical trials in damage control interventions are desperately needed to ensure that we are providing high-quality care to our patients. This will require increased funding for injury, a major public health burden in the United States. In the interim, publications should detail rates of and indications for damage control surgery and the context in which they are performed so that surgeons can better interpret appropriate use of these interventions.

References

1. Stone HH, Strom PR, Mullins RJ. Management of the major coagulopathy with onset during laparotomy. Ann Surg. 1983;197(5):532–5.
2. Rotondo MF, Schwab CW, McGonigal MD, Phillips GR, Fruchterman TM, Kauder DR, Latenser BA, Angood PA. 'Damage control': an approach for improved survival in exsanguinating penetrating abdominal trauma. J Trauma. 1993;35(3):375–82.
3. Moore EE. Staged laparotomy for the hypothermia, acidosis, and coagulopathy syndrome. Am J Surg. 1996;172(5):405–10.
4. Hatch QM, Osterhout LM, Podbielski J, Kozar RA, Wade CE, Holcomb JB, Cotton BA. Impact of closure at the first take back: complication burden and potential overutilization of damage control laparotomy. J Trauma. 2011;71(6):1503–11.
5. Higa G, Friese R, O'Keefe T, Wynne J, Bowlby P, Ziemba M, Latifi R, Kulvatunyou N, Rhee P. Damage control laparotomy: a vital tool once overused. J Trauma. 2010;69(1):53–9.
6. Roberts DJ, Bobrovitz N, Zygun DA, Ball CG, Kirkpatrick AW, Faris PD, Brohi K, D'Amours S, Fabian TC, Inaba K, Leppäniemi AK, Moore EE, Navsaria PH, Nicol AJ, Parry N, Stelfox HT. Indications for use of damage control surgery in civilian trauma patients: a content analysis and expert appropriateness rating study. Ann Surg. 2016;263(5):1018–27.
7. Roberts DJ, Zygun DA, Faris PD, Ball CG, Kirkpatrick AW, Stelfox HT. Indications for Trauma Damage Control Surgery International Study Group. Opinions of practicing surgeons on the appropriateness of published indications for use of damage control surgery in trauma patients: an international cross-sectional survey. J Am Coll Surg. 2016;223(3):515–29.
8. Pape HC, Rixen D, Morley J, Husebye EE, Mueller M, Dumont C, Gruner A, Oestern HJ, Bayeff-Filoff M, Garving C, Pardini D, van Griensven M, Krettek C, Giannoudis P, EPOFF Study Group. Impact of the method of initial stabilization for femoral shaft fractures in patients with multiple injuries at risk for complications (borderline patients). Ann Surg. 2007;246(3):491–9.
9. Pape HC, Grimme K, Van Griensven M, Sott AH, Giannoudis P, Morley J, Roise O, Ellingsen E, Hildebrand F, Wiese B, Krettek C, EPOFF Study Group. Impact of intramedullary instrumentation versus damage control for femoral fractures on immunoinflammatory parameters: prospective randomized analysis by the EPOFF Study Group. J Trauma. 2003;55(1):7–13.
10. Rixen D, Steinhausen E, Sauerland S, Lefering R, Maegele MG, Bouillon B, Grass G, Neugebauer EA, Members of the Damage Control Study Group. Randomized, controlled, two-arm, interventional, multicenter study on risk-adapted damage con-

trol orthopedic surgery of femur shaft fractures in multiple-trauma patients. Trials. 2016;17:47.
11. Nahm NJ, Vallier HA. Timing of definitive treatment of femoral shaft fractures in patients with multiple injuries: a systematic review of randomized and nonrandomized trials. J Trauma Acute Care Surg. 2012;73(5):1046–63.
12. Pape HC, Hildebrand F, Pertschy S, Zelle B, Garapati R, Grimme K, Krettek C, Reed RL 2nd. Changes in the management of femoral shaft fractures in polytrauma patients: from early total care to damage control orthopedic surgery. J Trauma. 2002;53(3):452–61.
13. Navarrete-Navarro P, Ruiz-Bailén M, Rivera-Fernández R, Guerrero-López F, Pola-Gallego-de-Guzmán MD, Vázquez-Mata G. Acute respiratory distress syndrome in trauma patients: ICU mortality and prediction factors. Intensive Care Med. 2000;26(11):1624–9.
14. Neal MD, Hoffman MK, Cuschieri J, Minei JP, Maier RV, Harbrecht BG, Billiar TR, Peitzman AB, Moore EE, Cohen MJ, Sperry JL. Crystalloid to packed red blood cell transfusion ratio in the massively transfused patient: when a little goes a long way. J Trauma Acute Care Surg. 2012;72(4):892–8.
15. Cirrochi R, Montedori A, Farinella E, Bonacini I, Tagliabue L, Abraha I. Damage control surgery for abdominal trauma. Cochrane Database Syst Rev. 2013;3:CD007438
16. Schreiber MA, Meier EN, Tisherman SA, Kerby JD, Newgard CD, Brasel K, Egan D, Witham W, Williams C, Daya M, Beeson J, McCully BH, Wheeler S, Kannas D, May S, McKnight B, Hoyt DB, Investigators ROC. A controlled resuscitation strategy is feasible and safe in hypotensive trauma patients: results of a prospective randomized pilot trial. J Trauma Acute Care Surg. 2015;78(4):687–95.
17. Holcomb JB, Tilley BC, Baraniuk S, Fox EE, Wade CE, Podbielski JM, DJ DJ, Brasel KJ, Bulger EM, Callcut RA, Cohen MJ, Cotton BA, Fabian TC, Inaba K, Kerby JD, Muskat P, O'Keeffe T, Rizoli S, Robinson BR, Scalea TM, Schreiber MA, Stein DM, Weinberg JA, Callum JL, Hess JR, Matijevic N, Miller CN, Pittet JF, Hoyt DB, Pearson GD, Leroux B, van Belle G, PROPPR Study Group. Ansfusion of plasma, platelets, and red blood cells in a 1:1:1 vs a 1:1:2 ratio and mortality in patients with severe trauma: the PROPPR randomized clinical trial. JAMA. 2015;313(5):471–82.
18. U.S. Food and Drug Administration, Code of Federal Regulations Title 21. Section 50.24, Exception from Informed Consent Requirements for Emergency Research [online]. Accessed 28 Aug 2016.
19. Stephens SW, Williams C, Gray R, Kerby JD, Wang HE. Preliminary experience with social media for community consultation and public disclosure in exception from informed consent trials. Circulation. 2013;128(3):267–70.
20. Stephens SW, Williams C, Gray R, Kerby JD, Wang HE, Bosarge PL. Using social media for community consultation and public disclosure in exception from informed consent. J Trauma Acute Care Surg. 2016;80(6):1005–9.
21. Freedman B. Equipoise and the ethics of clinical research. N Engl J Med. 1987;317(3):141–5.
22. Harvin JA, Kao LS, Liang MK, Adams SD, McNutt MK, Love JD, Moore LJ, Wade CE, Cotton BA, Holcomb JB. Decreasing the use of damage control laparotomy: a quality improvement project. J Am Coll Surg. 2017;225(2):200–9

Coagulation Perturbations After Severe Injury: Translational Approaches and the State of the Science

18

Mitchell Jay Cohen

Abstract

Despite evidence of acute traumatic coagulopathy hiding in plain site for decades, coagulopathy after trauma was thought to result from the iatrogenic effects of otherwise well-intentioned resuscitation. The luminary shock research of the late 1960s and early 1970s combined with advances in blood banking result in a cold red blood cell and crystalloid-based resuscitation practice which prevailed for decades. Indeed, the initial groundbreaking work on hemorrhagic shock revealed that shocked patients required both oxygen carrying capacity and blood flow (pressure) for survival [1–3]. While much of this early work was done in the era of whole blood, this was largely forgotten as a result of the contemporaneously timed move away from whole blood transfusion toward component therapy. Beginning in the mid-1970s, the blood banking community realized that they could component separate whole blood thereby taking a unit of whole blood and converting it to components; one unit of packed red blood cells (PRBCs) one unit of fresh frozen plasma (FFP) some part of a unit of platelets with the remainder becoming cryoprecipitate consisting of concentrated factors and fibrinogen. The white blood cells were spun or filtered off variably during the process. These changes which were initially made for resource allocation and financial reasons were solidified in the early 1980s by the emergence of HIV and concerns about the safety of the blood supply. Hence the new understanding from research on shock that our patients need oxygen carrying capacity and flow and left with components in the blood bank and crystalloid on the shelf our resuscitation practices evolved toward the delivery of large volumes of cold packed red blood cells and many liters of salt water. It was for decades common to resuscitate severely injured patients with multiple units of packed red blood cells and many liters of crystalloid with little to no attention paid to coagulation measures or any need for plasma or platelets. These resuscitation practices resulted in the creation of or exacerbation of iatrogenic coagulopathy characterized by dilution, hypothermia, and acidosis described below.

M.J. Cohen, M.D., F.A.C.S.
Department of Surgery, University of Colorado School of Medicine, Aurora, CO, USA
e-mail: mitchell.cohen@dhha.org

18.1 Introduction

Despite evidence of acute traumatic coagulopathy hiding in plain site for decades, coagulopathy after trauma was thought to result from the

J. Duchesne et al. (eds.), *Damage Control in Trauma Care*,
https://doi.org/10.1007/978-3-319-72607-6_18

iatrogenic effects of otherwise well-intentioned resuscitation. The luminary shock research of the late 1960s and early 1970s combined with advances in blood banking result in a cold red blood cell and crystalloid-based resuscitation practice which prevailed for decades. Indeed, the initial groundbreaking work on hemorrhagic shock revealed that shocked patients required both oxygen carrying capacity and blood flow (pressure) for survival [1–3]. While much of this early work was done in the era of whole blood, this was largely forgotten as a result of the contemporaneously timed move away from whole blood transfusion toward component therapy. Beginning in the mid-1970s, the blood banking community realized that they could component separate whole blood thereby taking a unit of whole blood and converting it to components; one unit of packed red blood cells (PRBCs) one unit of fresh frozen plasma (FFP) some part of a unit of platelets with the remainder becoming cryoprecipitate consisting of concentrated factors and fibrinogen. The white blood cells were spun or filtered off variably during the process. These changes which were initially made for resource allocation and financial reasons were solidified in the early 1980s by the emergence of HIV and concerns about the safety of the blood supply. Hence the new understanding from research on shock that our patients need oxygen carrying capacity and flow and left with components in the blood bank and crystalloid on the shelf our resuscitation practices evolved toward the delivery of large volumes of cold packed red blood cells and many liters of salt water. It was for decades common to resuscitate severely injured patients with multiple units of packed red blood cells and many liters of crystalloid with little to no attention paid to coagulation measures or any need for plasma or platelets. These resuscitation practices resulted in the creation of or exacerbation of iatrogenic coagulopathy characterized by dilution, hypothermia, and acidosis described below.

For many years, this was the mantra that any coagulopathy in trauma was a result of exogenous iatrogenic reasons which were unfortunate sequelae of our otherwise well-meant resuscitation. This mantra remained for many years until 2003 at which time Brohi and colleagues published their luminary paper defining acute traumatic coagulopathy [4]. Examining a retrospective dataset of injured patients brought by the helicopter service to the Royal London Hospital, investigators found that approximately one third of patients were coagulopathic upon arrival to the hospital. Patients who had impaired coagulation had a mortality rate of nearly 50% above a 10% baseline in those who had normal coagulation. Concurrently Macleod and colleagues published a similar characterization of patients with similar demographics, incidence, and outcomes [5]. Together these papers established that there existed an endogenous coagulopathy of trauma which occurred before or separate from the iatrogenic causes which had been previously thought to be the primary cause of coagulopathy after injury.

Based on these findings, several groups began the important work of characterizing and investigating mechanisms of coagulation perturbations after injury. Perhaps the first mechanistic characterization was an examination of 209 critically injured patients brought to San Francisco General Hospital. Investigators found that patients who were severely injured with an injury severity score >15 and shock (defined as a based deficit >−6) were coagulopathic with prolonged prothrombin and partial thromboplastin times [6, 7]. Patients with acute traumatic coagulopathy had significantly higher mortality rates and if they live higher rates of inflammatory complications including multiple organ failure, lung injury, and infection. Biochemical evaluation in this study and several other papers revealed several mechanistic insights. While this work evaluated multiple putative mechanistic phenotypes including factor depletion, impaired thrombin production, and compensatory anticoagulant pathways, this initial data suggested acute traumatic coagulopathy was associated with activation with protein C system which will be discussed in the section on acute traumatic coagulopathy below.

18.2 Iatrogenic Coagulopathy

While it is now understood that acute traumatic coagulopathy is an endogenous response to trauma and shock, our resuscitative practices and the dynamic development of the trauma patient over time also affect the coagulation milieu. As described in the introduction, for many years it was believed that the vicious triad of acidosis, hypothermia, and dilution were the only cause of coagulopathy after injury [8]. While this is now understood to be incorrect, each of these causes of coagulation disturbances (acidosis, hypothermia, and dilution) is important, and together they have been newly termed iatrogenic coagulopathy [8].

18.2.1 Hypothermia

After injury patients often become hypothermic from a combination of their injury, exposure in the prehospital and hospital environments (during rescue, resuscitation, and surgery), and the administration of large volumes of relatively cool resuscitation fluids. Because multiple techniques have been developed to mitigate hypothermia after trauma, as a result its incidence and severity have been lessened; even so this can be a vexing problem with implications for coagulation. Mechanisms for hypothermic coagulopathy include impaired protease function and impaired platelet function. Generally, thrombin production and function are impaired at temperatures below 33°C. While these disturbances have been well established in in vitro closed systems, effects in actual patients remain less well understood. Because most clotting assays including conventional clotting tests as well as viscoelastic testing are performed on plasma or whole blood rewarmed to 37°, any hypothermic perturbations are not seen clinically and in large characterization datasets. In addition to protease enzymatic activity, historical evidence also suggests that hypothermia adversely affects platelet function. Recent data however has shown that there is an endogenous platelet dysfunction of trauma affecting up to 50% of patients, which is likely more important than any hypothermic effects. In addition, new data suggests that platelet function is in fact preserved and possibly enhanced as temperature drops. That being said, the effects of hypothermia on coagulation are thought to be minor in comparison to the endogenous perturbations seen in ATC and relatively minor compared to the dilution of old-fashioned crystalloid-based resuscitation.

18.3 Dilutional

The final and perhaps most impactful of the triad of iatrogenic coagulopathy is dilutional coagulopathy (also termed resuscitation-associated coagulopathy). This dilution results from the (now fortunately) large-volume crystalloid-based resuscitation. In this scenario large volumes dilute coagulation factors which are already relatively depleted by cascade activation and loss from hemorrhage and are further diluted preventing clotting cascade propagation and thrombin and fibrin formation [9, 10]. Another cause of coagulation disturbances from dilution suggests that the reduction of hematocrit from blood loss replaced with crystalloid resulting in impaired platelet interaction with the growing fibrin plug resulting coagulopathy. Fortunately, in the era of plasma-based balanced resuscitation, there are much less dilution and resulting coagulation effects. Indeed while much effort has been spent on the debate of which resuscitation ratio (e.g., 1:1 vs. 1:2) is correct, this seems distracting from the salient mechanism which has curtailed historical dilutional coagulopathy. Instead of the particular ratio, the combination of a plasma-based blood product resuscitation with the often overlooked effect of a lack of large-volume crystalloid resuscitation has resulted in improved clotting and outcomes. While much of the world has gone to a plasma-based balanced ratio, some parts of Europe continue to utilize a starch-based fluid resuscitation regime which results in a fibrinogen bioavailability and dilutional coagulopathy. Indeed, their coagulopathic animal models and resultant publications are reflective of these clinical resuscitation policies making them unfortunately no longer relevant in 2017. Fortunately much of Europe and indeed the world is moving away from these resuscitation practices making dilutional coagulopathy much less prevalent.

18.4 Acute Traumatic Coagulopathy

As described above acute traumatic coagulopathy, which is also called trauma-induced coagulopathy (*these terms will be utilized interchangeably), was initially described by Brohi and colleagues in 2003. Subsequent to this significant work by multiple groups has elucidated and evaluated multiple mechanisms involved in ATC which will be described here.

18.4.1 Activated Protein C

Protein C is a serine protease which when activated from its inactive zymogen state in a proteolytic reaction involving (primarily) endothelial-bound thrombomodulin, thrombin and the endothelial protein C receptor [11, 12]. Once activated protein C exerts its anticoagulant effects through the proteolytic cleavage of factors Va and VIIIa. In addition, it prevents coagulation through working as a thrombin sink. Lastly it derepresses fibrinolysis by inhibiting PAI-1 which serves to free tPA resulting in increased lysis. Taken together activation of protein C binds thrombin and prevents clot from being formed while enhancing fibrinolysis. In trauma, these mechanisms have been extensively studied and characterized in multiple human studies and animal and in vivo models.

When severe injury is combined with tissue hypoperfusion, there is an activation of protein C to its activated form which results in proteolytic cleavage of factors Va and VIIIa as well as derepression of fibrinolysis from inhibition of PAI-1 and resultant increased activity of tPA. This protein C activation was initially described in polytrauma patients and has been corroborated in multiple human cohorts including in isolated TBI patients [7, 13]. Subsequent animal model and in vitro data have confirmed the initial clinical findings. Additional lab data suggests that the combination of thrombin production from tissue injury and thrombomodulin and endothelial protein C receptor expression at the endothelial surface from shock (tissue hypoperfusion) result in the necessary components for activation of this protein C. Patients with elevated activated protein C levels or conversely depleted protein C zymogen have increased bleeding, increased resuscitation needs, higher mortality, and when they survive increased inflammatory complications including ARDS, multiple organ failure, and infection. This last point is worth exploring as it highlights the crosstalk between coagulation and inflammation after injury. While it has considerable anticoagulant activity, APC is also profoundly cytoprotective with a signaling domain on the molecule separate from the protease domain which binds PAR-1 and results in anti-apoptosis, cleavage of extracellular histones, and reduced endothelial permeability. It seems plausible that activated protein C is being activated in high concentration after injury in an attempt to keep the host (patient) alive through the acute phase of injury. The unfortunate sequelae of too much of a good thing results in ATC. Later when a patient has survived through the initial acute phase to land in the ICU, the too much of a good thing is replaced by too little of a good thing with impaired cytoprotection and a resultant hypercoagulable state characterized by thrombotic risk and complications. This complex biology provides one example of the important crosstalk between inflammation and coagulation. This maladaptive protein C hypothesis would suggest that a combination of blocking the anticoagulant effect of APC and augmenting the cytoprotective effects would allow for a mitigation of coagulopathy while enhancing the beneficial inflammation-modulatory effects. The well-described failure of recombinant activated protein C (trade name Xigris) in septic shock was likely because of inappropriate dosing and poor patient selection. It was often described as the last very expensive therapeutic given patients just before they died and was taken off of the market due to this futility and the worry about bleeding risk. That being said the biological and clinical plausibility is extremely good, and the combination of blocking only the protease function (to mitigate ATC) has sound preclinical evidence. Recent development of engineered protein C molecules that have only the cytoprotective binding (with enhanced activity and no bleeding risk) by the group at Scripps provides the ability to test this in our injured patients in the near future.

While activation of the protein C system has been implicated in the acute coagulopathy of trauma, several other mechanisms have also been investigated. First is thrombin production and factor depletion. While it might seem obvious that factor depletion would be common after trauma and that repletion of factors via a plasma- or factor-based resuscitation would play a key role in mitigating coagulopathy, there is no evidence to support either of these theories. Several investigative groups have measured antigen and functional factor levels after injury, and while there is often a trend toward lower levels compared to uninjured controls, none of the measured factor levels drop low enough to result in a depletion coagulopathy characterized by impaired thrombin production [14, 15]. Of course, it is certainly possible that these low but not critically low factor levels are indeed depleted enough to cause a tissue-specific coagulopathy resulting in impaired clotting for what would be needed at the site of injury after a severe trauma however this remains an untested and outside of sophisticated animal model untestable theory. Speaking against this local or post trauma, situational coagulopathy is the always high thrombin production post trauma. In multiple animal models, thrombin production after injury remains high and does not seem to constitute a reason for impaired coagulation.

Along with factor levels, there are several other anticoagulant mechanisms separate from protein C including antithrombin and tissue factor pathway inhibitor. Each of these could potentially constitute an anticoagulant mechanism after injury; however, each has been interrogated and does not currently seem to be a contributor to coagulopathy after trauma.

18.4.2 Fibrinolysis and Fibrinolysis Shutdown

While impaired clot formation remains a centerpiece of impaired coagulation, fibrinolysis in all of its forms is emerging as a very important phenotype of post injury traumatic coagulopathy. From the first descriptions of acute traumatic coagulopathy, fibrinolysis has been integral. The initial characterizations of ATC and the subsequent protein C literature showed that there was not only an impairment in clot production but also enhanced fibrinolysis. While the initial characterization of fibrinolysis was quantified by fibrin split products, subsequent use of viscoelastic testing further quantified the prevalence and degree of fibrinolysis. Several groups quantified hyperfibrinolysis as defined by an LY30 of greater than 3 or 7.5% with varying amounts of prevalence in multiple studies using TEG and ROTEM. Brohi et al. subsequently measured plasmin and antiplasmin levels and quantified a higher prevalence of hyperfibrinolysis which was clinically significant and not seen with viscoelastic (ROTEM) measures.

An initial finding from the Colorado group suggested however that there was a U-shaped curve of fibrinolysis with patient cohorting into three distinct groups depending on their degree of lysis (from minimal to hyper). From this initial important work, the Colorado group identified that patients are separated into three distinct groups with a small group showing hyperfibrinolysis, a group with normal (or termed physiologic) fibrinolysis, and a newly described cohort with sub physiologic fibrinolysis which they termed fibrinolysis shutdown [16, 17]. Newly detailed assays using tPA challenge further delineated these and have detailed a newly emerging biology of fibrinolysis shutdown [18, 19].

18.5 Conclusion and Future Steps

The understanding of the underlying biology and physiology of acute traumatic coagulopathy has undergone tremendous advancement and a paradigm shift over the past decade. The realization and subsequent scientific evidence that traumatic coagulopathy exists as an endogenous biological and physiologic process combined temporally with the advancement of hemostatic resuscitation (which is covered elsewhere) have resulted in changes in resuscitation and tremendous documented mortality and morbidity reductions in the severely injured. Despite the lack of prospective randomized trials, the trauma community has digested the emerging science and redefined the state of care where resuscitative conduct is aimed at identifying and mitigating traumatic coagulopathy. From this move toward hemostatic resuscitation, lives have been saved and morbidity mitigated. While beneficial this one-size-fits-all approach to resuscitation clearly over-resuscitates some and under-resuscitates others. There unfortunately remains a lack of an individualized approach to phenotypic identification and personalized resuscitation. Fortunately, several groups have moved forward with a personalized medicine approach to trauma resuscitation, as an alternative to protocolized plasma-based resuscitation. Rizolli and colleagues studied TEG-based resuscitation against a 1:1-based resuscitation. Despite methodological issues including a relative small study and difficulties achieving the 1:1 ratio in the reference arm, there was a significant benefit to a targeted data-based resuscitation. Subsequently the group in Denver performed a larger prospective randomized prospective trial of TEG based vs. empiric care and showed a reduced mortality and morbidity in patients treated with TEG-based resuscitation. Taken together these indictments of a one-size-fits-all empiric treatment suggest that personalized tailoring of resuscitation provides a superior matching of need to treatment with incumbent saving of lives and reduction of unnecessary blood product transfusion. Finally, in a proof of concept, our group has recently reported the use of a dynamic model of coagulation for targeted treatment. In this work a mathematical model was fit to thrombin generation curves generated from ex vivo plasma from severely injured trauma patients. This in silico model could then with a limited number of parameters predict which factor treatments can normalize thrombin production [20]. Ultimately this work suggests a future where rather than giving large volumes of poorly characterized blood products we as a trauma community will provide in silico guided targeted treatment to place coagulation in the sweet spot for targeted treatment.

References

1. Carrico CJ, Coln CD, Lightfoot SA, Allsman A, Shires GT. Extracellular fluid volume replacement in hemorrhagic shock. Surg Forum. 1963;14: 10–2.
2. Shires T, Carrico CJ. Current status of the shock problem. Curr Probl Surg. 1966;3:3–67.
3. Shires T, Coln D, Carrico J, Lightfoot S. Fluid therapy in hemorrhagic shock. Arch Surg. 1964;88: 688–93.
4. Brohi K, Singh J, Heron M, Coats T. Acute traumatic coagulopathy. J Trauma. 2003;54(6):1127–30.
5. MacLeod JB, Lynn M, McKenney MG, Cohn SM, Murtha M. Early coagulopathy predicts mortality in trauma. J Trauma. 2003;55(1):39–44.
6. Brohi K, Cohen MJ, Davenport RA. Acute coagulopathy of trauma: mechanism, identification and effect. Curr Opin Crit Care. 2007;13(6):680–5.
7. Cohen MJ, Brohi K, Ganter MT, Manley GT, Mackersie RC, Pittet JF. Early coagulopathy after traumatic brain injury: the role of hypoperfusion and the protein C pathway. J Trauma. 2007;63(6): 1254–61; discussion 61–2
8. Cohen MJ, Kutcher M, Redick B, Nelson M, Call M, Knudson MM, et al. Clinical and mechanistic drivers of acute traumatic coagulopathy. J Trauma Acute Care Surg. 2013;75(1 Suppl 1):S40–7.
9. Kutcher ME, Ferguson AR, Cohen MJ. A principal component analysis of coagulation after trauma. J Trauma Acute Care Surg. 2013;74(5):1223–9; discussion 9–30
10. Kutcher ME, Howard BM, Sperry JL, Hubbard AE, Decker AL, Cuschieri J, et al. Evolving beyond the vicious triad: differential mediation of traumatic coagulopathy by injury, shock, and resuscitation. J Trauma Acute Care Surg. 2015;78(3): 516–23.

11. Esmon CT. The protein C pathway. Chest. 2003;124(3 Suppl):26S–32S.
12. Griffin JH, Zlokovic BV, Mosnier LO. Activated protein C: biased for translation. Blood. 2015;125(19):2898–907.
13. Cohen MJ, Call M, Nelson M, Calfee CS, Esmon CT, Brohi K, et al. Critical role of activated protein C in early coagulopathy and later organ failure, infection and death in trauma patients. Ann Surg. 2012;255(2):379–85.
14. Howard BM, Miyazawa BY, Dong W, Cedron WJ, Vilardi RF, Ruf W, et al. The tissue factor pathway mediates both activation of coagulation and coagulopathy after injury. J Trauma Acute Care Surg. 2015;79(6):1009–13; discussion 1014.
15. Johansson PI, Bochsen L, Stensballe J, Secher NH. Transfusion packages for massively bleeding patients: the effect on clot formation and stability as evaluated by Thrombelastograph (TEG). Transfus Apher Sci. 2008;39(1):3–8.
16. Moore HB, Moore EE, Gonzalez E, Chapman MP, Chin TL, Silliman CC, et al. Hyperfibrinolysis, physiologic fibrinolysis, and fibrinolysis shutdown: the spectrum of postinjury fibrinolysis and relevance to antifibrinolytic therapy. J Trauma Acute Care Surg. 2014;77(6):811–7; discussion 7
17. Moore HB, Moore EE, Liras IN, Gonzalez E, Harvin JA, Holcomb JB, et al. Acute fibrinolysis shutdown after injury occurs frequently and increases mortality: a multicenter evaluation of 2,540 severely injured patients. J Am Coll Surg. 2016;222(4):347–55.
18. Moore EE, Moore HB, Gonzalez E, Chapman MP, Hansen KC, Sauaia A, et al. Postinjury fibrinolysis shutdown: rationale for selective tranexamic acid. J Trauma Acute Care Surg. 2015;78(6 Suppl 1):S65–9.
19. Moore HB, Moore EE, Lawson PJ, Gonzalez E, Fragoso M, Morton AP, et al. Fibrinolysis shutdown phenotype masks changes in rodent coagulation in tissue injury versus hemorrhagic shock. Surgery. 2015;158(2):386–92.
20. Menezes AA, Vilardi RF, Arkin AP, Cohen MJ. Targeted clinical control of trauma patient coagulation through a thrombin dynamics model. Sci Transl Med. 2017;9(371)

Evolution of Resuscitation: What Is Damage Control Resuscitation?

19

Kyle J. Kalkwarf and John B. Holcomb

Abstract

The current treatment for massively bleeding patients is nearly identical to practices developed by physicians caring for thousands of injured combatants during World War I and II. After being forgotten for half a century, these techniques made a resurgence in the form of damage control resuscitation early in the twenty-first century, based on therapies employed during wars in Southwest Asia. The concepts include limiting crystalloid, whole blood, or balance blood component transfusions to achieve permissive hypotension, preventing hypothermia, and stopping bleeding as quickly as possible.

It will be tragic if medical historian can look back on the WWII period and write of it as a time when so much was learned and so little remembered.—Dr. Henry Beecher (1951) [1]

With the exception of a few cases of whole blood transfusion, including four during the Civil War, crystalloid was the standard of therapy for hemorrhage shock in the nineteenth century and the first two decades of the twentieth century [2–5]. However, the onset of World War I and the subsequent great influx of severely injured combatants caused Allied surgeons to deem crystalloid "unsatisfactory" for treating massive hemorrhage because of the increased bleeding it caused [6]. That knowledge, along with advances in blood typing and preservation techniques at the beginning of the twentieth century, allowed whole blood to become the standard of care during the final year of World War I [5, 7, 8]. This persisted for the next four decades until dried plasma was developed just prior to WWII, and it became the standard early resuscitation fluid for US military surgeons during the war. It was transfused to maintain a systolic blood pressure of 85 mm Hg along with appropriate skin color and warmth while readying whole blood and attempting to stop the bleeding [1, 9–11]. Surgeons learned that warming the patient to physiologic temperature and transfusing whole blood to achieve a lower than normal blood pressure resulted in the "most dramatic improvement" [12, 13].

In the early 1960s, research by leading civilian trauma surgeons seemed to indicate that infusing Ringer's lactate (LR) before whole blood improved survival for animals in hemorrhagic shock [14–19]. These models failed to take into account the chance for rebleeding from achieving a normal blood pressure and were not compared with whole blood resuscitation in scientific studies, but this did not prevent the adoption of crystalloids as a

K.J. Kalkwarf, M.D. • J.B. Holcomb, M.D. (✉)
Department of Surgery, McGovern Medical School, University of Texas Health Sciences Center, Houston, TX, USA
e-mail: john.holcomb@uth.tmc.edu

J. Duchesne et al. (eds.), *Damage Control in Trauma Care*,
https://doi.org/10.1007/978-3-319-72607-6_19

resuscitative fluid for bleeding casualties during the Vietnam War. An influential study published in the mid-1970s seemed to confirm the safety of crystalloid when it said that 1–2 l could be administered while waiting for whole blood to be cross-matched [20].

While increasing volumes of crystalloid were being incorporated into hemorrhagic shock resuscitation, advances in blood fractionation techniques permitted a unit of whole blood to be separated into separate units of red blood cells (RBCs), plasma, and platelets. This allowed for most patients requiring a blood transfusion to be treated with only the component in which they were deficient, thus conserving blood supplies while limiting exposure to potential pathogens and transfusion reactions [21–24]. At the time, experienced surgeons recommended moderation of crystalloid infusion and asserted that whole blood should be used to replace acute blood loss, but this did not prevent many busy trauma centers in the 1970s from exclusively infusing RBCs and LR in bleeding patients [18, 25–27].

The aggressive use of crystalloid and RBC resuscitation only grew in the last two decades of the twentieth century as studies proclaimed that transfusing platelets and plasma was not necessary until laboratory values demonstrated coagulopathy [28–31]. "Supranormal resuscitation" also became popular at this time because of subsequently refuted studies and HIV transmission was a concern for all blood transfusions [32–41].

19.1 Damage Control Resuscitation

At the beginning of the twenty-first century, complications resulting from large-volume crystalloid resuscitation, including cardiopulmonary dysfunction, abdominal compartment syndrome, multiple organ dysfunction syndrome, and mortality, were being identified and published [42, 43]. Coagulopathy was also identified in 25–33% of severely injured patients and was associated with increased mortality [44–49]. Observations of the clinical utility of whole blood were described from the 1993 Black Hawk Down episode [50]. As a result, the US military surgeons treating patients in Iraq and Afghanistan developed damage control resuscitation (DCR) as a way to mimic the lessons learned by Allied physicians treating thousands of combat casualties during the World Wars. DCR attempted to replicate the success of whole blood by transfusing balanced ratios of plasma and platelets to RBCs to achieve permissive hypotension while maintaining normal temperature and quickly stopping bleeding [51, 52]. This reduced the side effects associated with large-volume crystalloid infusion including dilutional coagulopathy, hypothermia from room temperature infusion, as well as increased inflammation, edema, and organ failure [53–58].

19.2 Limit Crystalloid

Large-volume crystalloid infusion worsens the "bloody vicious cycle" of coagulopathy, acidosis, and hypothermia by diluting clotting factors, cooling the patient, and worsening acidosis [27, 53, 54, 59, 60]. It also disrupts cellular mechanisms leading to inflammation and edema. This leads to increased mortality from cardiac, pulmonary, gastrointestinal, and immune system dysfunction as well as morbidity from decreased healing and increased incidences of anastomotic leak, abdominal compartment syndrome, and open abdomen [42, 43, 61–66, 56, 57–59]. Increased crystalloid resuscitation also results in more blood transfusions and more rapid clot breakdown (hyperfibrinolysis) [67–70].

19.3 Balanced Resuscitation

After implementing DCR in Iraq and Afghanistan, the military published their initial results with balanced resuscitation in 2007. The first retrospective trial showed improved survival for patients receiving higher ratios of plasma to RBCs [51]. These results were replicated in other military and civilian trials looking at both blunt and penetrating injuries [48, 71–78]. Similar results were found for balanced ratios of platelet transfusion [72, 79–83]. Civilian trauma centers quickly adopted balanced ratio massive resuscitation with 70–85% of level 1 centers now including it in their massive transfusion protocol, up from just a few centers a decade ago [84–86].

19.4 Survival Bias

A limitation to retrospective studies was highlighted in 2009 by a trial that examined the increased time required to thaw fresh frozen plasma (FFP) (93 min) for transfusion compared with RBCs (18 min) [87]. As a result, patients who survived ultimately received balance ratios of plasma, while those who died within the first few hours received RBCs but not other components which require longer to prepare. Prethawed plasma and never-frozen plasma are now available in more than 85% of surveyed trauma centers, to overcome the time required to thaw FFP [86, 88–93].

The PROPPR trial was a prospective, randomized, multicenter trial designed to evaluate the difference in outcomes between the two most common resuscitation ratios (1:1:1 and 1:1:2 (plasma/platelet/RBC)) [94]. While it did not show an improvement in 24 h or 30-day mortality, it did show the benefits of early balanced plasma and platelet resuscitation with decreased mortality at 3 h, decreased hemorrhagic death at 24 h, and increased median time to hemorrhage death [94–97]. PROPPR also showed no increase in complications for those treated with a 1:1:1 ratio, indicating that it is safe to transfuse higher ratios of plasma and platelets [94].

19.5 Whole Blood

While balance resuscitation was rapidly adopted in civilian trauma centers, the US military continued a long tradition of whole blood transfusions. Military physicians have safely transfused more than a million units of whole blood during wars over the past century, including more than 10,300 units of fresh whole blood to treat massively injured combatants in Iraq and Afghanistan [7, 8, 41, 98, 99]. Much of the transfused whole blood during these conflicts was provided by a walking blood bank of prescreened soldiers in rural settings. Retrospective reviews from these wars show improved 24-h and 30-day survival for massively transfused patients who received warm, fresh whole blood compared with those who received balanced ratios of blood components [100, 101]. This superiority is a result of the improved oxygen-carrying capacity, coagulation factors, platelet activity, flow characteristics, decreased dilution by storage solutions, and the superior hemostatic potential of whole blood compared to reconstituted component therapy [41, 98, 102].

19.6 Permissive Hypotension

In addition to replacing blood loss with whole blood or a balanced approximation, another component of damage control resuscitation is permissive hypotension. Originally described by World War I and II physicians, permissive hypotension contends that maintaining a lower than normal blood pressure decreases blood loss [9, 13]. The theory was confirmed by multiple animal models of uncontrolled hemorrhage [50, 103–107] and randomized trials in penetrating and blunt trauma patients [108–110].

19.7 Hypothermia

Hypothermia is common in severely injured trauma patients because of environmental exposure and infusion of room temperature fluids. It causes increased bleeding and mortality because of a reduction in coagulation enzyme activity and clot formation [27, 111–115]. Warming fluids and other rewarming techniques should be used to reverse these processes [57].

19.8 Stopping Hemorrhage

Rapid hemorrhage control is an important component of DCR because exsanguination is the leading cause of potentially survivable trauma deaths [116]. Tourniquets are effective for controlling extremity hemorrhage, and they have a low incidence of complications [117, 118]. Hemostatic dressings are effective for controlling compressible bleeding, but two-thirds of hemorrhagic deaths result from non-compressible torso trauma, so resuscitative endovascular balloon occlusion of the aorta (REBOA) has made a resurgence for quickly halting abdominal and pelvic hemorrhage with less morbidity than a resuscitative thoracotomy [116, 119–122]. Centers should implement a comprehensive hemorrhage control bundle, to begin prehospital and extend through the operating room [96].

19.9 Viscoelastic Hemostatic Assays

When bleeding slows, viscoelastic hemostatic assays (VHA), such as thromboelastography (TEG) and rotational thromboelastometry (ROTEM), can be used to guide resuscitation more precisely than fixed component ratios by evaluating clot formation, stability, and degradation as well as diagnose hypo- and hypercoagulable states [58, 123–126]. Rapid TEG is capable of predicting the need for component transfusions within 5 min, and a recent randomized control trial showed improved mortality and decreased blood component transfusions when comparing it with conventional coagulation tests [127, 128].

VHA also provide information on fibrinolysis, which is a spectrum of clot degradation ranging from hyperfibrinolysis with unmitigated hemorrhage to fibrinolysis shutdown causing excessive thrombus and subsequent organ dysfunction [129]. Fibrinolysis is diagnosed based on TEG LY30, and both extremes cause increased mortality [68, 129]. Administering tranexamic acid (TXA) within 3 h of injury reverses this laboratory abnormality, but it remains to be seen if this treatment for hyperfibrinolysis (LY30 > 3%) improves patient outcomes [130–132].

Conclusion

Cutting edge therapy for hemorrhage shock is nearly identical to the methods established while resuscitating thousands of critically wounded soldiers during WWI and WWII. The biggest difference is the currently accepted practice of balanced blood component therapy rather than whole blood, which was successfully used for half a century before being supplanted by crystalloid and RBCs, despite no comparison studies in uncontrolled hemorrhage. Because fractionated blood components are inferior to whole blood in oxygen-carrying capacity and coagulation, the best replacement for blood loss is almost assuredly whole blood. As a result, whole blood needs to be seriously evaluated as the therapy of choice for massively bleeding patients.

References

1. Beecher HK. Early care of the seriously wounded man. JAMA. 1951;145(4):193–200.
2. Jennings CE. The intra-venous injection of fluid for severe hæmorrhage. The Lancet. 1882;120(3081): 436–7.
3. Jennings CE. The intra-venous injection of fluid for severe haemorrhage. The Lancet. 1883;121(3102): 228–9.
4. Pye-Smith RJ. Sheffield public hospital and dispensary: five cases of intravenous injection of saline fluid for hæmorrhage and collapse. The Lancet. 1892;139(3582):913–5.
5. Schmidt PJ. Transfusion in America in the eighteenth and nineteenth centuries. N Engl J Med. 1968; 279(24):1319–20.
6. Fraser J, Cowell EM. Clinical study of blood pressure in wound conditions. JAMA. 1918;70
7. Spinella PC. Warm fresh whole blood transfusion for severe hemorrhage: US military and potential civilian applications. Crit Care Med. 2008;36(7):S340–5.
8. Hess JR, Thomas MJ. Blood use in war and disaster: lessons from the past century. Transfusion. 2003;43(11):1622–33.
9. Beecher HK. Preparation of battle casualties for surgery. Ann Surg. 1945;121(6):769–92.
10. Beecher HK. Resuscitation, and anesthesia for wounded men, the management of traumatic shock. Springfield. Charles C: Thomas; 1949.
11. Giangrande PL. The history of blood transfusion. Br J Haematol. 2000;100:758–67.
12. Robertson OH. Transfusion with preserved red blood cells. Br Med J. 1918;1(2999):691.
13. Cannon, Walter B. Traumatic Shock. New York: D. Appl Ther 1923.
14. Fogelman MJ, Wilson BJA. different concept of volume replacement in traumatic hypovolemia observations on injured man and animal. Am J Surg. 1960;99(5):694–701.
15. Shires T, Williams J, Brown F. Acute change in extracellular fluids associated with major surgical procedures. Ann Surg. 1961;154:803–10.

16. Shires T, Jackson DE. Postoperative salt tolerance. Arch Surg. 1962;84:703–6. PMID: 13912108
17. Wolfman EF, Neill SA, Heaps DK, Zuidema GD. Donor blood and isotonic salt solution. Effect on survival after hemorrhagic shock and operation. Arch Surg. 1963;86:869–73.
18. Shires T, Coln D, Carrico J, Lightfoot S. Fluid therapy in hemorrhagic shock. Arch Surg. 1964;88:688–93.
19. McClelland RN, Shires GT, Baxter CR, Coln CD, Carrico J. Balanced salt solution in the treatment of hemorrhagic shock. JAMA. 1967;199:830–4.
20. Carrico CJ, Canizaro PC, Shires GT. Fluid resuscitation following injury: rationale for the use of balanced salt solutions. Crit Care Med. 1976;4(2):46–54.
21. Davidsohn I. Speculation on future use of blood or blood component therapy. JAMA. 1967;202(10): 970–2.
22. Chaplin H Jr. Packed red blood cells. N Engl J Med. 1969;281(7):364–7.
23. Committee AMA. on Transfusion and Transplantation. Something old, something new. JAMA. 1970; 212(1):147.
24. Westphal RG. Rational alternatives to the use of whole blood. Ann Intern Med. 1972;76(6):987–90.
25. Moore FD, Shires G. Moderation. Ann Surg. 1967; 166:300–1.
26. Moore FD. Should blood be whole or in parts? N Engl J Med. 1969;280(6):327–8.
27. Kashuk JL, Moore EE, Millikan JS, Moore JB. Major Abdominal Vascular Trauma-A Unified Approach. Journal of Trauma and Acute Care Surgery. 1982 Aug 1;22(8):672–9. RJ Lowe in DiscussionKashuk JL, Moore EE, Millikan JS, Moore JB Major abdominal vascular trauma--a unified approach J Trauma 2008;65:261-270 RJ Lowe in Discussion
28. Counts RB, Haisch C, Simon TL, Maxwell NG, Heimbach DM, Carrico CJ. Hemostasis in massively transfused trauma patients. Ann Surg. 1979; 190(1):91–9.
29. Shackford SR, Virgilio RW, Peters RM. Whole blood versus packed-cell transfusions: a physiologic comparison. Ann Surg. 1981;193(3):337–40.
30. Lucas CE, Ledgerwood AM. Clinical significance of altered coagulation tests after massive transfusion for trauma. Am Surg. 1981;47(3):125–30.
31. Reed RL 2nd, Ciavarella D, Heimbach DM, Baron L, Pavlin E, Counts RB, Carrico CJ. Prophylactic platelet administration during massive transfusion. A prospective, randomized, double-blind clinical study. Ann Surg. 1986;203:40–8.
32. Bland R, Shoemaker WC, Shabot MM. Physiologic monitoring goals for the critically ill patient. Surg Gynecol Obstet. 1978;147(6):833–41.
33. Shoemaker WC, Appel PL, Kram HB, Waxman K, Lee TS. Prospective trial of supranormal values of survivors as therapeutic goals in high-risk surgical patients. Chest J. 1988;94(6):1176–86.
34. Fleming A, Bishop M, Shoemaker W, Appel P, Sufficool W, Kuvhenguwha A, Kennedy F, Wo CJ. Prospective trial of supranormal values as goals of resuscitation in severe trauma. Arch Surg. 1992;127:1175–9. Discussion 1179-1181
35. Bishop MH, Wo CCJ, Appel PL, et al. Relationship between supranormal circulatory values, time delays, and outcome in severely traumatized patients. Crit Care Med. 1993;21:56–60.
36. Boyd O, Grounds RM, Bennett ED. A randomized clinical trial of the effect of deliberate perioperative increase of oxygen delivery on mortality in high-risk surgical patients. JAMA. 1993;270(22):2699–707.
37. Bishop MH, Shoemaker WC, Appel PL, Meade P, Ordog GJ, Wasserberger J, Wo CJ, Rimle DA, Kram HB, Umali R. Prospective, randomized trial of survivor values of cardiac index, oxygen delivery, and oxygen consumption as resuscitation endpoints in severe trauma. J Trauma. 1995;38(5):780–7.
38. Gattinoni L, Brazzi L, Pelosi P, Latini R, Tognoni G, Pesenti A, Fumagalli RA. trial of goal-oriented hemodynamic therapy in critically ill patients. N Engl J Med. 1995;333(16):1025–32.
39. Velmahos GC, Demetriades D, Shoemaker WC, Chan LS, Tatevossian R, Wo CC, Vassiliu P, Cornwell EE III, Murray JA, Roth B, Belzberg H. Endpoints of resuscitation of critically injured patients: normal or supranormal?: a prospective randomized trial. Ann Surg. 2000;232(3):409–18.
40. Lee L, Moore EE, Hansen KC, Silliman CC, Chandler JG, Banerjee A. It's not your grandfather's field plasma. Surgery. 2013;153(6):857–60.
41. Spinella PC, Pidcoke HF, Strandenes G, Hervig T, Fisher A, Jenkins D, Yazer M, Stubbs J, Murdock A, Sailliol A, Ness PM. Whole blood for hemostatic resuscitation of major bleeding. Transfusion. 2016;56(S2):S190–202.
42. Brandstrup B, Tønnesen H, Beier-Holgersen R, Hjortsø E, Ørding H, Lindorff-Larsen K, Rasmussen MS, Lanng C, Wallin L, Iversen LH, Gramkow CS. Effects of intravenous fluid restriction on postoperative complications: comparison of two perioperative fluid regimens: a randomized assessor-blinded multicenter trial. Ann Surg. 2003;238(5):641.
43. Balogh Z, McKinley BA, Cocanour CS, Kozar RA, Valdivia A, Sailors RM, Moore FA. Supranormal trauma resuscitation causes more cases of abdominal compartment syndrome. Arch Surg. 2003;138:637–42.
44. Simmons RL, Collins JA, Heisterkamp CA 3rd, Mills DE, Andren R, Phillips LL. Coagulation disorders in combat casualties, I: acute changes after wounding. Ann Surg 1969;169(4):455–482.
45. MacLeod JB, Lynn M, McKenney MG, Cohn SM, Murtha M. Early coagulopathy predicts mortality in trauma. J Trauma. 2003;55(1):39–44.
46. Brohi K, Singh J, Heron M, Coats T. Acute traumatic coagulopathy. J Trauma. 2003;54:1127–30.
47. Niles SE, McLaughlin DF, Perkins JG, Wade CE, Li Y, Spinella PC, Holcomb JB. Increased mortality associated with the early coagulopathy of trauma in combat casualties. J Trauma Injury Infect Crit Care. 2008;64(6):1459–63. discussion 1463-5

48. Gunter OL Jr, BK A, Isbell JM, Mowery NT, Young PP, Cotton BA. Optimizing outcomes in damage control resuscitation: identifying blood product ratios associated with improved survival. J Trauma Injury Infect Crit Care. 2008;65(3):527–34.
49. Pidcoke HF, Aden JK, Mora AG, Borgman MA, Spinella PC, Dubick MA, Blackbourne LH, Cap AP. Ten-year analysis of transfusion in Operation Iraqi Freedom and Operation Enduring Freedom: increased plasma and platelet use correlates with improved survival. J Trauma Acute Care Surg. 2012;73(6):S445–52.
50. Mabry RL, Holcomb JB, Baker AM, Cloonan CC, Uhorchak JM, Perkins DE, Canfield AJ, Hagmann JH. United States army rangers in Somalia: an analysis of combat casualties on an urban battlefield. J Trauma Acute Care Surg. 2000;49(3):515–29.
51. Borgman MA, Spinella PC, Perkins JG, Grathwohl KW, Repine T, Beekley AC, Sebesta J, Jenkins D, Wade CE, Holcomb JB. The ratio of blood products transfused affects mortality in patients receiving massive transfusions at a combat support hospital. J Trauma. 2007;63(4):805–13.
52. Holcomb JB, Jenkins D, Rhee P, Johannigman J, Mahoney P, Mehta S, Cox ED, Gehrke MJ, Beilman GJ, Schreiber M, Flaherty SF. Damage control resuscitation: directly addressing the early coagulopathy of trauma. J Trauma Acute Care Surg. 2007;62(2):307–10.
53. Maegele M, Lefering R, Yucel N, Tjardes T, Rixen D, Paffrath T, Simanski C, Neugebauer E, Bouillon B. AG Polytrauma of the German Trauma Society (DGU). Early coagulopathy in multiple injury: an analysis from the German Trauma Registry on 8724 patients. Injury. 2007;38:298.
54. Tieu BH, Holcomb JB, Schreiber MA. Coagulopathy: its pathophysiology and treatment in the injured patient. World J Surg. 2007;31:1055–64.
55. Cotton BA, Au BK, Nunez TC, Gunter OL, Robertson AM, Young PP. Predefined massive transfusion protocols are associated with a reduction in organ failure and postinjury complications. J Trauma. 2009;66:41–8. discussion 48-49
56. Shah SK, Uray KS, Stewart RH, Laine GA, Cox CS. Resuscitation-induced intestinal edema and related dysfunction: state of the science. J Surg Res. 2011;166(1):120–30.
57. Duchesne JC, Kimonis K, Marr AB, Rennie KV, Wahl G, Wells JE, Islam TM, Meade P, Stuke L, Barbeau JM, Hunt JP, Baker CC, NE MS Jr. Damage control resuscitation in combination with damage control laparotomy: a survival advantage. J Trauma. 2010;69:46–52.
58. Feinman M, Cotton BA, Haut ER. Optimal fluid resuscitation in trauma: type, timing, and total. Curr Opin Crit Care. 2014;20(4):366–72.
59. Cotton BA, Reddy N, Hatch QM, LeFebvre E, Wade CE, Kozar RA, Gill BS, Albarado R, McNutt MK, Holcomb JB. Damage control resuscitation is associated with a reduction in resuscitation volumes and improvement in survival in 390 damage control laparotomy patients. Ann Surg. 2011;254(4):598–605.
60. Myburgh JA, Mythen MG. Resuscitation fluids. N Engl J Med. 2013;369:1243–51.
61. Lobo DN, Bostock KA, Neal KR, Perkins AC, Rowlands BJ, Allison SP. Effect of salt and water balance on recovery of gastrointestinal function after elective colonic resection: a randomized control trial. Lancet. 2002;359:1812–8.
62. Balogh Z, McKinley BA, Cocanour CS, Kozar RA, Holcomb JB, Ware DN, Moore FA. Secondary abdominal compartment syndrome is an elusive early complication of traumatic shock resuscitation. Am J Surg. 2002;184(6):538–43. discussion 543-4
63. Cotton BA, Guy JS, Morris JA Jr, Abumrad NA. The cellular, metabolic, and systemic consequences of aggressive fluid resuscitation strategies. Shock. 2006;26:115–21.
64. Ley EJ, Clond MA, Srour MK, Barnajian M, Mirocha J, Margulies DR, Salim A. Emergency department crystalloid resuscitation of 1.5 L or more is associated with increased mortality in elderly and nonelderly trauma patients. J Trauma. 2011;70:398–400.
65. Hatch QM, Osterhout LM, Podbielski J, Kozar RA, Wade CE, Holcomb JB, Cotton BA. Impact of closure at the first take back: complication burden and potential overutilization of damage control laparotomy. J Trauma. 2011;71(6):1503–11.
66. Schnüriger B, Inaba K, Wu T, Eberle BM, Belzberg H, Demetriades D. Crystalloids after primary colon resection and anastomosis at initial trauma laparotomy: excessive volumes are associated with anastomotic leakage. J Trauma Acute Care Surg. 2011;70(3):603–10.
67. Spinella PC, Perkins JG, Grathwohl KW, Repine T, Beekley AC, Sebesta J, Jenkins D, Azarow K, Holcomb JB. 31st CSH Research Working Group. Fresh whole blood transfusions in coalition military, foreign national, and enemy combatant patients during Operation Iraqi Freedom at a US combat support hospital. World J Surg. 2008;32(1):2–6.
68. Cotton BA, Harvin JA, Kostousouv V, Minei KM, Radwan ZA, Schöchl H, Wade CE, Holcomb JB, Matijevic N. Hyperfibrinolysis at admission is an uncommon but highly lethal event associated with shock and prehospital fluid administration. J Trauma Acute Care Surg. 2012;73(2):365–70. discussion 370
69. Duchesne JC, Heaney J, Guidry C, McSwain N Jr, Meade P, Cohen M, Schreiber M, Inaba K, Skiada D, Demetriades D, Holcomb J. Diluting the benefits of hemostatic resuscitation: a multi-institutional analysis. J Trauma Acute Care Surg. 2013;75(1):76–82.
70. Shrestha B, Holcomb JB, Camp EA, Del Junco DJ, Cotton BA, Albarado R, Gill BS, Kozar RA, Kao LS, McNutt MK, Moore LJ, Love JD, Tyson GH 3rd, Adams PR, Khan S, Wade CE. Damage-control resuscitation increases successful nonoperative management rates and survival after severe

blunt liver injury. J Trauma Acute Care Surg. 2015;78(2):336–41.
71. Spinella PC, Perkins JG, Grathwohl KW, Beekley AC, Niles SE, McLaughlin DF, Wade CE, Holcomb JB. Effect of plasma and red blood cell transfusions on survival in patients with combat related traumatic injuries. J Trauma. 2008;64(2 Suppl):S69–77. discussion S77–8
72. Holcomb JB, Wade CE, Michalek JE, Chisholm GB, Zarzabal LA, Schreiber MA, Gonzalez EA, Pomper GJ, Perkins JG, Spinella PC, Williams KL, Park MS. Increased plasma and platelet to red blood cell ratios improves outcome in 466 massively transfused civilian trauma patients. Ann Surg. 2008;248(3):447–58.
73. Duchesne JC, Hunt JP, Wahl G, Marr AB, Wang YZ, Weintraub SE, Wright MJ, McSwain NE Jr. Review of current blood transfusions strategies in a mature level I trauma center: were we wrong for the last 60 years. J Trauma. 2008;65:272–6. Discussion 276-278
74. Maegele M, Lefering R, Paffrath T, Tjardes T, Simanski C, Bouillon B. Working Group on Polytrauma of the German Society of Trauma Surgery (DGU). Red-blood-cell to plasma ratios transfused during massive transfusion are associated with mortality in severe multiple injury: a retrospective analysis from the Trauma Registry of the Deutsche Gesellschaft für Unfallchirurgie. Vox Sang. 2008;95(2):112–9.
75. Sperry JL, Ochoa JB, Gunn SR, Alarcon LH, Minei JP, Cuschieri J, Rosengart MR, Maier RV, Billiar TR, Peitzman AB, Moore EE. Inflammation the host response to injury investigators. An FFP:PRBC transfusion ratio >/=1:1.5 is associated with a lower risk of mortality after massive transfusion. J Trauma. 2008;65:986.
76. Teixeira PG, Inaba K, Shulman I, Salim A, Demetriades D, Brown C, Browder T, Green D, Rhee P. Impact of plasma transfusion in massively transfused trauma patients. J Trauma Injury Infect Crit Care. 2009;66(3):693–7.
77. Brown LM, Aro SO, Cohen MJ, Trauma Outcomes Group, Holcomb JB, Wade CE, Brasel KJ, Vercruysse G, MacLeod J, Dutton RP, Hess JR, Duchesne JC, NE MS, Muskat P, Johannigamn J, Cryer HM, Tillou A, Pittet JF, Knudson P, De Moya MA, Schreiber MA, Tieu B, Brundage S, Napolitano LM, Brunsvold M, Sihler KC, Beilman G, Peitzman AB, Zenait MS, Sperry J, Alarcon L, Croce MA, Minei JP, Kozar R, Gonzalez EA, Stewart RM, Cohn SM, Mickalek JE, Bulger EM, Cotton BA, Nunez TC, Ivatury R, Meredith JW, Miller P, Pomper GJ, Marin B. A high fresh frozen plasma: packed red blood cell transfusion ratio decreases mortality in all massively transfused trauma patients regardless of admission international normalized ratio. J Trauma. 2011;71(2 Suppl 3):S358–63.
78. Rowell SE, Barbosa RR, Diggs BS, Schreiber MA, Trauma Outcomes Group, Holcomb JB, Wade CE, Brasel KJ, Vercruysse G, MacLeod J, Dutton RP, Hess JR, Duchesne JC, NE MS, Muskat P, Johannigamn J, Cryer HM, Tillou A, Cohen MJ, Pittet JF, Knudson P, De Moya MA, Schreiber MA, Tieu B, Brundage S, Napolitano LM, Brunsvold M, Sihler KC, Beilman G, Peitzman AB, Zenait MS, Sperry J, Alarcon L, Croce MA, Minei JP, Kozar R, Gonzalez EA, Stewart RM, Cohn SM, Mickalek JE, Bulger EM, Cotton BA, Nunez TC, Ivatury R, Meredith JW, Miller P, Pomper GJ, Marin B. Effect of high product ratio massive transfusion on mortality in blunt and penetrating trauma patients. J Trauma. 2011;71(2 Suppl 3):S353–7.
79. Perkins JG, Cap AP, Spinella PC, Blackbourne LH, Grathwohl KW, Repine TB, Ketchum L, Waterman P, Lee RE, Beekley AC, Sebesta JA, Shorr AF, Wade CE, Holcomb JB. An evaluation of the impact of apheresis platelets used in the setting of massively transfused trauma patients. J Trauma. 2009;66:S77–85.
80. Zink KA, Sambasivan CN, Holcomb JB, Chisholm G, Schreiber MA. A high ratio of plasma and platelets to packed red blood cells in the first 6 hours of massive transfusion improves outcomes in a large multicenter study. Am J Surg. 2009;197(5):565–70. discussion 570
81. Inaba K, Branco BC, Rhee P, Blackbourne LH, Holcomb JB, Teixeira PG, Shulman I, Nelson J, Demetriades D. Impact of plasma transfusion in trauma patients who do not require massive transfusion. J Am Coll Surg. 2010;210(6):957–65.
82. Holcomb JB, Zarzabal LA, Michalek JE, Kozar RA, Spinella PC, Perkins JG, Matijevic N, Dong JF, Pati S, Wade CE, Trauma Outcomes Group, Holcomb JB, Wade CE, Cotton BA, Kozar RA, Brasel KJ, Vercruysse GA, JB ML, Dutton RP, Hess JR, Duchesne JC, NE MS, Muskat PC, Johannigamn JA, Cryer HM, Tillou A, Cohen MJ, Pittet JF, Knudson P, MA DM, Schreiber MA, Tieu BH, Brundage SI, Napolitano LM, Brunsvold ME, Sihler KC, Beilman GJ, Peitzman AB, Zenati MS, Sperry JL, Alarcon LH, Croce MA, Minei JP, Steward RM, Cohn SM, Michalek JE, Bulger EM, Nunez TC, Ivatury RR, Meredith JW, Miller PR, Pomper GJ, Marin B. Increased platelet:RBC ratios are associated with improved survival after massive transfusion. J Trauma. 2011;71(2 Suppl 3):S318–28.
83. Holcomb JB, del Junco DJ, Fox EE, Wade CE, Cohen MJ, Schreiber MA, Alarcon LH, Bai Y, Brasel KJ, Bulger EM, Cotton BA, Matijevic N, Muskat P, Myers JG, Phelan HA, White CE, Zhang J, Rahbar MH, PROMMTT Study Group. The prospective, observational, multicenter, major trauma transfusion (PROMMTT) study: comparative effectiveness of a time-varying treatment with competing risks. JAMA Surg. 201;148(2):127–36.
84. Malone DL, Hess JR, Fingerhut A. Massive transfusion practices around the globe and a suggestion for a common massive transfusion protocol. J Trauma. 2006;60(6 Suppl):S91–6.

85. Hess JR, Holcomb JB. Resuscitating properly. Transfusion. 2015;55(6):1362–4.
86. Treml AB, Gorlin JB, Dutton RP, Scavone BM. Massive transfusion protocols: a survey of academic medical centers in the United States. Anesth Anal. 2017;124(1):277–81.
87. Snyder CW, Weinberg JA, Jr MGG, Melton SM, George RL, Reiff DA, Cross JM, Hubbard-Brown J, Rue LW 3rd, Kerby JD. The relationship of blood product ratio to mortality: survival benefit or survival bias. J Trauma Injury Infect. Crit Care. 2009;66(2):358–62.
88. Zielinski MD, Johnson PM, Jenkins D, Goussous N, Stubbs JR. Emergency use of prethawed Group A plasma in trauma patients. J Trauma Acute Care Surg. 2013;74(1):69–75.
89. Matijevic N, Wang YW, Cotton BA, Hartwell E, Barbeau JM, Wade CE, Holcomb JB. Better hemostatic profiles of never-frozen liquid plasma compared with thawed fresh frozen plasma. J Trauma Acute Care Surg. 2013;74(1):84–90. discussion 90-1
90. Radwan ZA, Bai Y, Matijevic N, del Junco DJ, McCarthy JJ, Wade CE, Holcomb JB, Cotton BA. An emergency department thawed plasma protocol for severely injured patients. JAMA Surg. 2013; 148(2):170–5.
91. Holcomb JB, Pati S. Optimal trauma resuscitation with plasma as the primary resuscitative fluid: the surgeon's perspective. Hematology Am Soc Hematol Educ Program. 2013;2013:656–9.
92. Norii T, Crandall C, Terasaka Y. Survival of severe blunt trauma patients treated with resuscitative endovascular balloon occlusion of the aorta compared with propensity score-adjusted untreated patients. J Trauma Acute Care Surg. 2015;78(4):721–8.
93. Ho AM, Zamora JE, Holcomb JB, Ng CS, Karmakar MK, Dion PW. The many faces of survivor bias in observational studies on trauma resuscitation requiring massive transfusion. Ann Emerg Med. 2015;66(1):45–8.
94. Holcomb JB, Tilley BC, Baraniuk S, Fox EE, Wade CE, Podbielski JM, del Junco DJ, Brasel KJ, Bulger EM, Callcut RA, Cohen MJ, Cotton BA, Fabian TC, Inaba K, Kerby JD, Muskat P, O'Keeffe T, Rizoli S, Robinson BR, Scalea TM, Schreiber MA, Stein DM, Weinberg JA, Callum JL, Hess JR, Matijevic N, Miller CN, Pittet JF, Hoyt DB, Pearson GD, Leroux B, van Belle G, PROPPR Study Group. Transfusion of plasma, platelets, and red blood cells in a 1:1:1 vs a 1:1:2 ratio and mortality in patients with severe trauma: the PROPPR randomized clinical trial. JAMA. 2015;313(5):471–82.
95. Demetriades D, Kimbrell B, Salim A, Velmahos G, Rhee P, Preston C, Gruzinski G, Chan L. Trauma deaths in a mature urban trauma system: is "trimodal" distribution a valid concept? J Am Coll Surg. 2005;201(3):343–8.
96. Oyeniyi BT, Fox EE, Scerbo M, Tomasek JS, Wade CE, Holcomb JB. Trends in 1029 trauma deaths at a level 1 trauma center: Impact of a bleeding control bundle of care. Injury. 2016;3
97. Fox EE, Holcomb JB, Wade CE, Bulger EM, Tilley BC. On behalf of the PROPPR study group. Earlier endpoints are required for hemorrhagic shock trials among severely injured patients. Shock. [Submitted for publication].
98. Kauvar DS, Holcomb JB, Norris GC, Hess JR. Fresh whole blood transfusion: a controversial military practice. J Trauma. 2006;61(1):181–4.
99. Murdock AD, BersÈus O, Hervig T, Strandenes G, Lunde TH. Whole blood: the future of traumatic hemorrhagic shock resuscitation. Shock. 2014;41:62–9.
100. Spinella PC, Perkins JG, Grathwohl KW, Beekley AC, Holcomb JB. Warm fresh whole blood is independently associated with improved survival for patients with combat-related traumatic injuries. J Trauma Injury Infect Crit Care. 2009;66(4 Suppl):S69–76.
101. Holcomb JB, Spinella PC. Optimal use of blood in trauma patients. Biologicals. 2010;38(1):72–7.
102. Repine TB, Perkins JG, Kauvar DS, Blackborne L. The use of fresh whole blood in massive transfusion. J Trauma Injury Infect Crit Care. 2006;60(6 suppl):S59–69.
103. Kowalenko T, Stern S, Dronen S, Wang X. Improved outcome with hypotensive resuscitation of uncontrolled hemorrhagic shock in a swine model. J Trauma Acute Care Surg. 1992;33(3):349–53.
104. Burris D, Rhee P, Kaufmann C, Pikoulis E, Austin B, Eror A, DeBraux S, Guzzi L, Leppäniemi A. Controlled resuscitation for uncontrolled hemorrhagic shock. J Trauma. 1999;46:216–23.
105. Holmes JF, Sakles JC, Lewis G, Wisner DH. Effects of delaying fluid resuscitation on an injury to the systemic arterial vasculature. Acad Emerg Med. 2002;9:267–74.
106. Holcomb JB. Fluid resuscitation in modern combat casualty care: lessons learned from Somalia. J Trauma. 2003;54(5 Suppl):S46–51. Review
107. Sondeen JL, Coppes VG, Holcomb JB. Blood pressure at which rebleeding occurs after resuscitation in swine with aortic injury. J Trauma Injury Infect. Crit Care. 2003;54(5 suppl):S110–7.
108. Bickell WH, Wall MJ Jr, Pepe PE, Martin RR, Ginger VF, Allen MK, Mattox KL. Immediate versus delayed fluid resuscitation for hypotensive patients with penetrating torso injuries. N Engl J Med. 1994;331(17):1105–9.
109. Wall MJ Jr, Granchi TS, Liscum K, Aucar J, Mattox KL. Delayed versus immediate fluid resuscitation in patients with penetrating trauma: subgroup analysis. J Trauma. 1995;39:173.
110. Schreiber MA, Meier EN, Tisherman SA, Kerby JD, Newgard CD, Brasel K, Egan D, Witham W, Williams C, Daya M, Beeson J. A controlled resuscitation strategy is feasible and safe in hypotensive trauma patients: results of a prospective randomized pilot trial. J Trauma Acute Care Surg. 2015;78(4):687.

111. Jurkovich GJ, Greiser WB, Luterman A, Curreri PW. Hypothermia in trauma victims: an ominous predictor of survival. J Trauma. 1987;27(9):1019–24.
112. Ferrara A, MacArthur JD, Wright HK, Modlin IM, McMillen MA. Hypothermia and acidosis worsen coagulopathy in the patient requiring massive transfusion. Am J Surg. 1990;160:515–8.
113. Cosgriff NM, Ernest E, Sauaia A, Kenny-Moynihan M, Burch JM, Galloway B. Predicting life-threatening coagulopathy in the massively transfused patient: hypothermia and acidosis revisited. J Trauma Injury Infect Crit Care. 1997;42(5):857–62.
114. Martini WZ, Holcomb JB. Acidosis and coagulopathy: the differential effects on fibrinogen synthesis and breakdown in pigs. Ann Surg. 2007;246(5):831–5.
115. Hess JR, Brohi K, Dutton RP, Hauser CJ, Holcomb JB, Kluger Y, Mackway-Jones K, Parr MJ, Rizoli SB, Yukioka T, Hoyt DB, Bouillon B. The coagulopathy of trauma: a review of mechanisms. J Trauma. 2008 Oct;65(4):748–54.
116. Eastridge BJ, Mabry RL, Seguin P, Cantrell J, Tops T, Uribe P, Mallett O, Zubko T, Oetjen-Gerdes L, Rasmussen TE, Butler FK. Death on the battlefield (2001–2011): implications for the future of combat casualty care. J Trauma Acute Care Surg. 2012;73(6):S431–7.
117. Kragh JF Jr, Walters TJ, Baer DG, Fox CJ, Wade CE, Salinas J, Holcomb JB. Practical use of emergency tourniquets to stop bleeding in major limb trauma. J Trauma Acute Care Surg. 2008;64(2):S38–50.
118. Scerbo MH, Mumm JP, Gates K, Love JD, Wade CE, Holcomb JB, Cotton BA. Safety and appropriateness of tourniquets in 105 civilians. Prehosp Emerg Care. 2016;May 31:1–11. [Epub ahead of print]
119. Shina A, Lipsky AM, Nadler R, Levi M, Benov A, Ran Y, Yitzhak A, Glassberg E. Prehospital use of hemostatic dressings by the Israel Defense Forces Medical Corps: A case series of 122 patients. J Trauma Acute Care Surg. 2015;79(4):S204–9.
120. Inaba K, Siboni S, Resnick S, Zhu J, Wong MD, Haltmeier T, Benjamin E, Demetriades D. Tourniquet use for civilian extremity trauma. J Trauma Acute Care Surg. 2015;79(2):232–7. quiz 332-3
121. Moore LJ, Brenner M, Kozar RA, Pasley J, Wade CE, Baraniuk MS, Scalea T, Holcomb JB. Implementation of resuscitative endovascular balloon occlusion of the aorta as an alternative to resuscitative thoracotomy for noncompressible truncal hemorrhage. J Trauma Acute Care Surg. 2015;79(4):523–30. discussion 530-2
122. Morrison JJ, Galgon RE, Jansen JO, Cannon JW, Rasmussen TE, Eliason JLA. systematic review of the use of resuscitative endovascular balloon occlusion of the aorta in the management of hemorrhagic shock. J Trauma Acute Care Surg. 2016;80(2):324–34.
123. Spinella PC, Holcomb JB. Resuscitation and transfusion principles for traumatic hemorrhagic shock. Blood Rev. 2009;23(6):231–40.
124. Otton BA, Minei KM, Radwan ZA, Matijevic N, Pivalizza E, Podbielski J, Wade CE, Kozar RA, Holcomb JB. Admission rapid thrombelastography predicts development of pulmonary embolism in trauma patients. J Trauma Acute Care Surg. 2012;72(6):1470–5.
125. Holcomb JB, Minei KM, Scerbo ML, Radwan ZA, Wade CE, Kozar RA, Gill BS, Albarado R, McNutt MK, Khan S, Adams PR, McCarthy JJ, Cotton BA. Admission rapid thrombelastography can replace conventional coagulation tests in the emergency department: experience with 1974 consecutive trauma patients. Ann Surg. 2012;256(3):476–86.
126. Johansson PI, Stensballe J, Oliveri R, Wade CE, Ostrowski SR, Holcomb JB. How I treat patients with massive hemorrhage. Blood. 2014;124(20):3052–8.
127. Cotton BA, Faz G, Hatch QM, Radwan ZA, Podbielski J, Wade C, Kozar RA, Holcomb JB. Rapid thrombelastography delivers real-time results that predict transfusion within 1 hour of admission. J Trauma. 2011;71(2):407–14. discussion 414-7
128. Gonzalez E, Moore EE, Moore HB, Chapman MP, Chin TL, Ghasabyan A, Wohlauer MV, Barnett CC, Bensard DD, Biffl WL, Burlew CC, Johnson JL, Pieracci FM, Jurkovich GJ, Banerjee A, Silliman CC, Sauaia A. Goal-directed hemostatic resuscitation of trauma-induced coagulopathy: a pragmatic randomized clinical trial comparing a viscoelastic assay to conventional coagulation assays. Ann Surg. 2016;263(6):1051–9.
129. Moore EE, Moore HB, Gonzalez E, Sauaia A, Banerjee A, Silliman CC. Rationale for the selective administration of tranexamic acid to inhibit fibrinolysis in the severely injured patient. Transfusion. 2016;56(Suppl 2):S110–4.
130. CRASH-2 Trial Collaborators, Shakur H, Roberts I, Bautista R, Caballero J, Coats T, Dewan Y, El-Sayed H, Gogichaishvili T, Gupta S, Herrera J, Hunt B, Iribhogbe P, Izurieta M, Khamis H, Komolafe E, Marrero MA, Mejía-Mantilla J, Miranda J, Morales C, Olaomi O, Olldashi F, Perel P, Peto R, Ramana PV, Ravi RR, Yutthakasemsunt S. Effects of tranexamic acid on death, vascular occlusive events, and blood transfusion in trauma patients with significant haemorrhage (CRASH-2): a randomised, placebo-controlled trial. Lancet. 2010;376(9734):23–32.
131. CRASH-2 Collaborators, Roberts I, Shakur H, Afolabi A, Brohi K, Coats T, Dewan Y, Gando S, Guyatt G, Hunt BJ, Morales C, Perel P, Prieto-Merino D, Woolley T. The importance of early treatment with tranexamic acid in bleeding trauma patients: an exploratory analysis of the CRASH-2 randomised controlled trial. Lancet. 2011;377:1096–101.
132. Harvin JA, Peirce CA, Mims MM, Hudson JA, Podbielski JM, Wade CE, Holcomb JB, Cotton BA. The impact of tranexamic acid on mortality in injured patients with hyperfibrinolysis. J Trauma Acute Care Surg. 2015;78(5):905–11.

Adjuncts to Resuscitation

20

Ryan A. Lawless and Bryan A. Cotton

Abstract

Damage control resuscitation has been increasingly adopted and practiced over the last decade. The concepts used are not new to this era of medicine but are novel in combination. This chapter will focus on adjuncts to damage control resuscitation (DCR) including massive transfusion protocols, the "other" tenets of damage control resuscitation, hypertonic saline, tranexamic acid, pharmacologic resuscitation, Factor VIIa, and prothrombin complex, and viscoelastic testing.

Damage control resuscitation (DCR) is a treatment strategy targeting the conditions that potentiate hemorrhage in the traumatically injured patient [1]. The term originates from the US Navy in reference to the techniques used to salvage a damaged ship during conflict [2]. In the management of the hemorrhaging patient, DCR refers to an approach to resuscitation initially adopted to improve outcomes of patients undergoing an abbreviated laparotomy or other procedure due to grossly disturbed physiology. However, its early implementation and even adoption in the prehospital setting have resulted in many of these patients now undergoing definitive procedures as the initial operation. The three basic tenets of DCR include permissive hypotension, blood product resuscitation approximating whole blood, and minimizing use of crystalloid prior to surgical control of bleeding [3]. Ideally, this process begins in the prehospital setting and continues through the emergency room (ER) and operating room, and into the ICU, as needed.

Looking at the incorporation of the other two principles (permissive hypotension and minimizing crystalloids) into a mature trauma center already incorporating a transfusion strategy approaching whole blood, investigators found an improvement in survival among emergent laparotomy patients [4]. Cotton and colleagues evaluated 390 patients who underwent damage control laparotomy and were managed with a red blood cell:plasma:platelet ratio of 1:1:1. The investigators found that after adoption of permissive hypotension and minimal crystalloids in the ED and operating room, blood transfusions were reduced, patients arrived to the ICU with less coagulopathy and acidosis, and survival was increased 2.5-fold. Duke et al. investigated the combination of a restrictive fluid resuscitation strategy and DCR. They reported a significant reduction in preoperative and intraoperative crystalloid administration with improvements

R.A. Lawless, M.D.
The Department of Surgery, Denver Health Medical Center, The University of Colorado School of Medicine, Aurora, CO, USA

B.A. Cotton, M.D. (✉)
The Department of Surgery and the Center for Translational Injury Research, The McGovern Medical School at the University of Texas Health Science Center, Red Duke Trauma Institute at Memorial Hermann Hospital, Houston, TX, USA
e-mail: Bryan.A.Cotton@uth.tmc.edu

J. Duchesne et al. (eds.), *Damage Control in Trauma Care*,
https://doi.org/10.1007/978-3-319-72607-6_20

in hospital and ICU length of stay, a reduction in operative room mortality, and a resultant decrease in overall mortality [5].

20.1 Permissive Hypotension

The concept of permissive hypotension has been debated for years. Maintaining the patient's blood pressure high enough for adequate organ perfusion yet low enough as to avoid exsanguination is the goal. In 1918, Walter Cannon and John Fraser warned of the blood loss that could occur by elevating a patient's blood pressure before a surgeon was available [6]. The endpoint for resuscitation prior to the availability of a surgeon in their study was between 70 and 80 mmHg systolic blood pressure. In his document entitled "Surgery in World War II, General Surgery", Dr. Beecher stated that "*When the patient must wait for a considerable period, elevation of his systolic blood pressure to ~85 mmHg is all that is necessary*" and that "*…one should consider himself lucky if a systolic pressure of 80 mmHg to 85 mmHg can be achieved and then surgery undertaken*" [7]. However, human studies validated the data produced by animal studies have been few [8, 9].

In 2002, Dutton and colleagues conducted a randomized trial of hypotensive resuscitation [9]. A total of 110 patients were randomized on arrival to a resuscitation targeting a systolic blood pressure of 70 mmHg or a systolic of 100 mmHg. Each resuscitation strategy was continued until definitive hemostasis was achieved. While no survival difference was noted, the authors found that aiming for SBP of 70 mmHg (vs. >100 mmHg) was safe in patients arriving with evidence of hemorrhage. Carrick et al. recently evaluated a similar strategy in trauma patients undergoing a thoracotomy or laparotomy [10]. Aiming for mean arterial pressure of 50 or 65 mmHg, the investigators continued this goal throughout the operating room course. The authors found that while blood loss and transfusions were less in the hypotensive group (50 mmHg goal), this did not translate into an improvement in 30-day mortality. Both studies, however, were quite small and their results may reflect a type-II error. As well, the benefits of reduced hemorrhage outweigh the possible detrimental effects of organ ischemia and reperfusion injury [11].

20.2 Minimizing Crystalloids

Historically, large quantities of crystalloid and blood were advocated to replace the intravascular and extravascular fluid loss from hemorrhage. This strategy arose from studies in the 1950s and 1960s and was, until recently, endorsed by the American College of Surgeons Advanced Trauma Life Support (ATLS) course with the recommendation of 1–2 L of crystalloid during the initial management of trauma patients [12–14]. However, multiple studies have shown the detriments of aggressive crystalloid resuscitation including cardiac dysfunction, ARDS, multi-organ failure, and increases in mortality [15–21]. Moreover, the infusion of room temperature, high chloride containing fluid worsens hypothermia, acidosis, and coagulopathy [22]. Resuscitation to a normal blood pressure increases hemorrhage through the dilution of coagulation factors, displacement of tenuous clots, and decreases in blood viscosity leading to increased mortality [23–28].

Evaluating the impact of minimizing crystalloids in the clinical arena, Bickell and colleagues built on this extensive preclinical data by conducting a randomized trial of standard ATLS resuscitation (crystalloids) versus no fluid [27]. Patients presenting with hypotension (systolic ≤ 90 mmHg) and who had sustained penetrating torso injuries were randomized to one arm or the other beginning in the prehospital setting and the randomization resuscitation strategies were continued until the patient entered the operating room. Patients who received no fluid (delayed resuscitation) had lower mortality compared to those who received immediate fluid resuscitation. Two decades later, the Resuscitation Outcomes Consortium further investigated these two damage control resuscitation principles [29]. The investigators randomized study patients beginning in the prehospital setting to a systolic pressure of 70 mmHg and small boluses (250 mL) to maintain blood pressure goal, while the control group was randomized to

110 mmHg, received two liters initially, and additional fluid to maintain blood pressure target. Each protocol continued until hemorrhage control or 2 h after hospital arrival. The 24-h mortality for blunt trauma was significantly lower in the study arm compared to that observed in the control group (3% vs. 18%).

Assessment of Blood Consumption Score
ED systolic BP ED systolic blood pressure ≤ 90 mmHg
ED heart rate ≥ 120 beats per minutes
Penetrating Mechanism
Positive fluid on abdominal FAST

Fig. 20.1 Assessment of blood consumption score

20.3 Massive Transfusion Protocolization

The 1970s brought about the first discussions of massive transfusions (MT) and the associated 90% mortality rate [30]. However, the development of standardized delivery processes and protocolization of these MT processes would take another 30 years to arrive. With the implementation and maturation of these MT protocols, times to delivery of initial blood products, overall product utilization, and mortality were all significantly reduced [31, 32]. To put this in perspective, early improvements in hemorrhagic shock resuscitation (2000–2005) had reported mortalities for patients receiving a MT were 55–65% [33]. However, with increased adoption of MT protocols, mortality soon dropped to 45–50% by 2009. With further maturation and adoption of DCR tenets, MT mortalities continued to decrease to the current rates of 22–26% [34].

The layers of delay for blood product administration include the placement of the individual product orders, communication among providers, decisions regarding the products to transfuse, transportation of blood samples to the lab, and receipt and review of the lab values [35]. MT protocolization allows members of the trauma team to focus on managing the patient and their injuries and be less worried about choosing, obtaining, and transfusion of blood products. That said, establishing a massive transfusion protocol is not an easy task (Figs. 20.1, 20.2, 20.3 and 20.4). This is a multidisciplinary process involving the Emergency Medicine Physicians, Trauma Surgeons, Anesthesiologists, Hematologists, and Blood Bank. In 2008, Cotton et al. first demonstrated an improvement in mortality with the simple implementation of the MT process at their hospital [32]. In 2009, Riskin and colleagues also noted an improvement in mortality, which they attributed to improved communication with the blood bank and time to blood product availability [36]. In order for MT protocol to be effective, a center must have thawed or liquid plasma available for immediate delivery and transfusion [37–39]. Determining the content of the MTP cooler is highly debated in the literature to this day. In a recent randomized controlled trial, resuscitation of red blood cells:plasma:platelets in a ratio of 1:1:1 demonstrated a reduction in bleeding-related mortality [34]. However, overall mortality was not improved. No matter the take on the current literature, delivery of a standardized MT protocol and compliance with that protocol has been shown to improve outcomes in these patients [40, 41].

Once in place, knowing which patients will benefit from activation of the MT protocol can be difficult. Multiple scoring systems have been developed to identify patients that may benefit from a MT protocol [33]. While the predictive value of each of these scores is good, many of these include laboratory values that are not readily available upon the patient's arrival to the hospital making these scoring systems less useful. To address this, the Assessment of Blood Consumption (ABC) score was developed in 2009. It utilizes data readily available upon a patient's arrival to the hospital. The four components of the score are: ED systolic blood pressure ≤90 mmHg, ED heart rate ≥120 beats per minutes, penetrating mechanism, positive fluid on abdominal ultrasound evaluation. Each criterion consists of one point. Scores ≥2 indicate activation of the MT protocol (Fig. 20.1). While the ABC score overestimates the need for MT protocol with a positive predictive value of 50–55%, products can be returned and restocked. More importantly, the negative predic-

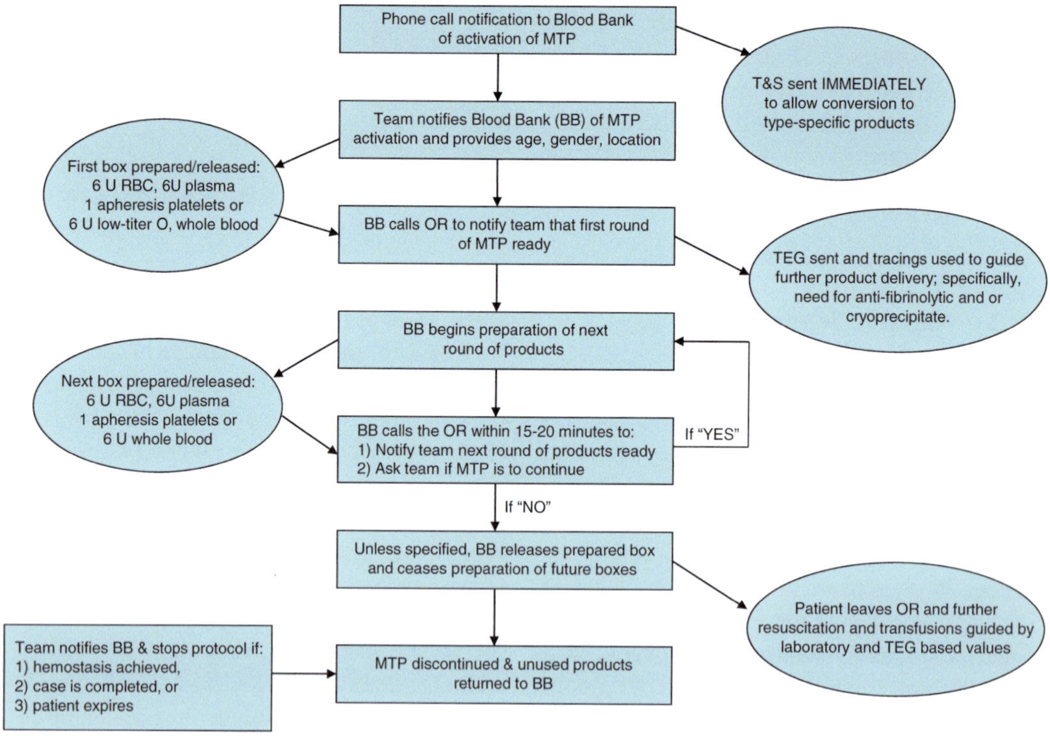

Fig. 20.2 Massive transfusion protocol at Memorial Hermann Hospital-Texas Trauma Institute

tive value for ABC is 95–96%; thereby minimizing those missed [39, 42, 43].

The ABC score is but one of many tools available to practitioners managing severely injured patients and should not replace a physician's discretion. Other clues to encourage activation of the MT protocol include persistent hemodynamic instability, active hemorrhage requiring surgical intervention, including interventional radiologic procedures, and the transfusion of non-crossmatched blood in the resuscitation bay [39]. A delay in identifying patients that require massive transfusion and delay in the initial cooler arrival, prolong the time to hemostasis and increase mortality [44, 45].

Once activated, the blood bank should immediately release MT coolers for transfusion approximately every 10–15 min. One simple rule: remain one cooler ahead of the current transfusion. Once the hemorrhage has been controlled and the patient is no longer hemodynamically unstable, the MT protocol can be discontinued. Laboratory indicators can be helpful in these situations and include hemoglobin levels, traditional coagulation tests, viscoelastic testing, platelet counts, and fibrinogen levels. The decision to terminate the MTP should be determined by the anesthesia and surgery teams jointly [39]. Compliance with the protocol is also essential for providing optimal care. Knowing when to activate and when to terminate the protocol can be guided by scoring tools and laboratory values. These values should assist, not replace, the judgment of the providers. The EAST guideline for damage control resuscitation recommends the development and implementation of a massive transfusion/DCR protocol in a multidisciplinary fashion with current literature and target blood product ratios. Furthermore, the same group endorses a high ratio MT/DCR strategy, if not whole blood [37].

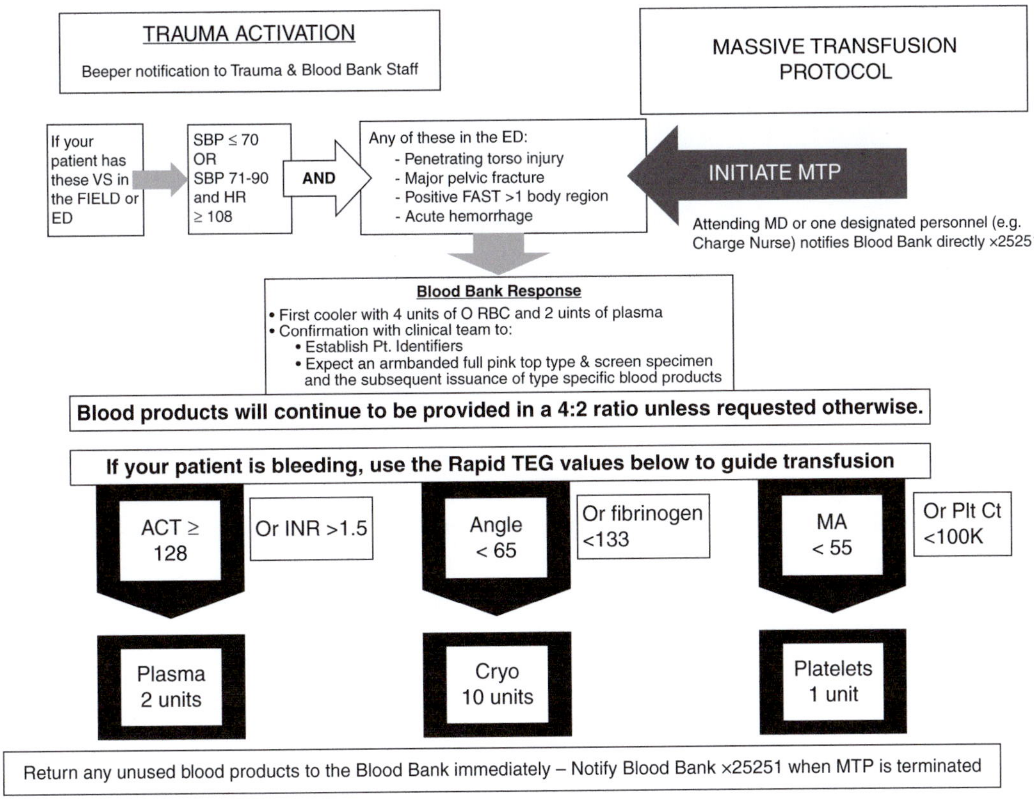

Fig. 20.3 r-TEG-based massive transfusion protocol at Denver HealthMedical Center

ACT ≥128	Transfuse plasma
r-value ≥1.1	Transfuse plasma
k-time ≥2.5	Transfuse plasma Add cryoprecipitate/fibrinogen if angle also abnormal
α-angle ≤60	Transfuse cryoprecipitate (or fibrinogen) Add platelets if mA is also abnormal
MA ≤55	Transfuse platelets Add cryoprecipitate/fibrinogen if angle also abnormal
LY-30 ≥3%	Administer tranexamic acid or amino-caproic acid

Fig. 20.4 r-TEG cut point values at Memorial Hermann Hospital-TexasTrauma Institute

20.4 Tranexamic Acid

The anti-fibrinolytic agent tranexamic acid (TXA) works by inhibiting the conversion of plasminogen to plasmin. In retrospective studies, administration of TXA to hemorrhaging patients has been associated with decreased mortality in both the civilian and military populations [46, 47]. It has also been shown to be a cost-effective adjunct for health care systems in poor and wealthy nations [48]. The identified window of benefit for the administration of TXA is within 3 h of injury [49]. However, TXA has failed to gain widespread acceptance and incorporation in the USA for multiple reasons. First, the large, multicenter, randomized trial of TXA in injured patients (CRASH-2) has several major methodological flaws. Also, whether TXA has any impact on trauma outcomes in a region already practicing DCR or a hospital with a MTP in place is unknown. The majority of patients enrolled in CRASH-2 were in low-income and middle-income countries where blood products, mature trauma centers, and experienced trauma teams are not readily available. Finally, how sick or injured (or uninjured) patients were in CRASH-2 is also a concern; less than half of patients (in either TXA or placebo groups) underwent an operation and only half received even one unit of blood.

In 2013, Napolitano et al. recommended TXA be used as part of a MTP in the following situations: (1) hyperfibrinolysis demonstrated on viscoelastic testing or (2) in patients with severe hemorrhagic shock (SBP ≤75 mmHg and a base deficit >5). Furthermore, given the increase in mortality seen with administration after 3 h, TXA should not be given when the time from injury is known or suspected to be greater than 3 h [50]. The current EAST guideline conditionally recommends TXA use as a hemostatic adjunct in the severely injured patient in the hospital setting only [37].

20.5 Fibrinogen Replacement

The case for the addition of fibrinogen, through either cryoprecipitate or fibrinogen concentrate, remains controversial. While in theory an argument can be easily made for its use in the bleeding patient, data in trauma and emergent cases is extremely lacking. The majority of data supporting its use is in the cardiac setting, and especially in those scenarios where intravascular support includes hydroxyethyl starches [51]. Hydroxyethyl starches reduce maximal clot firmness through a reduction in fibrinogen activity (as well as that of factors II, X, and XIII) [52]. One randomized trial of patients undergoing major aortic replacement surgery found a reduction in both red blood cell and plasma transfusions in patients receiving fibrinogen concentrate (compared to placebo) [53]. In the setting of trauma, Schochl et al. evaluated 131 patients who received fibrinogen concentrate guided by viscoelastic tests in the setting of bleeding [54]. The authors noted a significantly improved mortality compared to that predicted by the Trauma Related Injury Severity Score (TRISS) in patients who received fibrinogen concentrate during their initial resuscitation. As well, German investigators found that exsanguinating patients who received fibrinogen concentrate as part of their resuscitation had improved 6-h mortality (corresponding to the time of bleeding-related deaths [55]). The MATTERs II study, which was a retrospective study of UK and US military experience with combat injuries, evaluated the role of cryoprecipitate and tranexamic acid [56]. Investigators found that when patients received both cryoprecipitate and tranexamic acid as part of their care, mortality was half that of those who received neither (11.6 versus 23.6%). However, the PROMMTT investigators evaluated the impact of cryoprecipitate on bleeding patients from ten US Level-1 trauma centers and noted that its use varied greatly in their timing and use of cryoprecipitate in severely injured trauma patients [57]. However, the authors could not identify any association of cryoprecipitate use with in-hospital mortality. In addition, some have argued that routine replacement even in exsanguinating patients is unwarranted [58]. Opponents note that with early and more aggressive use of plasma, hypofibrinogenemia and/or fibrinogen dysfunction is uncommon. Given this, most would agree that randomized controlled studies in trauma are needed to determine if fibrinogen replacement is necessary. To that end, a randomized trial of fibrinogen replacement beginning in the prehospital setting, CRYOSTAT-2, will begin enrollment in 2017.

20.6 Prothrombin Complex Concentrate

Prothrombin complex concentrate (PCC) is a concentrated vitamin K-dependent coagulation factor product. It was originally approved for the treatment of hemophilia B and has been expanded to the reversal of vitamin K antagonist (VKA) effects. PCCs offer potential advantages over plasma including faster INR normalization in patients, delivery of smaller infusion volume, rapid administration, and no requirement for ABO blood-type matching.

All derived from pooled plasma and carry the possible risk of virus transmission. The 4-factor concentrates contain factors II, VII, IX, and X, while the 3-factor concentrates contain II, IX, and X. Sarode and colleagues conducted a multicenter, randomized trial in non-trauma, noncritical patients who were on warfarin and had need for urgent INR reversal [59]. The authors demonstrated that PCCs more rapidly reversed INR compared to plasma reversal, and did so with a similar adverse event profile. Studies in trauma are small and few [60]. However, some of these have noted effectiveness of PCC in the rapid reversal of VKA-related coagulopathy in trauma patients. Quick et al. demonstrated the safety and efficacy of PCC in the reversal of VKA-related coagulopathy in geriatric trauma patients [61]. Huynh et al. noted a more rapid correction of INR in patients on warfarin who sustained traumatic brain injury, with no differences in outcome. The utility of PCC incorporation into MT protocols or as a replacement for plasma in early resuscitation remains to be answered. Plasma provides volume expansion, acid-base buffering capacity, and high oncotic properties, all of which are beneficial in the patient with hemorrhagic shock, and none of which are present with PCCs [58]. In addition, plasma is effective in maintaining vascular endothelium integrity and clot stability, which has not yet been established for PCCs [62].

20.7 Recombinant Factor VIIa (rFVIIa)

Recombinant factor VIIa (rFVIIa) is currently approved for the treatment of hemophilia and has previously been advocated for the use in hemorrhaging trauma patients. It has been adopted and incorporated into many massive transfusion algorithms [63]. The rFVIIa is thought to activate the common coagulation pathway at pharmacologic doses [64]. Several retrospective studies show possible benefit in the use of rFVIIa as an adjunct to DCR by decreasing the overall need for blood transfusions, improvement in traditional coagulation tests, and hastening the resolution of bleeding [65–67]. However, randomized trials were less encouraging. Bouffard et al. published a randomized, placebo-controlled trial showing that patients suffering from blunt traumatic injury received less blood products with rFVIIa, but no benefit was seen in penetrating trauma [68]. Raobaikady et al. reported their randomized trial on the use of rFVIIa during pelvic reconstruction and noted no difference in transfusion requirements [69]. In

2010, the CONTROL trial evaluated the safety and efficacy of rFVIIa in a multinational randomized trial. There was no difference in survival between patients receiving rFVIIa and placebo, regardless of the mechanism of trauma. Similar to previous studies, rFVIIa decreased red blood cells and plasma transfusions and a trend toward less multi-organ failure was noted [70].

There was much early enthusiasm for the use of rFVIIa in the management of the bleeding patient. However, the popularity of DCR, with less crystalloid volume and earlier plasma and platelet transfusions, increased during the study periods for rVIIa. The current EAST guideline does not recommend for or against the use of rFVIIa as it does not appear to improve all-cause mortality and the only benefit is a possible reduction in the need for massive transfusion. They recommend further study to identify the optimal dose and timing for rFVIIa delivery [37].

20.8 Vasopressin

Arginine vasopressin (AVP) is an endogenous neurohypophyseal hormone released in response to changes in plasma osmolality and blood pressure [71]. Hypotension can stimulate the release of vasopressin as much as 40 times physiologic concentrations. Also, AVP clearance is prolonged leading to higher concentrations for a longer duration [72]. Its release is suppressed by elevations of norepinephrine and nitric oxide, which can be seen in hemorrhagic shock. Primarily, AVP works on the extracerebral arteriole V1 receptors leading to vasoconstriction. This causes an increase in systemic vascular resistance and a redistribution of blood flow from capacitance vessels in the periphery toward heart, brain, and kidneys [73]. However, this vasoconstriction is not as great in the coronary and renal system. AVP potentially has a vasodilatory effect on cerebral and renal vessels leading to improved blood flow [74].

The compensatory increase in endogenous vasopressin levels has been described in septic and hemorrhagic shock. Patients suffering from septic or hemorrhagic shock with a depressed endogenous AVP response show a significant increase in blood pressure with low-dose administration of AVP, while patients with a normal compensatory response did not show the same response to low-dose AVP administration [75, 76]. Animal models of liver injury associated hemorrhagic shock have shown decreased blood loss, increased mean arterial pressure, and significantly higher hemoglobin levels with vasopressin administration compared to standard crystalloid resuscitation [74]. AVP caused a shift in blood flow from the intra-abdominal injury leading to decreased blood loss. A temporary shunting of blood flow from the mesenteric vessels and profound peripheral vasoconstriction lead to restored perfusion of the liver and kidneys [74, 77]. Similar studies showed an increase in cardiac and cerebral blood flow following vasopressin administration secondary to cutaneous, muscular, adipose, gut vasoconstriction. The cardiovascular collapse and blood loss seen with crystalloid infusion was not demonstrated following AVP injection [78]. A randomized, placebo-controlled study (AVERT Shock) is currently underway to investigate the potential benefit of vasopressin administration during the early resuscitation of bleeding trauma patients [79].

20.9 Valproic Acid

Valproic acid (VPA) is a GABA-ergic medication used in the treatment of epilepsy, bipolar disorder, migraines, and neuropathic pain. There are multiple mechanisms of action that contribute to the biologic activity of VPA including the alteration of gene expression, the downregulation of enzymatic pathways, the enhancement of neurotransmission, and the stabilization of neuronal membranes [80–83]. Histone deacetylase has been implicated in the modulation of the lifespan of certain organisms through its effect on gene expression [84]. Hemorrhage and the resuscitation of hemorrhage have been shown to be associated with an imbalance in histone deacetylase (HDAC) and histone acetyltransferase (HAT) activity. The presence of shock induces changes in histone deacetylation which can be reversed with the infusion of VPA, a HDAC inhibitor. Animal models have shown that the cytoprotective and restorative effects occur with pretreatment and post-injury infusion of VPA [85–87]. This leads to improvement in early survival from near lethal hemorrhage. The survival advantage is likely due to better tolerance to the shock state by cells [88]. Further research needs to be performed in this area to investigate the utility of VPA in human trauma resuscitation.

20.10 Hypertonic Saline

The infusion of hypertonic saline has been described at multiple points during the management of the injured patient; from the point of injury, to specific injury management, to damage control resuscitation. Hypertonic saline infusion increases serum osmolality causing a shift of fluid volume from the intracellular to the extracellular space. This volume shift effectively increases preload, cardiac output, and mean arterial pressure [89]. Mazzoni et al. described an improvement in capillary endothelial swelling leading to an improvement in microcirculation with the infusion of hypertonic saline [90].

As described above, volume overload is detrimental to patients requiring management in damage control situations. It leads to the development of acute lung injury and acute respiratory distress syndrome, as well as to multisystem organ failure secondary to the cascade of inflammatory and immune responses associated with volume overload [91]. Hypertonic saline infusion allows for the rapid restoration of preload with less volume. Furthermore, the edema associated with resuscitation is attenuated leading to improved end organ perfusion [1]. Animal studies have shown that hypertonic saline infusion attenuates the proliferation of white blood cells, endothelial adhesion, and the expression of inflammatory markers in the lung and gut [92–94]. Rizoli and colleagues corroborated these findings by demonstrating a decreased neutrophil activation, decreased serum TNF-α levels, increased level of anti-inflammatory cytokines IL-1ra and IL-10, and attenuated norepinephrine surge associated with shock. This was demonstrated up to 24 h following injury [95]. Other animal studies have shown that hypertonic saline not only prevents, but reverses resuscitation-induced intestinal edema [96–98].

Duchesne et al. performed a retrospective comparison of low volume resuscitation with hypertonic saline and isotonic crystalloid infusion during the ICU phase of damage control resuscitation. They found a decrease in the volume infused, decreased ICU length of stay, lower prevalence of ARDS and multisystem organ failure, and a trend toward renal failure in the hypertonic saline group [91]. In 2013, Harvin and colleagues described a protocol of hypertonic saline (3% saline) infusion following damage control laparotomy with respect to primary fascial closure. They found that the isotonic crystalloid group received significantly more fluid compared to the hypertonic saline group; however, transfusions of blood products were similar. There were also similar rates of renal failure between the group. The investigators found that 100% of patients in the hypertonic saline group achieved primary fascial closure by post-damage control day 7 and a decreased time to fascial closure compared to 76% in the isotonic crystalloid group [99].

20.11 Viscoelastic Testing

Approximately 25% of severely injured patients have an established coagulopathy upon arrival to the emergency department [100, 101]. Prompt recognition and treatment of this cohort of patients is crucial. Most centers monitor five convention coagulation tests: prothrombin time (PT), international normalized ratio (INR), activated partial thromboplastin time (aPTT), platelet count, and fibrinogen levels. These tests are representative of a portion of the coagulation system. Utilization of these tests is limited by slow result times, poor association with clinical outcomes, and incomplete characterization of the complete coagulation system. Viscoelastic tests characterize the lifespan of a clot from the time to initial fibrin cross-linking to breakdown by fibrinolysis in a single assay [102]. The viscoelastic assays available are thromboelastography (TEG) (Haemonetics Corp, Niles, IN) and thromboelastometry (ROTEM) (TEM International, GmbH, Munich,

Germany). The rapid TEG (r-TEG) assay has been shown to be readily available within minutes of being drawn, correlates well with conventional coagulation tests, and is predictive of early transfusion necessity [103]. In 2012, Holcomb et al. found that r-TEG data was clinically superior to the five conventional coagulation assays and identified patients with an increased risk of early PRBC, plasma and platelet transfusions, and fibrinolysis. The authors suggested that admission conventional coagulation tests could be replaced with r-TEG [104]. Further investigation into specific TEG values found that the parameter of clot strength (G) provided a consistent, independent prediction of massive transfusion and coagulation-related mortality early in the resuscitation [105]. Most recently, Gonzalez et al. compared MTP goal-directed by TEG versus conventional coagulation tests. They found that using a goal directed, TEG-guided MTP improved survival and used less plasma and platelet transfusions during the early phase of resuscitation compared with conventional coagulation test directed MTP [106].

Conclusions

Damage control resuscitation has become increasingly adopted and practiced over the last 10 years. While many of the concepts used are not new, their application to early trauma resuscitation and their combination unique "cocktails" is novel, and the resultant improved outcomes applauded. This chapter evaluated many of these adjuncts to DCR including massive transfusion protocols, the less known and investigated DCR tenets, viscoelastic testing, hypertonic saline, tranexamic acid, Factor VIIa, and prothrombin complex.

In conjunction with early use of blood products (in ratios resembling whole blood), permissive hypotension and limited crystalloid administration are associated with reduced bleeding, less transfusions, and improved survival. Protocolization of the massive transfusion process, independent of ratios and products, is associated with improved survival. Use of viscoelastic testing to guide the resuscitation or bleeding patients appears to improve survival and reduce overall transfusion rates.

While VIIa and PCC appear to be of little use in the acute resuscitation of hemorrhage, TXA appears to improve survival in patients with penetrating mechanism, who are in profound shock, and receive the drug early after injury. Both hypertonic saline and vasopressin hold promise in the pursuit to limit fluid resuscitation and bleeding volume in hemorrhagic shock patients. Finally, use of valproic acid may not reduce bleeding but may allow for better tolerance of prolonged hemorrhagic shock, allowing for the delivery to appropriate levels of care for severely injured patients.

References

1. Duchesne J, McSwain N, Cotton B, Hunt J, Dellavolpe J, Lafaro K, et al. Damage control resuscitation: the new face of damage control. J Trauma. 2010;69:976–90.
2. Shapiro M, Jenkins DS, Rotondo M. Damage control: collective review. J Trauma. 2000;49:969–78.
3. Holcomb J, Jenkins D, Rhee P, Johannigman J, Mahoney P, Mehta S, et al. Damage control resuscitation: directly addressing the early coagulopathy of trauma. J Trauma. 2007;62:307–10.
4. Cotton B, Reedy N, Hatch Q, Podbielski J, McNutt M, Albarado R, et al. Damage control resuscitation reduces volumes and improves survival in 390 damage control laparotomy patients. Ann Surg. 2011;254:598–605.
5. Duke M, Guidry C, Guice J, Stuke L, Marr A, Hunt J, et al. Restrictive fluid resuscitation in combination with damage control resuscitation: time for adaptation. J Trauma. 2012;73:674–8.
6. Cannon WF. The preventative treatment of wound shock. JAMA. 1918;70:618.
7. Beecher H. Surgery in World War II, General surgery. In: Dot A, editor. Office of the Surgeon General Washington, DC: U.S. Government Printing Office; 1952:6.
8. Mapstone J, Roberts I, Evans P. Fluid resuscitation strategies: as systematic review of animal trials. J Trauma. 2003;55:571–89.
9. Dutton R, Mackenzie C, Scalea T. Hypotensive resuscitation during active hemorrhage: impact on in-hospital mortality. J Trauma. 2002;52:1141–6.
10. Carrick M, Morrison C, Tapia N, Leonard J, Suliburk J, Norman M, et al. Intraoperative hypotensive resuscitation for patients undergoing lapa-

rotomy or thoracotomy for trauma: early termination of a randomized prospective clinical trial. J Trauma. 2016;80:886–96.
11. Duchesne J, Kaplan L, Balogh Z, Malbrain M. Role of permissive hypotension, hypertonic resuscitation and the global increased permeability syndrome in patients with severe hemorrhage: adjuncts to damage control resuscitation to prevent intra-abdominal hypertension. Anaesthesiology Intensive Therapy. 2015;47:143–55.
12. Wiggers C. Physiology of shock. New York: Commonwealth Fund; 1950.
13. Shires G, Colin D, Carrico J, Lightfoot S. Fluid therapy in hemorrhagic shock. Arch Surg. 1964;88:688–93.
14. Committee on Trauma, American College of Surgeons. ATLS: advanced trauma life support: student course manual. 9th ed. Chicago, Il: American College of Surgeons; 2012.
15. Ng K, La C, Chan L. In vivo effect of haemodilution with saline on coagulation: a randomized controlled trial. Br J Anaesth. 2002;88:475–80.
16. Walker J, Criddle L. Pathophysiology and management of abdominal compartment syndrome. Am J Crit Care. 2003;12:367–71.
17. Rodas E, Malhotra A, Chhitwal R, Aboutanos M, Duane T, Ivatury R. Hyperacute abdominal compartment syndrome: an unrecognized complication of massive intraoperative resuscitation for extra-abdominal injuries. Am Surg. 2005;71:977–81.
18. Cotton B, Guy J, Morris J, Abumrad N. The cellular, metabolic, and systemic consequences of aggressive fluid resuscitation strategies. Shock. 2006;26: 115–21.
19. Schreiber M, Perkins J, Kiraly L, Underwood S, Wade C, Holcomb J. Early predictors of massive transfusion in combat casualties. J Am Coll Surg. 2007;205:541–5.
20. Tieu B, Holcomb J, Schreiber M. Coagulopathy: its pathophysiology and treatment in the injured patient. World J Surg. 2007;31:1055–64.
21. Balogh Z, McKinely B, Cocanour C, Kozar R, Holcomb J, Ware D, Moore F. Secondary abdominal compartment syndrome is an elusive early complication of traumatic shock resuscitation. Am J Surg. 2002;184:538–43.
22. Schreiber M. Coagulopathy in the trauma patient. Curr Opin Crit Care. 2005;11:590–7.
23. Stern S, Dronen S, Birrer P, Wang X. Effect of blood pressure on hemorrhage volume and survival in near-fatal hemorrhage model incorporating a vascular injury. Ann Emerg Med. 1993;22:155–63.
24. Kowalenko T, Stern S, Dronen S, Wang X. Improved outcome with hypotensive resuscitation of uncontrolled hemorrhagic shock in a swine model. J Trauma. 1992;33:349–53.
25. Riddez L, Johnson L, Hahn R. Central and regional hemodynamics during crystalloid fluid therapy after uncontrolled intra-abdominal bleeding. J Trauma. 1998;44:443–9.
26. Bickell W, Bruttig S, Millnamow G, O'Benar J, Wade C. The detrimental effects of intravenous crystalloid after aortotomy in swine. Surgery. 1991;110:529–36.
27. Bickell W, Wall M, Pepe P, Martin R, Ginger V, Allen M, Mattox K. Immediate versus delayed resuscitation for hypotensive trauma patients with penetrating torso injuries. N Engl J Med. 1994;331:1105–9.
28. Capone A, Safar P, Stezoski W, Tisherman S, Peitzman A. Improved outcome with fluid restriction in treatment of uncontrolled hemorrhagic shock. J Am Coll Surg. 1995;180:49–56.
29. Schreiber M, Meier E, Tisherman S, Kerby J, Newgard C, Brasel K, et al. A controlled resuscitation strategy is feasible and safe in hypotensive trauma patients: results of a prospective randomized pilot trial. J Trauma. 2015;78:687–97.
30. Wilson R, Mammen E, Walt A. Eight years if experience with massive blood transfusion. J Trauma. 1971;11:275–85.
31. O'keeffe T, Refaai M, Tchorz K, Forestner J, Sarode R. A massive transfusion protocol to decrease blood component use and costs. Arch Surg. 2008;143:686–91.
32. Cotton B, Gunter O, Isbell J, Au B, Robertson A, Morris J, et al. Damage control hematology: impact of a defined exsanguination protocol on mortality and blood utilization. J Trauma. 2008;64:117–8.
33. Cantle P, Cotton B. Prediction of massive transfusion. Crit Care Clin. 2017;33:71–84.
34. Holcomb J, Tilley B, Baraniuk S, Fox E, Wade C, Podbielski J, et al. Transfusion of plasma, platelets, and red blood cells in a 1:1:1 versus 1:1:2 ratio and mortality in patients with severe trauma: the PROPPR randomized clinical trial. JAMA. 2015;313:471–82.
35. Nunez T, Young P, Holcomb J, Cotton B. Creation, implementation, and maturation of a massive transfusion protocol for exsanguinating trauma patient. J Trauma. 2010;68:1498–505.
36. Riskin D, Tsai T, Riskin L, Hernandez-Boussard T, Purtill M, Maggio P, et al. Massive transfusion protocols: the role of aggressive resuscitation versus product ratio in mortality reduction. J Am Coll Surg. 2009;209:198–205.
37. Cannon J, Khan M, Raja A, Cohen M, Como J, Cotton B, et al. Damage control resuscitation in patients with severe traumatic hemorrhage: a practice management guideline from the Eastern Association for the Surgery of Trauma. J Trauma. 2017;82:605–17.
38. Radwan Z, Bai Y, Matijevic N, del Junco D, McCarthy J, Wade C, et al. An emergency department thawed plasma protocol for severely injured patients. JAMA Surg. 2013;148:170–5.
39. American College of Surgeons Committee on Trauma (nd). ACS TQIP massive transfusion in trauma guidelines. ACS TQIP Best Practice Guidelines: https://www.facs.org/quality-programs/trauma/tqip/best-practice. Accessed 1 Nov 2017.
40. Cotton B, Dossett L, Au B, Nunez T, Robertson A, Young P. Room for (performance) improvement:

provider-related factors associated with poor outcomes in massive transfusion. J Trauma. 2009;67:1004–12.
41. Baweezer M, Ahmed N, Izadi H, McFarlan A, Nathens A, Pavenski K. Compliance with massive transfusion protocol (MTP) impacts patient outcome. Injury. 2015;46:21–8.
42. Cotton B, Haut E, Dossett L, Shafi S, Au B, Nunez T, et al. Multicenter validation of a simplified score to predict massive transfusion. J Trauma. 2010;69:S33–9.
43. Nunez T, Voskrensky I, Dossett L, et al. Early prediction of massive transfusion in trauma: simple as ABC (assessment of blood consumption)? J Trauma. 2009;66:346–52.
44. Nunez T, Cotton B. Transfusion therapy in hemorrhagic shock. Curr Opin Crit Care. 2009;15:536–41.
45. Meyer D, Vincent L, Fox E, O'Keeffe T, Inaba K, Bulger E, et al. Every minute counts: time to delivery of initial massive transfusion cooler and its impact on mortality. J Trauma Acute Care Surg. 2017;83:19–24.
46. Morrison J, Dubose J, Rasmussen T, Midwinter M. Military application of tranexamic acid in trauma emergency resuscitation (MATTERs) study. Arch Surg. 2012;147:113–9.
47. Shakur H, Roberts I, Bautista R, Caballero J, Coats T, Dewan Y, et al. Effects of tranexamic acid on death, vascular occlusive events, and blood transfusion in trauma patients with significant hemorrhage (CRASH-2): a randomized, placebo-controlled trial. Lancet. 2010;376:23–32.
48. Guerriero C, cairns J, Perel P, Shakur H, Roberts I. Cost effectiveness analysis of administering tranexamic acid to bleeding trauma patients using evidence from the CRASH-2 trial. PLoS One. 2011;6:e18987.
49. Roberts I, Shakur H, Afolabi A, Brohi K, Coats T, Dewan Y, et al. The importance of early treatment with tranexamic acid in bleeding trauma patients: an exploratory analysis of the CRASH-2 randomised controlled trial. Lancet. 2011;377:1096–101.
50. Napolitano L, Cohen K, Cotton B, Schreiber M, Moore E. Tranexamic acid in trauma: how should we use it? J Trauma. 2013;74:1575–86.
51. Soloman C, Hagl C, Rahe-Meyer N. Time course of haemostatic effects of fibrinogen concentrate administration. Brit J Anaesth. 2013;110(6):947–56.
52. Fenger-Eriksen C, Tonnesen E, Ingerslev J, Sorensen B. Mechanisms of hydroxyethyl starch-induced dilutional coagulopathy. J Thromb Haemost. 2009;7:1099–105.
53. Rahe-Meyer N, Soloman C, Hanke A, Schmidt D, Lmoerzer D, Hochleitner G, et al. Effects of fibrinogen concentrate as first-line therapy during major aortic replacement surgery. Anesthesiology. 2013;118:40–50.
54. Schochl H, Neinbauer U, Hofer G, Voelckel W, Jambor C, Scharbert G, et al. Goal-directed coagulation management of major trauma patients using thromboelastometry (ROTEM)-guided administration of fibrinogen concentrate and prothrombin complex concentrate. Crit Care. 2010;14(2):R55.
55. Wafaisade A, Lefering R, Maegele M, Brockamp T, Mutschler M, Lendemans S, et al. Administration of fibrinogen concentrate in exsanguinating trauma patients is associated with improved survival at 6 hours but not at discharge. J Trauma Acute Care Surg. 2013;74:387–95.
56. Morrison J, Ross J, DuBose J, Jansen J, Midwinter M, Rasmussen T. Association of cryoprecipitate and tranexamic acid with improved survival following wartime injury. JAMA Surg. 2013;148(3):218–25.
57. Holcomb J, Fox E, Zhang X, White N, Wade C, Cotton B, et al. Cryoprecipitate use in the PROMMTT study. J Trauma Acute Care Surg. 2013;75:S31–9.
58. Young P, Cotton B. A window of opportunity: the aggressive use of plasma in early resuscitation. Transfusion. 2011;51:1880–2.
59. Sarode R, Milling T, Refaai M, Mangione A, Schneider A, Durn B, Goldstein J. Efficacy and safety of a 4-factor prothrombin complex concentrate in patients on vitamin antagonists presenting with major bleeding: a randomized, plasma-controlled, phase IIIb study. Circulation. 2013;128(11):1234–43.
60. Matsushima K, Benjamin E, Demetriades D. Prothrombin complex concentrate in trauma patients. Am J Surg. 2015;209:413–7.
61. Quick J, Bartels A, Coughenour J, Barnes S. Experience with prothrombin complex for the emergent reversal of anticoagulation in rural geriatric trauma patients. Surgery. 2012;152:722–8.
62. Pati S, Matijevic N, Doursout M, Ko T, Cao Y, Deng X, et al. Protective effects of fresh frozen plasma on vascular endothelial permeability, coagulation, and resuscitation after hemorrhagic shock are time dependent and diminish between days 0 and 5 after thaw. J Trauma. 2010;69:S55–63.
63. Holcomb J. Damage control resuscitation. J Trauma. 2007;62:S36–7.
64. Franchini M, Lippi G, Guidi G. The use of recombinant activated factor VII in platelet-associated bleeding. Hematology. 2008;13:41–5.
65. Benharash P, Bongard F, Putnam B. Use of recombinant factor VIIa for adjunctive hemorrhage control in trauma and surgical patients. Am Surg. 2005;71:776–80.
66. Dutton R, Hess J, scalea T. Recombinant factor VIIa for hemorrhage control: early experience in critically ill trauma patients. J Clin Anesth. 2003;15:184–8.
67. Khan A, Parry J, Crowley W, McAllen K, Davis A, Bonnell B, Hoogeboom J. Recombinant factor VIIa for the treatment of severe postoperative and traumatic hemorrhage. Am J Surg. 2005;189:331–4.
68. Boffard K, Riou B, Warren B, Choong P, Rizoli S, Rossaint R, et al. Recombinant factor VIIa as adjunctive therapy for bleeding control in severely injured trauma patients: two parallel randomized, placebo-

controlled, double-blinded clinical trials. J Trauma. 2005;59:8–15.
69. Raobaikady R, Redman J, Ball J, Maloney G, Grounds R. Use of activated recombinant coagulation factor VII in patients undergoing reconstruction surgery for traumatic fracture of pelvis or pelvis and acetabulum: a double-blind, randomized, placebo-controlled trial. Br J Anesth. 2005;94:586–91.
70. Hauser, C., Boffard, K., Dutton, R., Bernard, G., Croce, M., Holcomb, J., … Group, C. S. Results of the CONTROL trial: efficacy and safety of recombinant activated factor VII in the management of refractory traumatic hemorrhage. J Trauma. 2010;69:489–500.
71. Cossu A, Mura P, de Giudici L, Puddu D, Pasin L, Evangelista M, et al. Vasopressin in hemorrhagic shock: a systematic review and meta-analysis of randomized animal trials. BioMed Res Int. 2014;2014:9. epub
72. Errington E, Rocha E. Vasopressin clearance and secretion during haemorrhage in normal dogs and in dogs with experimental diabetes insipidus. J Physiol. 1972;227:395–418.
73. Forrest P. Vasopressin and shock. Anaesth Intensive Care. 2001;29:463–72.
74. Stadlbauer K, Wagner-Berger H, Raedler C, Voelckel W, Wenzel V, Krismer A, et al. Vasopressin, but not fluid resuscitation, enhances survival in a liver trauma model with uncontrolled and otherwise lethal hemorrhagic shock in pigs. Anesthesiology. 2003;98:699–704.
75. Cohn S. Potential benefit of vasopressin in resuscitation of hemorrhagic shock. J Trauma. 2007;62:S56–7.
76. Robin J, Oliver J, Landry D. Vasopressin deficiency in the syndrome of irreversible shock. J Trauma. 2003; 54:S149–54.
77. Voelckel W, Raedler C, Wenzel V, Lindner K, Krismer A, Schmittinger C, et al. Arginine vasopressin, but not epinephrine, improves survival in uncontrolled hemorrhagic shock after liver trauma in pigs. Crit Care Med. 2003;31:1160–5.
78. Stadlbauer K, Wagner-Berger H, Krismer A, Voelckel W, Konigsrainer A, Lindner K, Wenzel V. Vasopressin improves survival in a porcine model of abdominal vascular injury. Crit Care. 2007;11:R81.
79. https://clinicaltrials.gov/ct2/show/NCT01611935.
80. Blaheta R, Cinatl J. Anti-tumor mechanisms if valproate: a novel role for an old drug. Med Res Rev. 2002;22:492–511.
81. Kouzarides T. Acetylation: a regulatory modification to rival phosphorylation? EMBO J. 2000;19:1176–9.
82. Phiel C, Zhang F, Huang E, Guenther M, Lazar M, Klein P. Histone deacetylase is a direct target of valproic acid, a potent anticonvulsant, mood stabilizer, and teratogen. J Biol Chem. 2001;276:36,734–41.
83. Berger S. Gene activation by histone and factor acetyltransferase. Curr Opin Cell Biol. 1999;11:336–41.
84. Chang K, Min K. Regulation of lifespan by histone deacetylase. Ageing Res Rev. 2002;1:313–26.
85. Lin T, Alam H, Chen H, Britten-Webb J, Rhee P, Kirkpatrick J, Koustova E. Cardiac histones are substrates of histone deacetylase activity in hemorrhagic shock and resuscitation. Surgery. 2006;139:365–76.
86. Gonzalez E, Chen E, Munuve R, Mehrani T, Britten-Webb J, Nadel A, et al. Valproic acid prevents hemorrhage-associated lethality and affects the acetylation patterns of cardiac histones. Shock. 2006;25:395–401.
87. Shultz C, Sailhamer E, Li Y, Liu B, Tabbara M, Butt M, et al. Surviving blood loss without fluid resuscitation. J Trauma. 2008;64:629–40.
88. Alam H, Shuja F, Butt M, Duggan M, Li Y, Zacharias N, et al. Surviving blood loss without blood transfusion in a swine poly-trauma model. Surgery. 2009;146:325–33.
89. Chappell D, Jacob M, Hofmann-Kiefer K, Conzen P, Rehm M. A rational approach to perioperative fluid management. Anesthesiology. 2008;109:723–40.
90. Mazzoni M, Borgstrom P, Arfors K, Intaglietta M. Dynamic fluid redistribution in hyperosmolar resuscitation of hypovolemic hemorrhage. Am J Physiol. 1988;255(3):H629–37.
91. Duchesne J, Simms E, Guidry C, Duke M, Beeson E, McSwain N, Cotton B. Damage control immunoregulation: is there a role for low-volume hypertonic saline resuscitation in patients managed with damage control surgery? American. Surgeon. 2012;78:962–8.
92. Pascual J, Khawaja K, Chaudry P, Christou N. Hypertonic saline and the microcirculation. J Trauma. 2003;54(suppl):S133–40.
93. Deree J, de Campos TS, Loomis W, Hoyt D, Coimbra R. Hypertonic saline and pentoxifylline attenuates gut injury after hemorrhagic shock. Journal of Trauma. 2007;62:818–27.
94. Deree J, Martins J, Leedom A, Lamon B, Putnam J, de Campos T, et al. Hypertonic saline and pentoxifylline reduces hemorrhagic shock resuscitation-induced pulmonary inflammation through attenuation of neutrophil degranulation and proinflammatory mediator synthesis. J Trauma. 2007;62:104–11.
95. Rizoli S, Rhind S, Shek P, Inaba K, Filips D, Tien H, et al. The immunomodulatory effects of hypertonic saline resuscitation in patients sustaining traumatic hemorrhagic shock: a randomized, controlled, double-blinded trial. Ann Surg. 2006;243:47–57.
96. Attuwaybi B, Kozar R, Gates K, Moore-Olufemi S, Sato N, Weisbrodt N, Moore F. Hypertonic saline prevents inflammation, injury, and impaired intestinal transit after gut ischemia/reperfusion by inducing heme oxygenase-1 enzyme. J Trauma. 2004;56:749–58.
97. Attuwaybi B, Kozar R, Moore-Olufemi S, Sato N, Hassoun H, Weisbrodt N, Moore F. Heme oxygenase-1 induction by hemin protects against gut ischemia/reperfusion injury. J Surg Res. 2004;118:53–7.
98. Gonzalez E, Kozar R, Suliburk J, Weisborodt N, Mercer D, Moore F. Conventional dose hypertonic saline provides optimal gut protection and limits

remote organ injury after gut ischemia reperfusion. J Trauma. 2006;61:66–73.

99. Harvin J, Mims M, Duchesne J, Cox C, Wade C, Holcomb J, Cotton B. Chasing 100%: the use of hypertonic saline to improve early primary fascial closure after damage control laparotomy. J Trauma. 2013;74:426–30.
100. MacLeod J, Jynn M, McKenny M, Cohn S, Murtha M. Early coagulopathy predicts mortality in trauma. J Trauma. 2003;55:39–44.
101. Moore E, Moore F, Fabian T, Bernard A, Fulda G, Hoyt D. Human polymerized hemoglobin for the treatment of hemorrhagic shock when blood is unavailable: the USA multicenter trial. J Am Coll Surg. 2009;208:1–13.
102. Gonzalez E, Pieracci F, Moore E, Kashuk J. Coagulation abnormalities in the trauma patient: the role of point-of-care thromboelastography. Semin Thromb Hemost. 2010;36:723–37.
103. Cotton B, Faz G, Hatch Q, Radwan Z, Podbielski J, Wade C, et al. Rapid thromboelastography delivers real-time results that predict transfusion within 1 hour of admission. J Trauma. 2011;71:407–17.
104. Holcomb J, Minei K, Scerbo M, Radwan Z, Wade C, Kozar R, et al. Admission rapid thromboelastography can replace conventional coagulation tests in the emergency department. Ann Surg. 2012;256:1–11.
105. Pezold M, Moore E, Wohlauer M, Sauaia A, Gonzalez E, Banerjee A, Silliman C. Viscoelastic clot strength predicts coagulation-related mortality within 15 minutes. Surgery. 2012;151:48–54.
106. Gonzalez E, Moore E, Moore H, Chapman M, Chin T, Ghasabyan A, et al. Goal-directed hemostatic resuscitation of trauma induced coagulopathy: a pragmatic randomized clinical trial comparing a viscoelastic assay to conventional coagulation assays. Ann Surg. 2016;263:1051–9.

Damage Control in the Austere Environment

21

D.M. Nott

Abstract

Before the concept of damage control, patients admitted with severe injuries following significant blood loss would spend hours on the operating table to anatomically correct their injuries. The long operating time spent resecting livers, anastomosing bowel, bringing out stomas, and closing tense abdomens would inevitably lead to patients dying on the operating table or in the recovery ward.

21.1 Introduction

Before the concept of damage control, patients admitted with severe injuries following significant blood loss would spend hours on the operating table to anatomically correct their injuries. The long operating time spent resecting livers, anastomosing bowel, bringing out stomas, and closing tense abdomens would inevitably lead to patients dying on the operating table or in the recovery ward.

Twenty years ago, the term "damage control"(DC) described an abdominal staged procedure that reduced postoperative deaths in patients with exsanguinating hemorrhage [1]. Rather than addressing anatomy, it addressed the physiology that resulted from coagulopathy, hypothermia, and acidosis. The onus was to stop bleeding and sepsis as quickly as possible, followed by transfer to the intensive care unit for warming and normalization of the physiological parameters of temperature and coagulation during which the abdomen was left open to reduce the effects of abdominal compartment syndrome (ACS). Upon restoration of physiology, the patient returned to the operating theater, and packs were removed and bowel continuity established and the abdomen closed.

21.2 Damage Control Resuscitation

The recent conflicts in Iraq and Afghanistan have produced a change in the way DC is currently practiced. It is known that 30% of trauma patients who have significant blood loss are also coagulopathic and hypothermic [2, 3]. Rather than resuscitating patients and then performing DC, resuscitation must therefore begin either in the prehospital setting or immediately on arrival. This resuscitation became known as damage control resuscitation (DCR). Rather than elevate the blood pressure to normal values, the blood pressure was maintained to a level that would allow perfusion of the heart, kidneys, liver, and brain which equates to around 80 mm Hg. A concerted

D.M. Nott, O.B.E., D.Sc., M.D., F.R.C.S.
Imperial College, London, UK
e-mail: d.nott@imperial.ac.uk

J. Duchesne et al. (eds.), *Damage Control in Trauma Care*,
https://doi.org/10.1007/978-3-319-72607-6_21

effort was made to replace like with like, and so blood and blood products replaced blood loss. Limiting the amount of crystalloid is necessary to reduce third space overload which can lead to tissue edema and dilution of coagulation factors. So, DCR consists of hypotensive resuscitation and hemostatic resuscitation using blood components, given in a 1:1:1 ratio of packed red cells, fresh frozen plasma, and platelets [4], with severely limiting the use of crystalloids. Hypothermia which is caused by anaerobic respiration due to the initial tissue hypoxia is addressed by increasing the inflow temperature to 39C and giving blood and blood products at an average flow rate of 500 mL/min using a level one infuser. The coagulopathy is addressed by thromboelastography [5] and more coagulation products given as necessary. If the physiology can be normalized during the operation, then a discussion between anesthetist and surgeon can decide whether to stage or complete the operation.

The advances in DC gained have been widely adopted by civilian trauma centers throughout UK and the world. However, these advances require a significant amount of infrastructure. The question is whether these principles can be applied to patients with similar injuries in an austere environment or does one accept a significantly higher mortality.

21.3 Humanitarian Austere Damage Control Resuscitation

In the summer of 2012 at a field hospital in the Northern Syria, the initial decision to perform DC was based on the ATLS category of class 3 and class 4 shock, pertaining to a loss of between 1500 mL and more than 2 L of blood. Because there was no accurate way of measuring, all patients in this category were assumed to be hypothermic and coagulopathic. Resuscitation began with warmed crystalloid solution to improve the cardiac output. The temperature of the intravenous fluids was around 40 °C. This was achieved, by placing bags of fresh whole blood (FWB) and crystalloid solution in a bucket of hot water warmed by a kettle. To assess the correct temperature, it was assumed that if the operator's hands could not tolerate the water in the bucket for more than 30 s, then the temperature was higher than 43 °C and if the operator could for around a minute or so, then this would equate to a temperature of around 42 °C and the bags of crystalloid and blood placed in the bucket for around 5 min or so. Minimal amounts of crystalloid were infused calibrated to the radial pulse. Hemoglobin was measured using a hemoglobinometer and oxygen saturation with a probe placed on a digit.

Following an improvement in blood pressure or maintenance of a radial pulse, all patients received one unit of warm FWB, which was typed, crossmatched, and tested for hepatitis B and C and HIV. It is known that FWB improves cardiac output, microcirculatory hemodynamics, and oxygen consumption and may correct coagulopathy more efficiently because of increased function and concentration of platelets and plasma. It has been shown that one unit of FWB may be equivalent to ten pools of platelets [6, 7].

Resuscitative surgical skills were used to arrest non-compressible bleeding, and all arterial injuries were shunted as quickly as possible. The clotting time was assessed by a colleague using blood tilted in a syringe until it had signs of clotting. Solid organs that were bleeding or had the potential to rebleed were removed, and omentum was packed into liver injuries. At the same time, warm saline was poured into the abdomen using bags of saline that were warmed in the bucket.

21.4 Physiological Monitoring

There is no instrumentation available to measure pH and acid base balance in this environment. However, we have known from animal studies that there is a critical amount of oxygen in the blood that prevents anaerobic respiration. This depends on maintaining a good cardiac output and having enough oxygen in the red cells to maintain aerobic respiration. Many studies have shown that the critical hemoglobin level to maintain oxygen delivery to tissues during hemorrhage is 5 g/dL and above but only if the cardiac output can be maintained [8, 9]. A hemoglobin of 6 g/dL was therefore chosen as the cutoff for further whole blood administration as previous work has shown.

Strict damage control principles were applied, and the operation was curtailed as soon as possible and the abdomen packed with counted swabs and the abdominal skin closed with a running suture. All patients were extubated and put on a normal ward with a nasogastric tube and urinary catheter. Following a period of anything up to but not exceeding 36 h, when deemed to be physiologically normal, patients were brought back to the operating theater and the bowel anastomosis completed, and if there is a vascular injury, the vascular shunt is removed and a vascular reconstruction attempted.

21.5 Abdominal Closure

Twenty years ago, laparostomy was necessary because of the high incidence of ACS due to crystalloid extravasation. Modern DC resuscitation using blood and components has significantly reduced this requirement [10] In this environment, however, because of lack of blood, a significant amount of crystalloid must be given to maintain a reasonable cardiac output, which increases the risk of ACS. It is important that the surgeon anticipates this risk as there is no provision for laparostomy.

Any noticeable edema of the small or large bowel, tightness in closure, and doughy feeling of the abdominal wall were cues for ACS. In these cases, a component separation was performed on both sides of the abdominal wall. This technique involves releasing the external oblique from the anterior rectus sheath aponeurosis. This allowed on average a further 14 cm of laxity of the anterior abdominal wall for further expansion and subsequent reduction of intra-abdominal pressure.

There were no hard and fast rules relating to bowel anastomosis: all small bowel anastomoses were closed, most right colonic anastomoses were closed, and all left-sided colon injuries were treated by either anastomosis and defunctioning ileostomy or Hartmann's procedure. These can easily be brought out in abdominal wall which has undergone component separation.

Although many more patients were treated, 61 patients fell into the category of requiring DC based on exsanguinating hemorrhage. To the whole team's credit, not one patient died during this time. This included adults and children. Of the 61 patients, 15% had an Hb around 5 g/dL. Postoperatively, oxygen saturation gave an indication of acidosis and fluid requirements, a low oxygen saturation implying shift of the oxygen dissociation curve to the right. Close observation of the urine output in the first 2–3 days was as important as the initial surgery and all related to the continuing restoration of physiology.

This study performed in the Medecins Sans Frontieres hospital in Atmeh, Northern Syria, in 2012, has been tried and tested subsequently in well over 300 patients in Aleppo in 2013 and 2014 with excellent results.

References

1. Rotondo MF, Schwab CW, McGonigal MD, Phillips GR, Fruchterman TM, Kauder DR, et al. Damage control: an approach for improved Survival in exsanguinating penetrating abdominal injury. J Trauma. 1993;35:375–83.
2. Jurkovich GJ, Greiser WB, Luterman A, Curreri PW. Hypothermia in trauma victims: an ominous predictor of survival. J Trauma. 1987;27:1019–24.
3. Brohi K, Singh J, Heron M, Coats T. Acute traumatic coagulopathy. J Trauma. 2003;54:1127–30.
4. Gunter OL, Brigham K, Isbell JM, Mowery NT, Young PP, Cotton BA. J Trauma. 2008;65:527–34.
5. Doran CM, Woolley T, Midwinter MJ. Feasibility of using rotational thromboelastography to assess coagulation status of combat casualties in a deployed setting. J Trauma. 2010;69:540–8.
6. Mohr R, Martinowitz U, Lavee J, Amroch D, Ramot B, Goor DA. The haemostatic effect of transfusing fresh whole blood versus platelet concentrates after cardiac operations. J Thorac Cardiovasc Surg. 1998;96:530–4.
7. Spinella PC, Perkins JG, Grathwolhl KW, Beekley AC, Holcomb JB. Warm fresh whole blood is independently associated with improved survival for patients with combat related traumatic injuries. J Trauma. 2009;66:S69–76.
8. Weoskopf RB, Viele MK, Feiner J, Kelley S, Lieberman J, Noorani M, et al. Human cardiovascular and metabolic response to acute, severe isovolaemic anaemia. JAMA. 1998;27:217–22.
9. Cain SM. Oxygen delivery and uptake in dogs during anaemia and hypoxic hypoxaemia. J Appl Physiol. 1977;42:228–34.
10. Schreiber MA. The beginning of the end for damage control surgery. Brit J Surg. 2012;99:10–1.

22 Damage Control Surgery and the Boston Marathon Bombing

David R. King

Abstract

The practice of trauma surgery in the aftermath of the Boston Marathon bombing took place within the walls of the multiple Boston Level I trauma centers, as well as several adjacent community hospitals. The approach to these patients reflected the general philosophy of rapid damage control, abbreviated surgery, frequent returns to the operating room in a staged fashion, and high-ratio blood transfusions. The real lesson for surgeons, however, is learned from careful examination of the prehospital treatment of the injuries resulting from the two improvised explosive devices detonated on Boylston Street during the running of the 117th Boston Marathon at 14:49 on April 15, 2013: damage control starts at the point of wounding.

D.R. King, M.D., F.A.C.S.
Division of Trauma, Emergency Surgery, and Surgical Critical Care, Harvard Medical School, Boston, MA, USA

Massachusetts General Hospital and Harvard Medical School, Boston, MA, USA
e-mail: dking3@mgh.harvard.edu

22.1 Preface

The practice of trauma surgery in the aftermath of the Boston Marathon bombing took place within the walls of the multiple Boston Level I trauma centers, as well as several adjacent community hospitals. The approach to these patients reflected the general philosophy of rapid damage control, abbreviated surgery, frequent returns to the operating room in a staged fashion, and high-ratio blood transfusions. The real lesson for surgeons, however, is learned from careful examination of the prehospital treatment of the injuries resulting from the two improvised explosive devices detonated on Boylston Street during the running of the 117th Boston Marathon at 14:49 on April 15, 2013: damage control starts at the point of wounding.

As a surgeon, soldier, Bostonian, 50+-time chronic marathoner, and participant of the 117th Boston Marathon (3:12 marathon, roughly an hour before the blasts), I will forever remember the events of that day and how they altered our city in perpetuity. I remember those who died (29-year-old Krystle Campbell, 23-year-old Lu Lingzi, 8-year-old Martin Richard, and 27-year-old Sean Collier) and celebrate those who lived: the survivors. This chapter is dedicated to the survivors of the Boston Marathon bombing.

J. Duchesne et al. (eds.), *Damage Control in Trauma Care*,
https://doi.org/10.1007/978-3-319-72607-6_22

22.2 History Repeats Itself

Described in antiquity, tourniquets have been used to control extremity bleeding during amputations. This evolved to encompass the use of tourniquets as a first aid maneuver for extremity bleeding. The merits of tourniquet use as a first aid hemorrhage control maneuver have been repeatedly debated, mostly based on historical battlefield experiences that traditionally condemned the practice for its dreaded limb-threatening complications [1, 2]. Data collected throughout the most recent decade and a half of war in Iraq and Afghanistan [3, 4], however, have caused physicians, first responders, and policymakers to reconsider previously held beliefs around tourniquet use in the prehospital management of severely bleeding extremities [1]. This contemporary military wartime experience demonstrates that while improvised tourniquets are rarely effective, the ubiquitous availability and early use of commercial, purpose-designed tourniquets reduce death rates from extremity wound exsanguination [5–8]. The Boston Marathon bombing was the first major, modern US terrorist event with multiple, severe, warlike, lower extremity injuries [9] resulting from dismounted improvised explosive devices. Mass casualty events with multiple, severe extremity injuries are common on the battlefield but uncommon in the homeland. In Boston, trained medical professionals, civilian first responders, and nonmedical bystanders rushed to aid the injured, mostly attending to extremity wounds [10, 11].

22.3 The Bombing

Two ground-level improvised explosive devices were detonated on Boylston Street during the running of the 117th Boston Marathon, at 14:49:43 and 14:49:57 on April 15, 2013. Two hundred forty-three injured patients presented with a myriad of injuries (Fig. 22.1). Of the total population of 243 injured casualties, 152 patients presented to the emergency department (ED) within 24 h of the explosions, of which 66 patients were suffering from at least one extremity injury. In those patients with an extremity injury. Figure 22.2 depicts the additional injury burden among all patients presenting with extremity injuries.

Of the 66 patients with extremity injury, 4 patients had upper extremities affected, 56 patients had only lower extremities affected, and 6 patients had combined upper and lower extremity injuries. There were 17 lower extremity traumatic amputations (LETA) in 15 patients, of whom 10 suffered below-knee traumatic amputation (BKA), 3 suffered above-knee traumatic amputation (AKA), 1 patient suffered bilateral BKA, and 1 suffered a BKA and an AKA.

There were additionally 10 patients with severe soft tissue injury (without traumatic amputation) having 12 lower extremities with 14 major vascular injuries (MVI). Seven of the latter were arterial (one femoral, two popliteal, and four other named arteries), and seven were venous (one femoral, three popliteal, and three other named veins). Two lower extremities had combined arteriovenous injuries (one combined femoral arteriovenous and one combined popliteal arteriovenous injuries). The burden of extremity injury is presented in Fig. 22.3.

Of all 66 patients with extremity injuries, 29 (44%) were recognized and documented as having life-threatening extremity exsanguination at the point of injury, including all 15 (100%) LETA patients, 7 of 10 (70%) MVI patients, and 7 of 41 (11%) non-LETA and non-MVI patients with other massive soft tissue and open long-bone fractures.

Among the 29 patients with recognized exsanguination, 27 tourniquets were applied at the point of injury: 94% of the LETA extremities, 42% of the lower extremities with major vascular injuries, and 6 of the 7 additional extremities with major soft tissue injury. No patient had more than one tourniquet per extremity, and no junctional injuries with significant hemorrhage were identified. Of the 16 LETA patients with tourniquets, 4 had improvised tourniquets applied by EMS, 7 had improvised tourniquets applied by non-EMS responders (some of whom had known medical training but were not acting as part of the

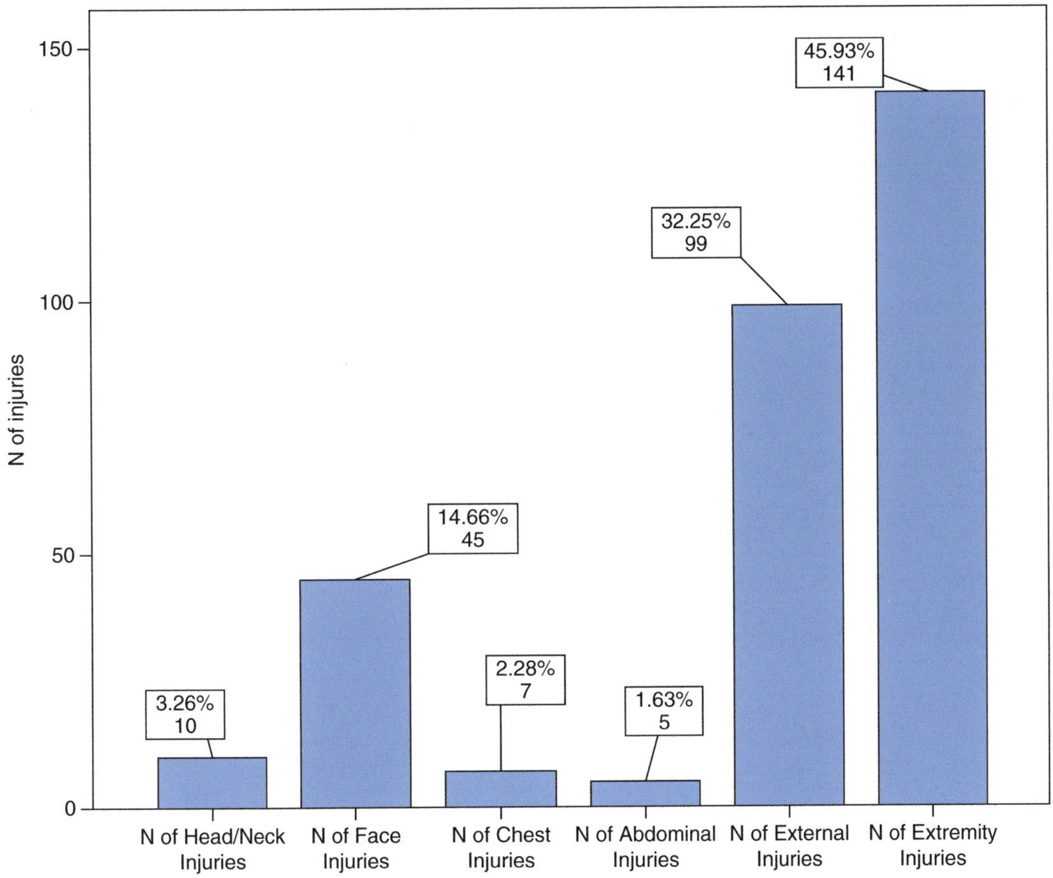

Fig. 22.1 Distribution of total injuries per body region among all 243 presenting patients

official Boston EMS response, including physicians, off-duty soldiers, etc.), and 5 had improvised tourniquets of unknown origin. Of the five lower extremities with MVI, two had improvised tourniquets applied by EMS, two had improvised tourniquets applied by non-EMS responders, and one had an improvised tourniquet of unknown origin. Of the six additional extremities with major soft tissue injury and exsanguination, four had improvised tourniquets applied by EMS, and two had improvised tourniquets of unknown origin. Figures 22.4 and 22.5 reflect the sources of the tourniquets recovered. In total, 37% of tourniquets were applied by EMS. Eight limbs presented to the ED with life-threatening exsanguination and had no prehospital tourniquet in place on arrival.

All tourniquets were improvised, including those applied by EMS, and no commercially available and purpose-designed tourniquets were identified. A review of photography and video from the scene response demonstrates a single extremity with soft tissue injury (but not a LETA) identified with a combat application tourniquet (CAT) in place. We have no knowledge of this patient's trauma burden or outcome. At the Massachusetts General Hospital, all six improvised tourniquets encountered were venous tourniquets and required replacement with a CAT tourniquet to prevent ongoing extremity exsanguination and effect hemostasis upon arrival in the ED. Similar reports exist from other Boston hospitals. The most commonly encountered EMS tourniquet was an improvised tourniquet consisting of rubber tubing and a Kelly clamp (Fig. 22.6). Among the 66 patients with extremity injuries, mortality was 0%.

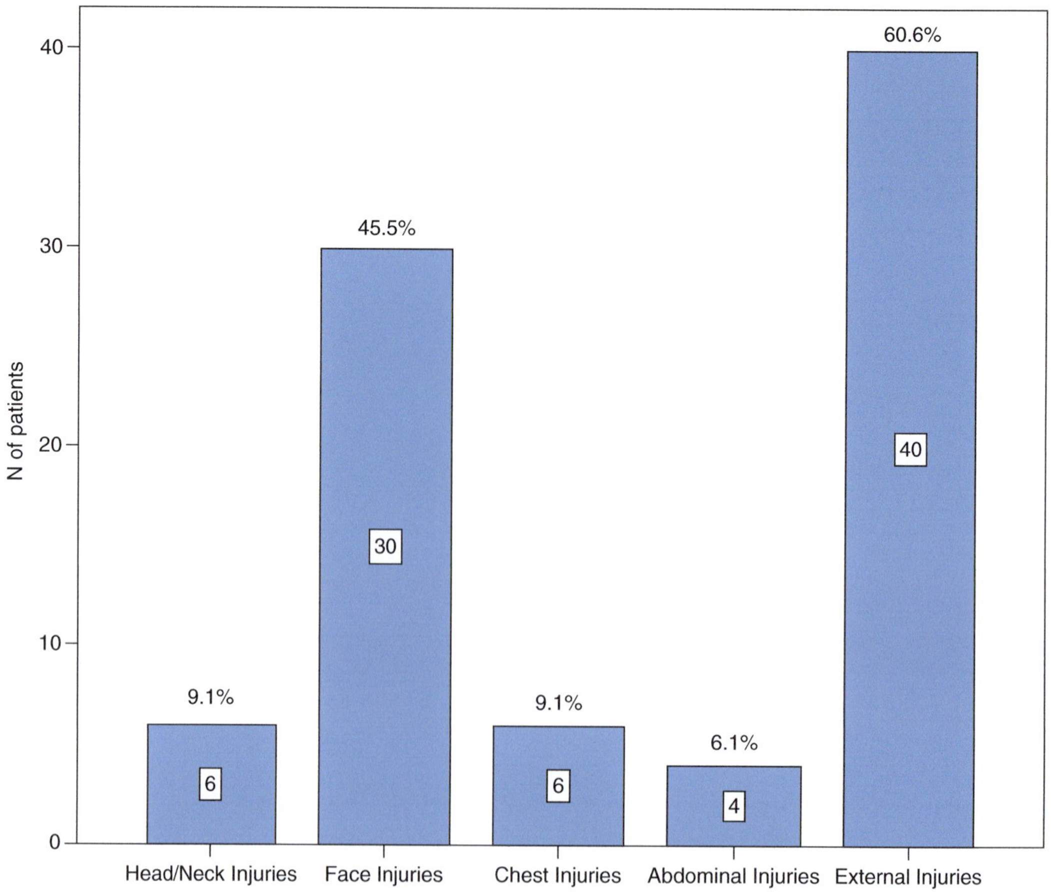

Fig. 22.2 Distribution of non-extremity injuries per body region among the 66 patients with extremity injuries

22.4 Analysis of the Unthinkable

Although the Boston Marathon bombing was not the first terrorist event in the United States, it was the first modern event to create mass casualties with a pattern of severe lower extremity blast injury commonly seen on the battlefield from improvised explosive devices. The Boston experience demonstrated the nearly universal use of improvised tourniquets as a primary prehospital and presurgical attempt at hemostatic intervention for life-threatening extremity hemorrhage: an attempt at damage control that largely failed. A recent study conducted in Boston describes the city's informal tourniquet protocol and use of the commonly seen improvised tourniquet after the bombing; however, this manuscript conspicuously omits data regarding effectiveness of the improvised tourniquet or why this device was specifically selected over others [12]. Recent data derived from military experience does not support the use of improvised tourniquets as best practice, as multiple studies [3–8] have consistently reported superior hemostatic results with the use of commercial, purpose-designed tourniquets. Our collective military experience has also established the hemostatic superiority of the commercially available devices by directly comparing them to improvised devices [13–15]. As a result, US combat personnel are now trained in self- and buddy application of these purpose-designed tourniquets [1, 3–8], and each US military service member carries at least one CAT tourniquet (often two). The translation of this military posture (general availability of tourniquets and widespread training on how to apply

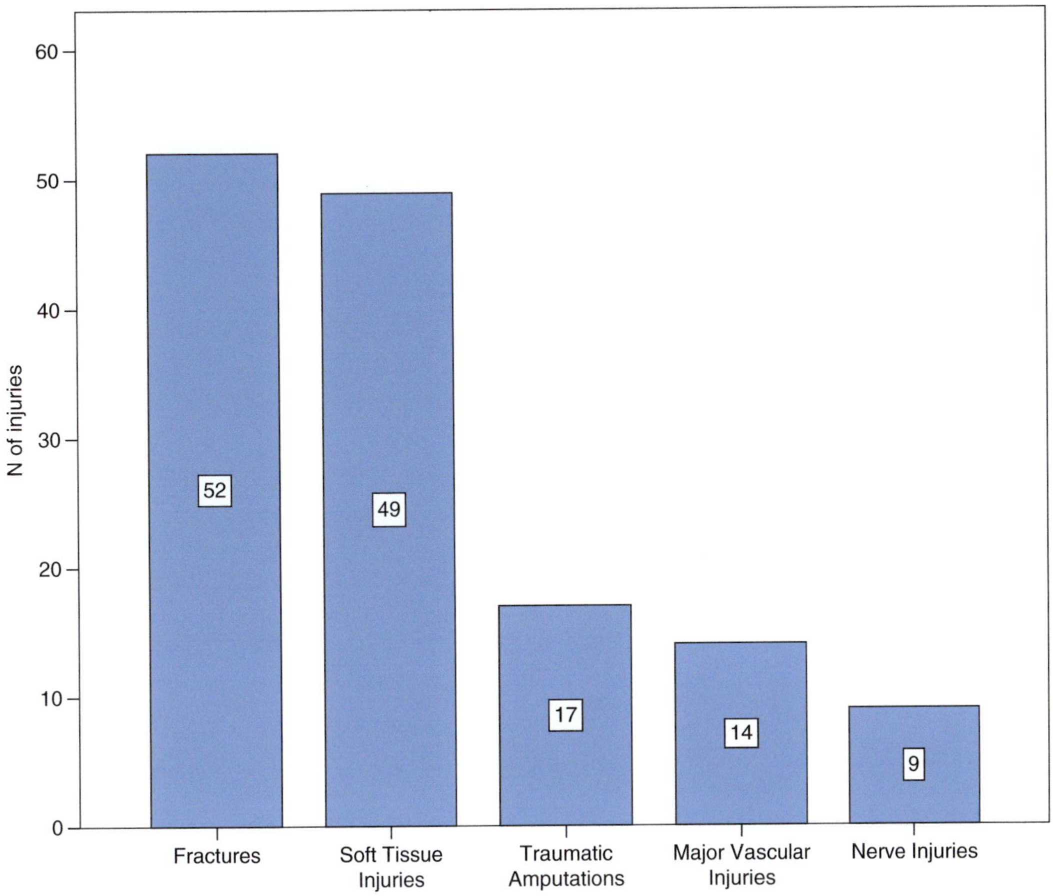

Fig. 22.3 Distribution of extremity injuries by type among the 66 patients with injured limbs

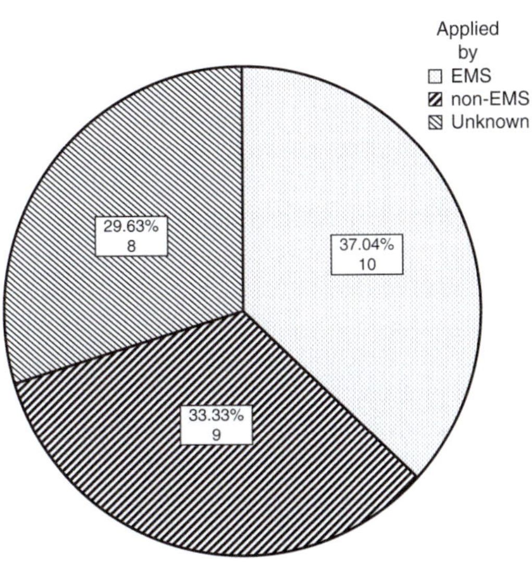

Fig. 22.4 Sources of the 27 tourniquets

them correctly) to the homeland has not been realized, unlike other battlefield lessons such as early use of anti-fibrinolytics, high-ratio transfusion, and abbreviated surgery, which have gained far more translational traction in the homeland [16]. Had translation been more successful, one may have expected far more than a single commercial tourniquet identified after the bombing. Damage control should start at the point of wounding.

Additional evidence from the civilian community [15, 17] demonstrates an obvious deficiency in the translation of the military's extremity hemorrhage control posture. A retrospective study on trauma registries at two large Level I trauma centers in Canada [15] revealed that of 190 patients who suffered isolated extremity injuries with arterial injury, only 4 patients had

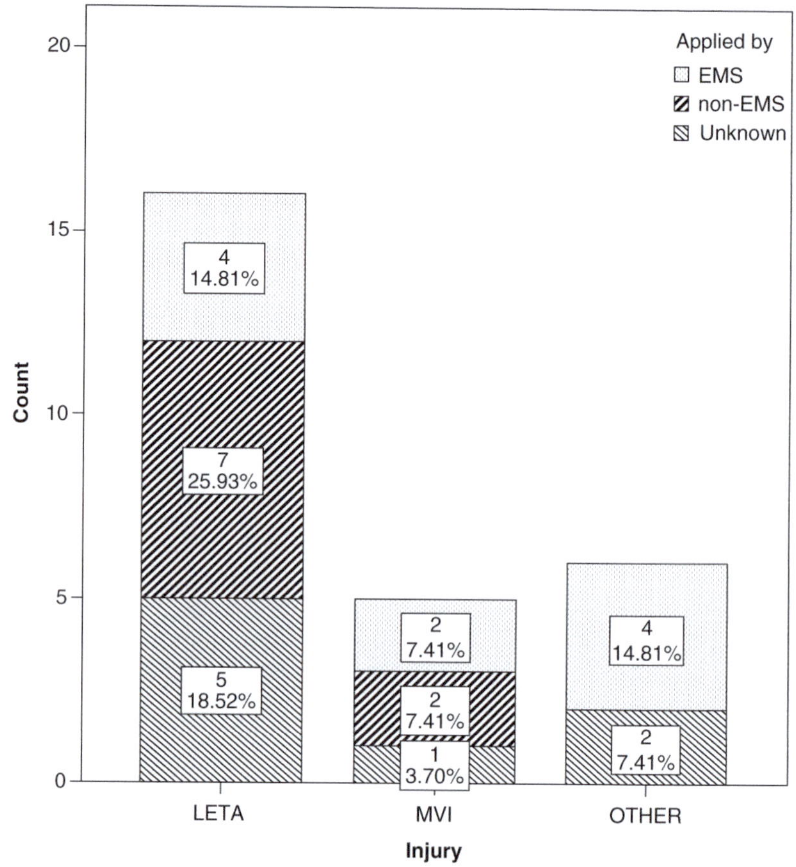

Fig. 22.5 Sources of the 27 tourniquets among 66 patients with extremity injury categorized by injury type

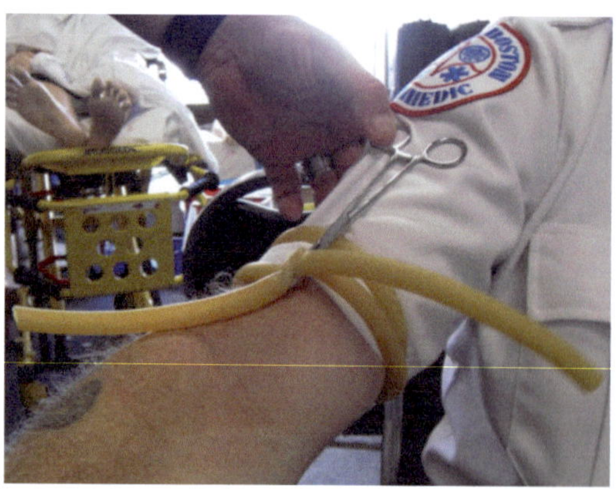

Fig. 22.6 Typical EMS improvised tourniquet

a tourniquet present upon arrival. Those were all improvised tourniquets (necktie, belt, or handkerchief) applied by police or bystanders. In the non-tourniquet group, six deaths were recorded as a direct result of exsanguination. While statistically significant differences were difficult to observe given the small number of patients who received a prehospital tourniquet, this study highlights the profound absence of systematic use of tourniquets in the prehospital environment. Following this, the 2012 Adult Traumatic Hemorrhage Control Protocol was introduced to all EMS providers in the province of Alberta, Canada—a protocol that advises the use of a Combat Application Tourniquet for uncontrolled extremity bleeding and completes the translation of battlefield lessons to the homeland. Each state in the United States should consider adopting a similar protocol.

Although it is certainly possible to improvise an effective arterial tourniquet, the data suggests this is uncommonly done appropriately, especially under stress [4, 10–17]. An improvised tourniquet should be (1) wide enough to compress arterial and venous vasculature without creating pressure necrosis of the skin or neurapraxia (as may occur with narrow tourniquets, such as rubber tubing) and (2) have a device attached to create a mechanical advantage to generate adequate circumferential pressure (such as a windlass). The improvised tourniquets used in Boston met only the second of these two fundamental criteria. It is important to note that as materials science and tourniquet technology advances, it may be possible to create an effective arterial tourniquet device without a windlass [18, 19].

While full translation of the military posture regarding extremity hemorrhage control and tourniquet use may be ideal, one must accept that, in the setting of sudden disaster, tourniquets will continue to be improvised despite all efforts at translation by policy-makers. Improvised tourniquets, and the temporary hemorrhage control they offer, will always be used in mass casualty scenarios, and their role should not be entirely discounted. An improvised venous tourniquet can provide temporary hemorrhage control [3, 5, 6]; however, a comprehensive review of emergency tourniquet use recently highlighted the significance of unintentional venous tourniquets as potentially deadly [2], particularly in the minutes following initial bleeding control. The experience in Boston, with apparent, initial, hemostasis with improvised tourniquets at point of injury, supports this notion and appears to echo that of known paradoxical bleeding after venous tourniquet application. Venous tourniquets can create initial adequate hemorrhage control that soon worsens, as a time-dependent function, until hemorrhage control is lost and supplanted by paradoxical hemorrhage, the worsening of hemorrhage than if no tourniquet were used at all [3]. Perhaps an educational campaign to teach the correct way to apply a purpose-designed tourniquet, as well as how to improvise an effective arterial tourniquet, may be appropriate since it is nearly certain that limbs will have improvised tourniquets applied after the next, unfortunate, bombing in the homeland. Several studies suggest that adequate training can be minimal (less than a minute) and still result in trainees who can apply effective tourniquets [18, 19].

Despite some possible limitations with respect to prehospital extremity hemorrhage control, there were no in-hospital deaths. The mean transport time from point of injury to ED was 24 min, substantially faster than the range of commonly reported evacuation times in the military and civilian literature, which could vary from well under 1 h to over 2 h after time of wounding, depending on the setting and circumstances [10, 13, 20–23]. The high number of Boston area metropolitan trauma centers all colocated in a very small geographic area near the Boston Marathon finish line likely contributed to this rapid evacuation time, as well as the robust medical infrastructure already in place at the finish line for the expected event-related illnesses.

The Boston bombing experience suggests that (1) instances of multiple exsanguinating extremity injuries, like battlefield wounds, can occur in the homeland and (2) improvised tourniquets likely provided initial hemorrhage control, but the absence of purpose-designed devices in the bombing response likely created cases of paradoxical bleeding. When contrasted to the wealth of evidence gathered from the last decade of military experience, these findings call for a reconsideration of our practices. We recommend that all EMS services translate a military posture with an extremity hemorrhage control protocol that emphasizes appropriate training with liberal availability of commercial, purpose-designed tourniquets. Proper tourniquet application techniques should be presented in the Advanced Trauma Life Support and Prehospital Trauma Life Support training manuals, among others. Several notable organizations, including the Hartford Consensus and the American College of Surgeons, are recommending translation and adoption of military posture toward prehospital extremity hemorrhage control [24, 25]. Physician leaders and policy-makers should insist on translation of a prehospital extremity hemorrhage control posture similar to the ubiquitous adoption and presence of automated external defibrillators in nearly every ambulance, federal building, cafeteria, and other public gathering area in the United States. Damage control should start at the point of wounding.

22.5 By the Numbers

Although much attention has been given to the obvious absence of purpose-made tourniquets in the Boston bombing response, other lessons were also learned of significant importance. For sake of completeness, the entire list of lessons learned is presented here:

1. *No tourniquets or advanced topical hemostatic agents were available.* Unfortunately, this is a posture that was poorly translated to the homeland from the battlefield.
2. *Improvised tourniquets do not work.* Although we must not discourage bystanders from responding to disaster to aid the injured, we must also be intellectually honest and recognize that (despite the lay press reporting) the improvised tourniquets applied on Boylston were likely not arterial tourniquets. Improvisation of an arterial tourniquet is a skill set that can be taught and should be widely incorporated into general first aid classes.
3. *There was no formal tourniquet training or protocol.* If purpose-made tourniquets had been available, proper training to ensure correct application is necessary. The Committee on Tactical Combat Casualty Care publishes guidelines regarding tourniquet use, and formal training and written protocols are widely available. These should be adopted as permanent part of every first responder's educational curriculum.
4. *There was too much "stay and play" in the medical tent at the finish line.* While the finish line medical tent instantly became the de facto triage area after the bombing, the transport times recorded for many severely injured patients was over an hour. By either design or by a matter of mass confusion, some patients remained in the medical tent for an extended period. In a city with five Level I trauma centers, and hundreds of patients with surgical injuries, patients should be moved to hospitals in a swifter fashion.
5. *Electronic medical record systems are slow.* For some patients, electronic registration in the ED became a bottleneck for fastest care. In most cases, patients cannot even receive a single unit of blood without an assigned medical record number. During a mass casualty event, this electronic registration system becomes bogged down and slow, sometimes limiting expediency of care. Hospitals should create a contingency plan to have preassigned mass casualty medical record numbers or implement a system capable of rapid registration of hundreds of patients.
6. *Sequential medical record numbers are dangerous.* Assigning patients sequential medical record numbers in simple escalating numerical fashion creates an unacceptable margin of error since there will be many simultaneous patients with medical record numbers differing by only a single digit (1234567, 1234568, 1234569, etc.). This creates an unacceptable environment for a potential clerical error, single keystroke mistake, that would potentially result in a surgeon looking at the hemoglobin value of the wrong patient or (worse yet) ordering tests or procedures on the wrong patient. Medical record numbers during disasters should vary widely to prevent this error.
7. *The most visually stimulating injury is often not the most life-threatening one.* The Boston bombing patients arrived with extremely devastating, and visually stimulating, limb injuries. These injuries, despite their appearance, were easily controlled with tourniquets. Some patients also had coexisting intracavitary hemorrhage. This can often be overlooked when the clinician inappropriately focused on the limb injury and neglects a complete trauma evaluation, particularly of the peritoneal and thoracic cavities. Once an effective tourniquet is in place, the limb injury becomes (temporarily) forgettable.
8. *Don't Go Home Just Yet: The tertiary trauma survey is extremely important.* In disasters, it is a common urge to "take a break" once each patient's index operation is complete, and all the bleeding and contamination is controlled. This, however, is a mistake. Once the initial surgery is done, the entire trauma team must reassemble to go over each patient again, in

exceptional detail. The purpose of this is twofold. First, the entire team needs to understand each patient's condition and status, so appropriate planning for operative take-backs, additional imaging, and other interventions can be planned and prioritized. Second, small injuries are commonly missed and will only be identified by a careful tertiary survey. Although most of our patients had non-life-threatening ruptured tympanic membranes, for example, these were largely not identified until post trauma day 2 on a careful tertiary exam. This is, of course, an appropriate injury to miss on initial evaluation in a mass casualty situation; however, failure to recognize and treat this injury (and others like it) could result in long-term disability.

22.6 In a Nutshell

After the Boston Marathon bombings, extremity exsanguination at point of injury was either left untreated or treated with an improvised tourniquet in the prehospital environment. An effective, prehospital extremity hemorrhage control posture should be translated to all civilian first responders in the United States and should mirror the military's posture toward extremity bleeding control. Physician leaders and policymakers must support this initiative. The prehospital response to extremity exsanguination after the Boston Marathon bombing demonstrates that our current practice is an approach, lost in translation, from the battlefield to the homeland [11]. Within the United States, wide adoption of this lesson is also lacking [26].

22.7 Damage Control Starts at the Point of Injury

Emergent, effective extremity bleeding control begins at the point of injury in the prehospital environment. Ubiquitous training and presence of appropriate tourniquets, as well as advanced topical hemostatic bandages for managing junctional hemorrhage, constitute field damage control maneuvers. A low-volume (or NO volume) fluid restrictive resuscitation strategy should be adopted. Triage must be rapid, and medical providers must accept that the triage process will be imperfect. Patients who are triaged as emergent may, in fact, not be dying. Other patients triaged as non-emergent may unexpectedly deteriorate. Frequent re-triage is required and may alter initial triage decisions.

In the emergency department, patients should be re-triaged by a senior surgeon or senior emergency medicine physician. Utilization of the operating rooms is a finite resource, and only patients who truly need a lifesaving operation should be triaged straight to the operating room. Care decisions should be made regarding axial imaging studies as many of these studies are initially unnecessary. A plain chest X-ray and a focused abdominal ultrasound exam is often the only imaging required to make an informed in-hospital triage decision.

Patients waiting for less-than-emergent surgery should receive minimal crystalloid therapy. If resuscitation is required, volume expansion with a transfusion strategy that approximates fresh whole blood should be utilized. For many hospitals, this means adopting a strategy of high-ratio transfusion of packed red blood cells/plasma/platelets. When possible, all fluids and blood products should be warmed to normal body temperature. Anti-fibrinolytics should be liberally administered. For patients with limb injuries that have a tourniquet in place and are waiting for surgery, tourniquet conversion should be considered if time and manpower permit.

In the operating room, only hemorrhage control and contamination control are desired. Abbreviated surgery, vascular shunts, bowel stapled and left in discontinuity, and temporary abdominal closures should dominate the landscape. Ideally, only warmed blood and blood products should be administered during damage control surgery. The operating room should be made as warm as possible; the surgeon should become exceedingly uncomfortable with the temperature in the room. When in doubt, all body cavities should be surgically interrogated. Bilateral tube thoracostomy, pericardial window, and laparotomy are the imaging methods of choice during damage control in disasters.

Patients should be rapidly transferred to the intensive care unit and the operating room reset for the next patient. Once all index operations are complete, the entire team should reassemble to re-triage and regroup resources. If the disaster is expected to become protracted, rest and sleep cycles should be instituted so that human resources do not become all simultaneously exhausted.

22.8 Epilogue

The Boston Marathon bombing solidified multiple lessons for our city. First, damage control starts at the point of injury. No one should die from a preventable cause of death such as limb exsanguination. Second, triage becomes the most important decision that is made on the scene of a disaster. That decision should be revisited often following initial triage of all casualties. Third, re-triage at the hospital is important to prevent inappropriate utilization of human and physical plant infrastructure on patients who are not truly dying. Finally, abbreviated surgery with attention to high-ratio transfusion, use of anti-fibrinolytics, vascular shunts, contamination control, and temporary abdominal (or chest) closure are necessary.

References

1. Welling DR, McKay PL, Rasmussen TE, Rich NMA. Brief history of the tourniquet. J Vasc Surg. 2012;55(1):286–90.
2. Kragh JF Jr, Swan KG, Smith DC, Mabry RL, Blackbourne LH. Historical review of emergency tourniquet use to stop bleeding. Am J Surg. 2012;203(2):242–52.
3. Kragh JF Jr, O'Neill ML, Walters TJ, Dubick MA, Baer DG, Wade CE, Holcomb JB, Blackbourne LH. Minor morbidity with emergency tourniquet use to stop bleeding in severe limb trauma: research, history, and reconciling advocates and abolitionists. Mil Med. 2011;176(7):817–23.
4. King DR, van der Wilden G, Kragh JF Jr, Blackbourne LH. Forward assessment of 79 prehospital battlefield tourniquets used in the current war. J Spec Oper Med. 2012;12(4):33–8.
5. Beekley AC, Sebesta JA, Blackbourne LH, Herbert GS, Kauvar DS, Baer DG, Walters TJ, Mullenix PS, Holcomb JB, 31st Combat Support Hospital Research Group. Prehospital tourniquet use in Operation Iraqi Freedom: effect on hemorrhage control and outcomes. J Trauma. 2008;64(2 Suppl):S28–37.
6. Kragh JF Jr, Walters TJ, Baer DG, Fox CJ, Wade CE, Salinas J, Holcomb JB. Survival with emergency tourniquet use to stop bleeding in major limb trauma. Ann Surg. 2009;249(1):1–7.
7. Kragh JF Jr, Littrel ML, Jones JA, Walters TJ, Baer DG, Wade CE, Holcomb JB. Battle casualty survival with emergency tourniquet use to stop limb bleeding. J Emerg Med. 2011;41(6):590–7.
8. Lakstein D, Blumenfeld A, Sokolov T, Lin G, Bssorai R, Lynn M, Ben-Abraham R. Tourniquets for hemorrhage control on the battlefield: a 4-year accumulated experience. J Trauma. 2003;54(5 Suppl):S221–5.
9. Kapur GB, Hutson HR, Davis MA, Rice PL. The United States twenty-year experience with bombing incidents: implications for terrorism preparedness and medical response. J Trauma. 2005;59(6):1436–44.
10. Gates JD, Arabian S, Biddinger P, Blansfield J, Burke P, Chung S, Fischer J, Friedman F, Gervasini A, Goralnick E, Gupta A, Larentzakis A, McMahon M, Mella J, Michaud Y, Mooney D, Rabinovici R, Sweet D, Ulrich A, Velmahos G, Weber C, Yaffe MB. The initial response to the Boston marathon bombing: lessons learned to prepare for the next disaster. Ann Surg. 2014;260(6):960–6.
11. King DR, Larentzakis A, Ramly EP. Tourniquet use at the Boston Marathon bombing: lost in translation. Boston Trauma Collaborative. J Trauma Acute Care Surg. 2015;78(3):594–9.
12. Kalish J, Burke P, Feldman J, Agarwal S, Glantz A, Moyer P, Serino R, Hirsch E. The return of tourniquets. Original research evaluates the effectiveness of prehospital tourniquets for civilian penetrating extremity injuries. JEMS. 2008;33(8):44–6. 49-50, 52, 54.
13. D'Alleyrand JCG, Dutton RP, Pollak AN. Extrapolation of battlefield resuscitative care to the civilian setting. J Surg Orthop Adv. 2010;19(1):62–9.
14. Evaluation of self-applied tourniquets for combat applications, second phase. 2013. http://archive.rubicon-foundation.org/xmlui/handle/123456789/6870?show=full. Accessed 19 Sep 2013.
15. Passos E, Dingley B, Smith A, Engels PT, Ball CG, Faidi S, Nathens A, Tien H, Canadian Trauma Trials Collaborative. Tourniquet use for peripheral vascular injuries in the civilian setting. Injury. 2014;45(3):573–7.

16. Duchesne JC, Islam TM, Stuke L, Timmer JR, Barbeau JM, Marr AB, Hunt JP, Dellavolpe JD, Wahl G, Greiffenstein P, Steeb GE, McGinness C, Baker CC, McSwain NE Jr. Hemostatic resuscitation during surgery improves survival in patients with traumatic-induced coagulopathy. J Trauma. 2009;67(1):33–7. discussion 37-9.
17. Dorlac WC, DeBakey ME, Holcomb JB, Fagan SP, Kwong KL, Dorlac GR, Schreiber MA, Persse DE, Moore FA, Mattox KL. Mortality from isolated civilian penetrating extremity injury. J Trauma. 2005;59(1):217–22.
18. Wall PL, Duevel DC, Hassan MB, Welander JD, Sahr SM, Buising CM. Tourniquets and occlusion: the pressure of design. Mil Med. 2013;178(5):578–87.
19. Wall PL, Welander JD, Singh A, Sidwell RA, Buising CM. Stretch and wrap style tourniquet effectiveness with minimal training. Mil Med. 2012;177(11):1366–73.
20. Ingalls N, Zonies D, Bailey JA, Martin KD, Iddins BO, Carlton PK, Hanseman D, Branson R, Dorlac W, Johannigman JA. review of the first 10 years of critical care aeromedical transport during Operation Iraqi Freedom and Operation Enduring Freedom: the importance of evacuation timing. JAMA Surg. 2014;149(8):807–13.
21. Ball CG, Williams BH, Tallah C, Salomone JP, Feliciano DV. The impact of shorter prehospital transport times on outcomes in patients with abdominal vascular injuries. J Trauma Manag Outcomes. 2013;7(1):11.
22. Crandall M, Sharp D, Unger E, Straus D, Brasel K, Hsia R, Esposito T. Trauma deserts: distance from a trauma center, transport times, and mortality from gunshot wounds in Chicago. Am J Public Health. 2013;103(6):1103–9.
23. Bulger EM, Guffey D, Guyette FX, MacDonald RD, Brasel K, Kerby JD, Minei JP, Warden C, Rizoli S, Morrison LJ, Nichol G, Resuscitation Outcomes Consortium Investigators. Impact of prehospital mode of transport after severe injury: a multicenter evaluation from the Resuscitation Outcomes Consortium. J Trauma Acute Care Surg. 2012;72(3):567–73. discussion 573-5
24. Jacobs LM, NE MS Jr, Rotondo MF, Wade D, Fabbri W, Eastman AL, Butler FK Jr, Sinclair J, Joint Committee to Create a National Policy to Enhance Survivability from Mass Casualty Shooting Events. Improving survival from active shooter events: the Hartford Consensus. J Trauma Acute Care Surg. 2013;74(6):1399–400.
25. Bulger EM, Snyder D, Schoelles K, Gotschall C, Dawson D, Lang E, Sanddal ND, Butler FK, Fallat M, Taillac P, White L, Salomone JP, Seifarth W, Betzner MJ, Johannigman J, Mc Swain N Jr. An evidence-based prehospital guideline for external hemorrhage control: American College of Surgeons Committee on Trauma. Prehosp Emerg Care. 2014;18(2):163–73.
26. Ramly E, Runyan G, King DR. The state of the union. J Trauma Acute Care Surg. 2016;80(5):787–91.

23 The Open Abdomen in Damage Control Surgery

Jeff Garner and Rao R. Ivatury

Abstract

The open abdomen is an integral part of the damage control surgical philosophy although it does present its own physiological penalties; it is therefore vital that as much attention is paid to the management of the open abdomen as the other aspects of DCS and the surgeon must have a full range of techniques at their command. The predominant reason for an open abdomen in DCS is to avoid the deleterious effects of raised intra-abdominal pressure such as reduced splanchnic and renal blood supply, splinting of the diaphragm with reduced tidal volume and reduced venous return.

When the abdomen is left open, the muscle fibres shorten and retract, and the viscera begin to adhere to the underside of the abdominal wall, so the key to open abdomen management is a temporary abdominal closure that minimises loss of domain and prevents adhesion formation. A variety of techniques are available, and the method chosen should reflect the local availability of equipment and skills of the surgeon. Silo methods such as the Bogota bag should only be used if nothing else is available as the techniques of choice are some sort of medial fascial traction and topical negative pressure dressings either individually or preferably in combination.

The outcomes following temporary abdominal closure are highly variable, but definitive fascial closure rates of up to 90% are achievable; complications include failure to achieve fascial closure, fistulation and subsequent incisional hernia aside from mortality which is largely attributable to the underlying traumatic injuries.

23.1 Introduction

The open abdomen (OA) has become a sine qua non of damage control surgery (DCS); it is a key tenet of the damage control philosophy and a major stage of the practical proceedings. This chapter explores the rationale for it, the penalties for failing to manage it properly and most importantly the techniques for temporary abdominal closure which, for many practical reasons, are another essential facet of OA management. Long before the pathophysiology of the abdominal compartment syndrome (ACS) or the benefits of DCS had been elucidated, surgeons had wrestled

J. Garner, M.D., F.R.C.S. (✉)
The Rotherham NHS Foundation Trust, Rotherham, South Yorkshire, UK

R.R. Ivatury, M.D, F.A.C.S., F.C.C.M.
Virginia Commonwealth University, Richmond, VA, USA

J. Duchesne et al. (eds.), *Damage Control in Trauma Care*,
https://doi.org/10.1007/978-3-319-72607-6_23

with the fact that some abdomens couldn't or shouldn't be closed; it was the British WW2 surgeon Ogilvie in the 1940s who described suturing stout cotton cloth to the edges of the fascial defect to 'prevent retraction of the edges of the gap, keeps the intestinal contents from protruding … and allows the abdominal wall to be used as a whole in respiration' [1] in what was clearly the forerunner of mesh-mediated fascial traction.

This chapter is concerned with the open abdomen following damage control laparotomy for trauma, but it should be remembered that in many parts of the world, DCS or abbreviated laparotomy with an OA takes places much more commonly for other indications, primarily the septic abdomen, infected pancreatic necrosis, following abdominal aortic aneurysm repair, or necrotizing abdominal wall infections [2]. This variety of indications leads to significant heterogeneity when considering the available data for techniques and outcomes.

The indications for an open abdomen are now well established and may be summarised as one of three scenarios: OA to reduce intra-abdominal pressure in ACS or prophylactically left open in a situation where significant intra-abdominal hypertension could be anticipated, in cases where repeated entry into the abdominal cavity (often to clear septic foci) are required or where there has been loss of abdominal wall substance precluding direct closure. It is also clear that failure to achieve definitive fascial closure after DCS is associated with longer hospital stay, decreased function and quality of life, increased costs from delayed reconstruction and increased complications [3].

Table 23.1 Definitions of intra-abdominal hypertension and abdominal compartment syndrome

Intra-abdominal hypertension (IAH)		Sustained or repeated pathological elevation of intra-abdominal pressure above 12 mmHg (graded I–IV)
	I	12–15 mmHg
	II	16–20 mmHg
	III	21–25 mmHg
	IV	>25 mmHg
Abdominal compartment syndrome (ACS)		Sustained IAH >20 mmHg associated with new organ dysfunction or failure
	Primary ACS	ACS as a result of pathology within the abdominopelvic cavity
	Secondary ACS	ACS in the absence of abdominopelvic pathology
	Recurrent ACS	Recurrent ACS after previous medical or surgical treatment of ACS

23.2 The Abdominal Compartment Syndrome

Just like any other closed fascial compartment in the body, an uncontrolled rise in intra-compartmental pressure above a certain level has deleterious physiological effects. The normal intra-abdominal pressure is normally zero or slightly below, is normally of the order of 5–7 mm Hg in the critically ill patient (from oedema and ileus) and may increase slowly over time without physiological penalty to 10–15 mm Hg in certain non-pathological states such as obesity and pregnancy [4]. Increases in pressure to above 12 mm Hg are termed intra-abdominal hypertension [4] and when coupled with physiological consequences are termed the abdominal compartment syndrome. The World Society for the Abdominal Compartment Syndrome (WSACS) has updated their widely accepted published definitions which allow uniform reporting [5] (Table 23.1).

Intra-abdominal pressure should be measured at end expiration in the supine position with a transducer zeroed to the level of the midaxillary line. The recommended technique is with a bladder transducer after instillation of 25 mL of sterile saline [5].

Raised intra-compartmental pressure heralds a panoply of physiologic problems.

23.2.1 Cardiovascular

IAH reduces cardiac output due to decreased flow in the inferior vena cava from direct compression, reduced superior vena caval return due to increased intrathoracic pressures and a marked increase in afterload. A spuriously elevated central venous pressure may thus suggest that the patient is hypervolemic [6].

23.2.2 Respiratory

The splinting of the diaphragms reduces pulmonary compliance, total lung capacity and functional residual capacity with increased airway pressure leading to significant increases in thoracic resistance to ventilation with hypercarbia and hypoxia [4]. Prior haemorrhage and resuscitation in an animal model exacerbate the thoracic sequelae of IAH [7].

23.2.3 Abdominal

Direct renal vessel compression from IAH leads to worsening oliguria unresponsive to volume expansion or vasopressors; increased renal vascular resistance and sodium and water retention are also implicated [8]. Reductions in all intra-abdominal circulations are noted with IAH resulting in a gut mucosal metabolic acidosis, bowel ischemia and bacterial translocation [9] contributing to sepsis and multi-organ failure. The reduction in blood flow also extends to the abdominal wall vasculature leading to decreased compliance which may contribute to difficulties in direct fascial closure, coupled with increased risks of wound infection and dehiscence [10]. The mortality rate for ACS is up to 50% even if subsequently decompressed [11].

In DCS for trauma, the risk factors that make an open abdomen sensible are multifactorial. It is known that major injury per se (even remote from the abdomen) and abdominal surgery are risks, as are hypothermia, massive fluid resuscitation and polytransfusion, hypotension and shock [5]. There is undoubtedly a huge systemic inflammatory response syndrome (SIRS) response to major trauma and is postulated that this pro-inflammatory cytokine drive will contribute to the necessity for an open abdomen [12]. A recent randomised trial of two different vacuum temporary abdominal closures showed a difference in mortality outcome between the two closures, but this was not mediated by differences in cytokine clearance however [13].

23.3 The Open Abdomen

In the context of DCS for trauma, the abdomen will be left open through the midline, but for other indications, such as secondary ACS for severe pancreatitis, decompression through transverse incisions has been reported with success [14]. Facilitation of accurate communication and comparison of research methodology have been achieved by the publication of an accepted grading system of the open abdomen; first produced in 2009, the definitions were revised in 2013 to take greater account of the impact of enterocutaneous fistulation (ECF), which in the context of the open abdomen is often termed enteroatmospheric fistulation (EAF) [15] (Table 23.2).

On a practical level, it is clear that in the context of an open abdomen, the aim of management

Table 23.2 Recognised grading of the open abdomen [15]

1		*No fixation*
	A	Clean, no fixation
	B	Contaminated, no fixation
	C	Enteric leak, no fixation
2		*Developing fixation*
	A	Clean, developing fixation
	B	Contaminated, developing fixation
	C	Enteric leak, developing fixation
3		*Frozen abdomen*
	A	Clean, frozen abdomen
	B	Contaminated, frozen abdomen
4		Established enteroatmospheric fistula

is to commence the OA in as low a grade as possible and then to subsequently prevent deterioration down the grades.

23.3.1 Penalties for an Open Abdomen

Whilst closing an abdomen under undue tension has clear physiologic penalties which can be obviated by leaving the fascia apart, the open abdomen has its own distinct and significant penalties. Decompression of the ACS abdomen generates second hit phenomena such as ischemia-reperfusion and residual intra-abdominal sepsis which will contribute further to the SIRS response [16]. The OA patient is, by definition, critically ill, and attention must be paid to minimising the additional impacts of the open abdomen.

The OA exposes a large area of viscera to the atmosphere, and fluid and temperature losses are considerable. These patients have usually been aggressively resuscitated, and there is significant egress of residual abdominal fluid washout and transudation from the exposed gut; this makes managing fluid and electrolyte balance difficult, contributes to marked cooling and presents significant nursing and skin care issues. The open abdomen loses protein, and an additional 2 g of nitrogen per litre of abdominal fluid lost is required to try and maintain nitrogen balance [17]. It is also a particularly catabolic state with marked capillary leakage [18].

The open abdomen is inherently fistulogenic, and development of an EAF represents the most catastrophic complication, aside from mortality, of an open abdomen (Fig. 23.1). The exact causes are unclear but are likely to include abrasion and trauma from handling and desiccation making the gut more friable. Anastomotic suture/staple lines are particularly at risk of dehiscence.

Within 12 h of fascial separation, there is shortening of the fascial fibres and lateral retraction leading to an inexorable loss of domain; in addition, adhesions begin to form almost immediately between the viscera and the underside of the abdominal wall, especially in the face of denudement of the peritoneal lining of the abdominal wall, and it is these two key factors—loss of domain and visceral adhesions—that limit or prevent delayed abdominal wall closure after the initial laparotomy.

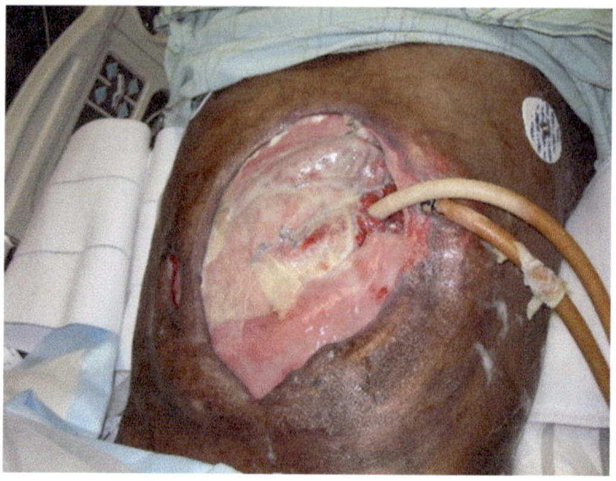

Fig. 23.1 Enteroatmospheric fistulation as a result of an open abdomen for trauma

So whilst it is clear that the open abdomen will avoid the penalties of an abdominal compartment syndrome, leaving the abdomen completely ‘open’ is also suboptimal, not least because of the nursing issues of repeated turns for skin care when the viscera are unrestrained. The corollary then is that some form of temporary abdominal closure (TAC) is a necessary adjunct to the open abdomen; the evidence for which form of temporary abdominal closure is best applied to an OA is only now becoming clear, balancing as it does the needs to provide the best definitive fascial closure rate at the earliest opportunity with the least complication profile and at affordable cost, and this is, in part, determined by the indication for the open abdomen in the first place.

23.4 Temporary Abdominal Closures

Before considering what the ideal TAC would look like, it is important to consider the goals that

Table 23.3 The goals for temporary abdominal closure [2]

Cover and protect abdominal contents	Prevent evisceration
Prevent or treat ACS	Help manage fluid
Not damage fascia	Minimize loss of domain
Facilitate reoperation and abdominal exploration	Keep patient dry with intact skin
Prevent adhesion formation	Remove infectious material

Table 23.4 Characteristics of the ideal temporary abdominal closure [19]

Universally available	Easy and fast to apply
Porous	Controls fluid loss
Prevents ACS	Leaves fascia and skin intact
Not reactive to bowel or other organs	Easy to remove and to replace
Maintains peritoneal cavity sterility	Inexpensive

the 'ideal TAC' would achieve. It must obviate or minimise the two features that will limit subsequent definitive closure, i.e. domain loss and visceral adhesions, it must maintain physiological stability as much as is possible in the critically ill patient, it must facilitate nursing and intensive therapy care, and it should not limit later reconstructive options. These goals are summarised in Table 23.3 [2].

These admirable goals are surprisingly difficult to achieve in the unique environment of the open abdomen, given the heterogeneity of its aetiologies, and as such the requirements of the ideal TAC are wide-ranging (Table 23.4) [19].

No TAC fulfils all these criteria, and so the choice of TAC is dependent on local availability of products, the costs and financial constraints of the healthcare system, the skills of the surgeons managing the abdomen and local policies and procedures. It is thus useful to have a working knowledge of a variety of techniques, of which there a multitude available as both homemade solutions and commercial products. Over time, a number of these techniques have been combined but are described as individual methods here for ease of understanding.

23.4.1 Skin Suture/Towel Clips

There may be some occasions where it is clear to the operating surgeon that subsequent definitive abdominal closure is likely to be possible at the first relook laparotomy, and so a simple skin-only closure may be contemplated. This is unlikely to be the case following DCL for trauma. Multiple towel clip closure looks impressive but is hampered by the lack of availability of towel clips these days, interference with subsequent imaging, damage to the skin and evisceration (Fig. 23.2); a continuous running suture closure is swift, cheap and easily reversible, limits fluid and heat loss and does not damage the fascia but must be converted to definitive fascial closure within approximately 24 h before fascial retraction and visceral adhesions prevent this. It has a reasonable rate of later definitive fascial closure [20]. There is a significant risk of recurrent ACS with this technique however (13–36%) [21], and it has largely been abandoned and is not recommended after trauma DCL.

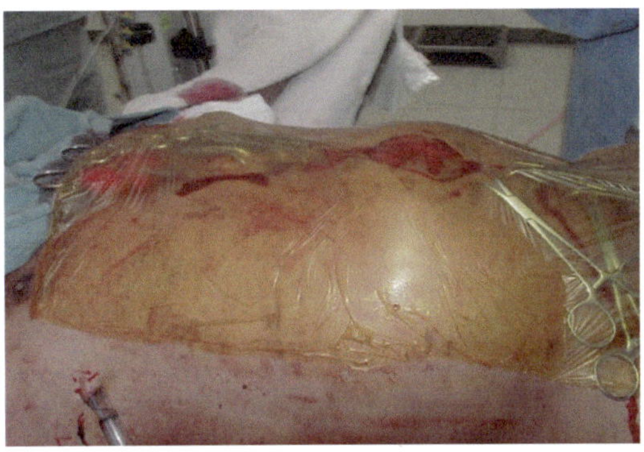

Fig. 23.2 Towel clip closure (skin only)

23.4.2 The Bogota Bag/Silo Technique

This is simple and quick and is probably the most widely known TAC technique but fails to fulfil many of the goals or characteristics of the ideal. An inert sterile material—typically an opened out saline i.v. bag—is sutured to either the fascial edges or the skin edge. It increases the domain for the oedematous gut to reside in, but only temporarily (Fig. 23.3). There is a 16% incidence of recurrent ACS with this technique. If sutured to the fascia, it may damage it and decrease the chance of successful definitive closure at a later stage as it needs to be removed and reapplied at each relaparotomy or, if applied to the skin edge to maintain fascial integrity, does little to prevent fascial retraction. The Bogota bag is rarely watertight, and abdominal fluid typically leaks profusely out between the retaining sutures complicating nursing skin care and may even exacerbate hypothermia by pooled fluid on the bed cooling the patient. There is also the risk of evisceration between the sutures. The outcomes for the Bogota bag technique in terms of definitive fascial closure are worse than for other techniques, but it is appreciated that its ease and simplicity are attractive to the inexperienced surgeon in the middle of the night, as it will allow the patient to be transferred off the operating table to the ITU, at which point it is imperative that a more experienced colleague is involved to further manage the abdominal wall.

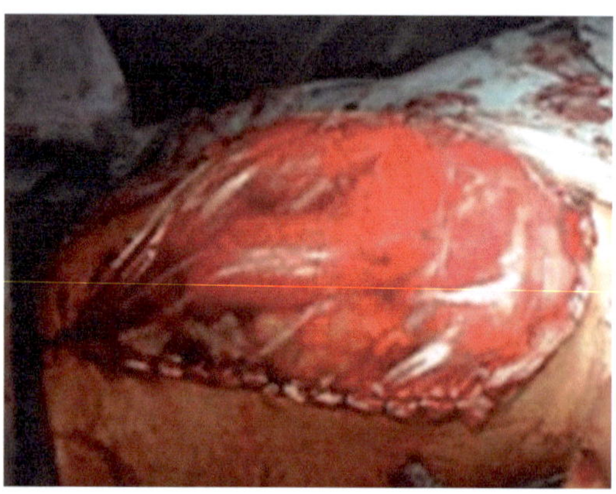

Fig. 23.3 An opened out saline i.v. bag opened out and sutured to the fascial edges to provide a temporary increase in domain—the Bogota bag

23.4.3 Opsite® Sandwich

A variety of variations on a theme have been described for this technique, and it has been combined with other techniques to increase its utility. In essence, one or two laparotomy pads are laid out on the sticky side of an adhesive sterile drape sheet and covered with another. This sterile towel sandwich can then be tucked into the paracolic gutters between the viscera and the abdominal wall to prevent adhesions. Fenestration of the sticky drapes, two suction drains on top and coverage with a third adherent drape over the whole open abdominal cavity also allows for egress of some abdominal fluid [22]. It is cheap and easy to apply although the sticky drapes can be a little too sticky at times and it prevents adhesions; unfortunately it does not counteract the loss of domain, and fluid removal is variable and usually insufficient.

23.4.4 Mesh

Mesh use for TAC can be permanent or temporary, and the mesh itself may be a permanent or absorbable synthetic or a biologic sutured to the fascial edges as a bridge. Implantation of permanent synthetic meshes as definitive bridged closure of the defect is associated with unacceptably high rates of enterocutaneous fistulation and should be avoided—they may be used as one form of dynamic fascial traction however (see below). An absorbable mesh such as polyglactin may sit safely on top of the exposed GI tract, will restrain the viscera and may impart some form of medialisation force on the separated fascia. If the visceral oedema subsides sufficiently to allow direct fascial closure, then the mesh may be

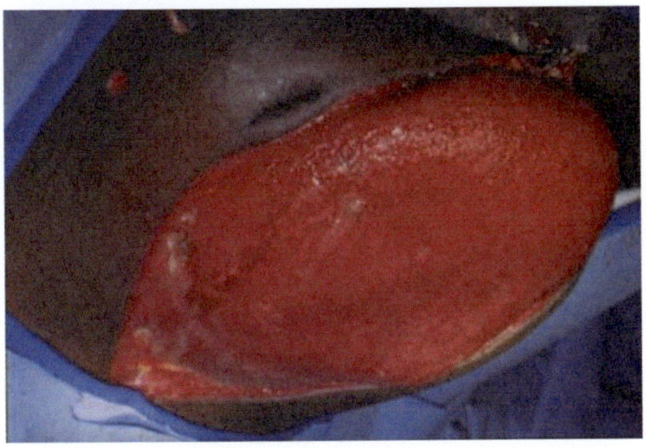

Fig. 23.4 A polyglactin mesh engulfed in granulation tissue across a laparostomy; this will subsequently receive a split-thickness skin graft to complete epithelialisation

removed, but often it has begun to become engulfed in granulation tissue on top of the gut, at which point it can be left in situ to stabilise the abdominal wall until the laparostomy is solidly granulated and can be then split skin grafted as planned ventral hernia management (Fig. 23.4).

23.4.5 Negative Pressure Wound Therapy (NPWT)

Originally described by Brock and Barker in 1995 [23], the homemade vacuum pack (Barker or VacPac) has now been largely superseded by a variety of commercial products, but all have the same essential components. A fenestrated sterile plastic sheet is used to envelope the viscera and prevent adhesions to the underside of the abdominal wall; the fascial defect is filled with laparotomy pads or specialised polyurethane sponges and the abdomen sealed with self-adhesive drapes and a negative pressure applied by either closed suction drains (which can be applied to wall suction) or to a self-contained commercial vacuum machine.

Both the home-grown methods and commercial systems prevent adhesions, control fluid egress and provide inward force on fascia to prevent lateral traction; the commercial systems also make claims for reduced bacterial translocation and increased neovascularisation, thereby aiding healing, which have been described in animal models and in non-OA applications [24, 25]. The commercial systems are costly in comparison to homemade systems, but there is evidence of improved outcomes [13]; lingering doubts about increased risk of fistulation with commercial NPWT now seem to have been addressed [26].

23.4.6 Dynamic Fascial Traction

Dynamic fascial traction (DFT) can be instituted by a variety of methods and is now commonly coupled with some form of NPWT to further improve outcomes. The original description was of a patented hook and burr device (the Wittmann Patch) sutured to the fascial edges and approximated under moderate tension to provide inward tension. As abdominal oedema subsided, the burr was unhooked, trimmed and pulled in a little further until the fascia eventually met in the midline at which stage the patch was removed and the fascial closure completed as part of the staged abdominal repair (STAR) procedure [27]. As the technique developed, a sterile plastic sheet to wrap the viscera and prevent adhesions and NPWT to manage fluid egress were added. Originally described with bedside tightening of the mesh, the presence of the fenestrated plastic sheet now means that a return to theatre for changing of the sheet is required. Two variations of this technique have been described. As the Wittmann Patch is an expensive commercial product, an alternative cheaper homemade version involves suturing a heavyweight polypropylene mesh to the fascia on either side and suturing them together under tension in the midline with a heavy nonabsorbable suture. This can then be undone, the meshes trimmed and resutured as oedema subsides (Fig. 23.5). Arguments against the use of permanent synthetic meshes in the open abdomen (with their increased risk of fistulation) are countered by the fact that a sterile fenestrated

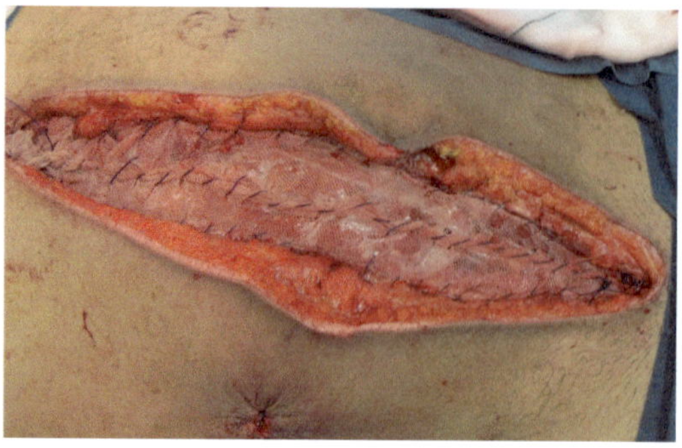

Fig. 23.5 Mesh-mediated fascial traction following an abdominal gunshot wound

drape protects the viscera from the mesh and that the mesh itself is removed when fascial approximation is achieved and the midline is ready to be closed definitively [28].

A further variant is the abdominal reapproximation anchor system (ABRA system), which passes a series of elastomer strings through the full thickness of the abdominal wall on either side and allows gradually increasing tension to approximate the fascial midline [29].

23.5 Outcomes of TAC

Given the multiplicity of TACs available, many of which are used in combination, and the variety of indications, it is extremely difficult if not impossible to examine the literature and state categorically what 'the best' temporary abdominal closure is; considerations such as costs and availability, surgeon skills and indication all influence the choice of TAC. However, a series of consensus meetings and systematic reviews have slowly shed light on this issue.

23.5.1 Definitions

Whilst Table 23.3 outlines the goals of a temporary abdominal closure, the three main end-points for evidential studies are mortality (which is of course highly dependent on the indication), rates of fascial closure and complications. Three definitions are useful here (Table 23.5).

Table 23.5 Definitions of eventual outcomes of the abdominal wall

Definitive fascial closure	Fascia to fascia closure of the midline wound—this may be *early* (within 8 days of primary laparotomy) or *delayed* (after 8 days but within the first hospitalisation) [2, 30]. This closure may be reinforced by a mesh
Partial fascial closure/bridged repair	Where there is only partial fascia to fascia apposition (or none at all) and the remainder of the defect is bridged by a prosthetic material
Planned ventral hernia	Discharge from hospital with a fascial defect covered by only skin, skin graft or chronic granulation tissue with an expectation to return for delayed reconstruction

A Medline search for 'open abdomen' yields nearly 6000 articles, yet there are only 5 randomised trials comparing different methods of wound closure [13, 31–34] meaning that despite the enormous volumes, there remains a poor quality evidence base. What can be said as a generalisation is that definitive fascial closure rates are higher after trauma indications for OA than sepsis [35] and complication rates (especially fistulation) are higher following OA for septic indications than trauma whichever TAC is employed [36].

One specific data set deserves examination. The American Association for the Surgery of Trauma (AAST) Open Abdomen registry was a prospectively maintained database that enrolled posttraumatic DCL open abdomens across 14 Level 1 US trauma centres in 2010 and 2011. Reporting on approximately 500 patients with posttraumatic open abdomens, this data reveal important findings. The overall definitive primary fascial closure rate was 59.1% in those who survived more than 48 hours from injury which ranged from 33.4% to 72.2% across the 14 centres. Independent predictors of failure to achieve DFC were increased numbers of relook laparotomies, intra-abdominal abscess formation, bloodstream infections, acute renal failure, ECF formation and an injury severity score (ISS) >15. It is unclear though whether increasing ISS contributes to increasing rates of failure to achieve DFC. Mortality rates were significantly higher in those who did not achieve fascial closure [37]. Median time to first take-back laparotomy was 36 h, but every hour's delay in returning to the operating room beyond 24 h was associated with a 1.1% decrease in the odds of achieving primary fascial closure; there was also a tendency to increased intra-abdominal complications beyond 48 h to first take-back [38].

Furthermore, increased numbers of take-backs were associated with an increased rate of ECF/IAS. DuBose et al. reported the rates of enteric fistula in this dataset as 5.2% (1.2% in those with DFC compared to 12.8% in those without) [37], but multivariate analysis revealed that those that did suffer ECF or intra-abdominal sepsis (IAS) had almost double the number of relook laparotomies, a greater rate of colonic resection and increased fluid resuscitation volumes [39].

From this trauma-specific, prospectively accrued data, it is clear that open abdomen management, of whatever technique, must strive to achieve definitive fascial closure at the earliest opportunity with the smallest numbers of take-backs whilst maintaining the patient in the best physiological shape as possible. This dataset does not however identify which TAC technique is best suited to that task.

A series of systematic reviews and meta-analysis have been performed with surprisingly wide variation in inclusion criteria and methodology, coupled with varying proportions of the different techniques as some became more popular or commercially available; all largely conclude the same things. Boele van Hensbroek et al. reviewed TAC for all indications including 51 studies (19 purely trauma) and 3169 patients [40] and identified that the highest DFC rates and lowest mortality rates were with the Wittmann Patch (90% and 17%, respectively) followed by dynamic retention sutures (85% and 23%) and vacuum-assisted closure (60% and 18%).

Three years later, Quyn et al. [36] described a 76.3% DFC rate for the Wittmann Patch in trauma cases compared to 68.8% for VAC; fistula rates were 6.8% and 7.3%, respectively. Navsaria et al.'s series reported their own patients but also a systematic review of commercial NPWT applications in series where the septic patients were in the minority and most were trauma patients—overall DFC rate was 63.7% with a 2.7% fistula rate [41]. Cirocchi et al.'s systematic review only included one fifth of trauma patients and showed no statistical difference in DFC or fistula rates between those who received NPWT and those who didn't; mortality was however lower in those receiving NPWT [42]. The 'International Consensus Conference on the Management of the Open Abdomen in Trauma' which took place in 2014 and published its outcomes in 2016 [43] focussed specifically on post-trauma DCL open abdomens and made a series of evidence-based recommendations. Chief amongst these was the strong recommendation for the use of NPWT for the management of the open abdomen to evacuate fluid, potentially lessen the intraperitoneal cytokine load, simplify nursing care and prevent fascial retraction. They went on to recommend that DFC is achieved as early as possible in the course of OA management and reference the recommendation of Atema et al.'s [44] systematic review of non-trauma OA which highlighted NPWT in combination with a dynamic fascial traction system as being the optimal method of ensuring DFC at approximately 73%.

The landscape of delayed abdominal reconstruction has been revolutionised by the popularisation of component separation techniques, and so it is unsurprising that they should now form part of the armamentarium of the surgeon managing the open abdomen acutely. Reports are scarce, but Chiara recommends acute component separation for defects of between 7 and 20 cm after OA management, and Sharrock et al.'s meta-analysis [45] also gives credence to this as a viable technique, but this seems to be based on a single paper which on inspection does not appear to utilise the technique. It has been used in three burn patients with ACS with apparent successful OA closure [46].

23.6 Worries over Fistulation with NPWT

The abiding worry about widespread adoption of NPWT for OA management has been that of increased fistulation rates when vacuum is used when compared to other treatment modalities. The randomized trial of polyglactin 910 mesh versus NPWT revealed a (nonsignificant) difference in fistula rates of 5% vs. 21% [34]; averaged rates of perhaps 5.7% for homemade vacuum [40] have potentially been extrapolated across all NPWT techniques causing disquiet. A UK nationwide registry of open abdomen management showed no difference in enteric fistula rates between those who received NPWT and those who didn't (14.4% vs. 9.1%), but it did show a lower rate of DFC in the NPWT patients (41.1% vs. 60.1%) [26]; it should be noted that this cohort primarily underwent OA management for septic indications rather than following trauma. The International Consensus opinion is that 'OA and NPWT do not harm intestinal anastomoses as long as these are buried deeply in the abdominal cavity' [43].

23.7 Longer-Term Outcomes

In common with much of the literature on incisional hernia repair, long-term outcome reporting following OA management is scarce. Brandl et al. described the outcome after OA for a variety of indications and with a variety of TAC techniques which was a 35% incisional hernia rate in 112 patients who achieved DFC during their initial hospitalisation at a median of 26 months after discharge. Worryingly two thirds of their patients had the midline fascia closed with a rapidly absorbable suture (polyglactin) [47]. In 55 OA patients treated according to a protocolised mesh-mediated fascial traction and NPWT regimen, 74% achieved DFC; follow-up of 34 patients for a mean of 46 months again identified a 35% incisional hernia rate; increased numbers of take-backs during the initial hospitalisation were predictive of incisional hernia [48]. Interestingly, a comparison of trauma-DCL patients who survived to discharge identified longer hospital stay, increased infectious complications, higher rates of enteric fistula and more laparotomies in those who left with planned ventral hernia, but after delayed reconstruction a median of 9 months later, rates of return to normal social and work activities were the same between primary DFC and reconstructed patients; there was no difference in subsequent incisional hernia rates [49].

23.8 Nutrition

It is clear that an open abdomen presents a significant catabolic state, and so consideration must be given to the nutritional requirements of the OA patient, and enteral nutrition (EN) should be started as soon as possible in all patients with more than 75 cm of usable small bowel from the duodenojejunal flexure [43]. Allied to the benefits in reducing the catabolic drain from the exposed viscera, early EN was associated with higher DFC rates (albeit after more operations and a longer time period), decreased mortality and complication rates in those trauma-OA patients without bowel injury; no such benefits were apparent when there was bowel injury [50].

23.9 Paediatric Studies

There is an understandable paucity of literature regarding traumatic open abdominal management in children, although paediatric surgeons have their own experiences of dealing with abdominal wall defects from omphalocele and gastroschisis management. IAH or ACS occurs in approximately 10% of patients admitted to a paediatric ICU, but it seems that medical therapy can avert the progression from IAH to ACS [51]. Gutierrez and Gollin described 25 patients with OA over a four and a half-year period, but only four were from trauma. All were managed with NPWT, 9 died and 14 achieved definitive fascial closure [52]. Given the increased elasticity and compliance of the paediatric abdominal wall, it may be reasonable to simply institute NPWT should the need arise and avoid fascial traction devices to avoid any potential damage to the abdominal wall itself.

23.10 Summary

The indications for an open abdomen after trauma-DCL are now well established and are those situations where direct closure of the abdomen would place the patient at risk of intra-abdominal hypertension and where further access to the abdomen is expected or there has been loss of the abdominal wall. Open abdomen management should incorporate the application of a suitable temporary abdominal closure. The choice of TAC depends on the resource constraints of the healthcare system and the available facilities and skills of the surgeon; the aim should be to maximise early definitive fascial closure with the lowest possible rates of complications—especially enterocutaneous fistulation. The technique of choice is a dynamic fascial traction method coupled with negative pressure wound therapy via a commercial device.

It is clear that the early institution of active management of the abdominal wall leads to better outcomes, and if an inexperienced surgeon performs the initial open abdomen laparotomy, early involvement of someone experienced in the ongoing management of the open abdomen should be instituted.

References

1. Ogilvie WH. The late complications of abdominal war wounds. Lancet. 1940;2:253–6.
2. Vargo D, Richardson D, Campbell A, et al. Management of the open abdomen: from initial operation to definitive closure. Am Surg. 2009;75(11):S1–S22.
3. Cheatham ML, Safcsak K, Llerena LE, Morrow CE Jr, Block EF. Long-term physical, mental and functional consequences of abdominal decompression. J Trauma. 2004;56:237–41.
4. Malbrain MLNG, Cheatham ML, Kirkpatrick A, et al. Results from an international conference of experts on intra-abdominal hypertension and abdominal compartment syndrome. Definitions. Intensive Care Med. 2006;32:1722–32.
5. Kirkpatrick AW, Roberts DJ, De Waele J, et al. Intra-abdominal hypertension and the abdominal compartment syndrome: updated consensus definitions and clinical practice guidelines from the World Society of the Abdominal Compartment Syndrome. Intensive Care Med. 2013;39(7):1190–206.
6. Saggi BH, Sugerman HJ, Ivatury RR, et al. Abdominal compartment syndrome. J Trauma. 1998;45(3):597–609.
7. Simon RJ, Friedlander MH, Ivatury RR, et al. Hemorrhage lowers the threshold for intra-abdominal hypertension-induced pulmonary dysfunction. J Trauma. 1997;42(3):398–403.
8. Sugrue M, Buist D, Hurihan F, et al. Prospective study of intra-abdominal hypertension and renal function after laparotomy. Br J Surg. 1995;82:235–8.
9. Doty JM, Oda J, Ivatury RR, et al. the effects of hemodynamic shock and increased intra-abdominal pressure on bacterial translocation. J Trauma. 2002;52(1):13–7.
10. Diebel L, Saxe J, Dulchavsky S. Effect of intra-abdominal pressure on abdominal wall blood flow. Am Surg. 1992;58:573–6.
11. Hong JJ, Cohn SM, Perez JM, Dolich MO, Brown M, McKenney MG. Prospective study of the incidence and outcome of intra-abdominal hypertension and the abdominal compartment syndrome. Br J Surg. 2002;89(5):591–6.
12. Chen J, Ren J, Zhang W, Li J. Open versus closed abdomen treatment on liver function in rats with sepsis and abdominal compartment syndrome. J Trauma. 2011;71(5):1319–25.
13. Kirkpatrick AW, Roberts DJ, Faris PD, et al. Active negative pressure peritoneal therapy after abbreviated laparotomy. Ann Surg. 2015;262:38–46.
14. Leppaniemi A, Mentula P, Hienonen P, Kemppainen E. Transverse laparotomy is feasible and effective in the treatment of abdominal compartment syndrome in severe acute pancreatitis. WJES. 2008;3:6. https://doi.org/10.1186/1749-7922-3-6.
15. Björck M, Kirkpatrick AW, Cheatham M, Kaplan M, Leppäniemi A, De Waele JJ. Amended classification of the open abdomen. Scand J Surg. 2016;105(1):5–10.
16. Rezende-Neto JB, Moore EE, Melo de Andrade MV, et al. Systemic inflammatory response secondary to abdominal compartment syndrome: stage for multiple organ failure. J Trauma. 2002;53:1121–8.
17. Cheatham ML, Safcsak K, Brzezinski SJ, et al. Nitrogen balance, protein loss and the open abdomen. Crit Care Med. 2007;35:127–31.
18. Huang Q, Ki J, Lau W-Y. Techniques for abdominal wall closure after damage control laparotomy: from temporary closure to early/delayed fascial closure: a review. Gastro Res Prac. 2016;2016:15. https://doi.org/10.1155/2016/2073260.
19. de Waele JJ, Leppaniemi AK. Temporary abdominal closure techniques. Am Surg. 2011;77:S46–50.
20. Tremblay LN, Felciiano DV, Schmidt J, et al. Skin only or silo closure in the critically ill patient with an open abdomen. Am J Surg. 2001;182:670–5.

21. Regner JL, Kobayashi L, Coimbra R. Surgical strategies for management of the open abdomen. World J Surg. 2012;36:497–510.
22. Wilde JM, Loudon MA. Modified Opsite® sandwich for temporary abdominal closure: a non-traumatic experience. Ann R Coll Surg Engl. 2007;89:57–61.
23. Brock WB, Barker DE, Burns RP. Temporary closure of open abdominal wounds: the vacuum pack. Am Surg. 1995;61:30–5.
24. Chen SZ, Li J, Li XY, et al. Effects of vacuum-assisted closure on wound microcirculation: an experimental study. Asian J Surg. 2005;28:211–7.
25. Moues CM, Vos CM, Bend GJ, et al. Bacterial load in relation to vacuum-assisted closure wound therapy: a prospective randomized trial. Wound Repair Regen. 2004;12:11–7.
26. Carlson GL, Patrick H, Amin AI, et al. Management of the open abdomen: a national study of clinical outcomes and safety of negative pressure wound therapy. Ann Surg. 2013;257(6):1154–9.
27. Wittman DH. Staged abdominal repair: development and current practice of an advanced operative technique for diffuse suppurative peritonitis. Acta Chir Austricaca. 2000;32:171–8.
28. Petersson U, Acosta S, Bjorck M. Vacuum-assisted wound closure and mesh-mediated fascial traction: a novel technique for late closure of the open abdomen. World J Surg. 2007;31:2133–7.
29. Reamer MW, Yelle J-D, Reitsma B, Doumit G, Allen MA, Bell MS. Management of open abdominal wounds with a dynamic fascial closure system. Can J Surg. 2008;51(3):209–14.
30. Diaz JJ Jr, Dutton WD, Ott MM, et al. Eastern association for the surgery of trauma: a review of the management of the open abdomen: part 2 "Management of the open abdomen". J Trauma. 2011;71(2):502–12.
31. Rencuzogullari A, Dalci K, Eray IC, et al. Comparison of early surgical alternatives in the management of the open abdomen: a randomised controlled study. Ulus Travma Acil Cerrahi Derg. 2015;21(3):168–74.
32. Long KL, Hamilton DA, Davenport DL, Bernanrd AC, Kearney PA, Chang PKA. prospective controlled evaluation of the abdominal reapproximation anchor abdominal wall closure system in combination with VAC therapy compared to VAC alone in the management of an open abdomen. Am Surg. 2014;80(6):567–71.
33. Correa JC, Meija DA, Duque N, Montoya JM, Uribe CM. Managing the open abdomen: negative pressure closure versus mesh-mediated fascial traction closure: a randomized trial. Hernia. 2016;20(2):221–9.
34. Bee TK, Croce MA, Magnotti LJ, et al. Temporary abdominal closure techniques: a prospective randomized trial comparing polyglactin 910 mesh and vacuum-assisted closure. J Trauma. 2008;65(2):337–42.
35. Bruhin A, Ferreira F, Chariker M, Smith J, Runkel N. Systematic review and evidence based recommendations for the use of negative pressure wound therapy in the open abdomen. Int J Surg. 2014;12:1105–14.
36. Quyn AJ, Johnston C, Hall D, et al. The open abdomen and temporary abdominal closure systems: historical evolution and systematic review. Colorectal Dis. 2012;14(8):e429–38.
37. DuBose JJ, Scalea TM, Holcomb JB, et al. Open abdominal management after damage-control laparotomy for trauma: a prospective observational American association for the surgery of trauma multicentre study. J Trauma Acute Care Surg. 2013;74:113–22.
38. Pommerening MJ, DuBose JJ, Zielinski MD, et al. Time to first take-back operation predicts successful primary fascial closure in patients undergoing damage control laparotomy. Surgery. 2014;156:431–8.
39. Bradley MJ, DuBose JJ, Scalea TM, et al. Independent predictors of enteric fistula and abdominal sepsis after damage control laparotomy: results from the prospective AAST open abdomen registry. JAMA Surg. 2013;148(10):947–54.
40. Boele van Hensbroek P, Wind J, Dijkgraaf MGW, Busch ORC, Goslings JC. Temporary closure of the open abdomen: a systematic review on delayed primary fascial closure in patients with an open abdomen. World J Surg. 2009;33:199–207.
41. Navsaria P, Nicol A, Hudson D, Cockwill J, Smith J. Negative pressure wound therapy management of the "open abdomen" following trauma: a prospective study and systematic review. World J Emerg Surg. 2013;8:4.
42. Cirocchi R, Birindelli A, Biffl WL, et al. What is the effectiveness of the negative pressure wound therapy (NPWT) in patients treated with open abdomen technique? A systematic review and meta-analysis. J Trauma Acute Care Surg. 2016;81:575–84.
43. Chiara O, Cimbanassi S, Biffl W, et al. International consensus conference on open abdomen in trauma. J Trauma Acute Care Surg. 2016;80:173–83.
44. Atema JJ, Gans SL, Boermeester MA. Systematic review and meta-analysis of the open abdomen and temporary abdominal closure techniques in non-trauma patients. World J Surg. 2015;39:912–25.
45. Sharrock AE, Barker T, Yuen HM, Rickard R, Tai N. Management and closure of the open abdomen after damage control laparotomy for trauma. A systematic review and meta-analysis. Injury. 2016;47:296–306.
46. Poulakidas S, Kowal-Vern A. Component separation technique for abdominal wall reconstruction in burn patients with decompressive laparotomies. *J Trauma*. 2009;67:1435–8.
47. Brandl A, Laimer E, Perathoner A, Zitt M, Pratschke J, Kafka-Ritsch R. Incisional hernia rate after open abdomen treatment with negative pressure and delayed primary fascia closure. Hernia. 2014;18:105–11.
48. Willms A, Schaaf S, Schwab R, et al. Abdominal wall integrity after open abdomen: long-term results of vacuum-assisted wound closure and mesh-mediated fascial traction (VAWCM). Hernia. 2016;20:849–58.

49. Zosa BM, Como JJ, Kelly KB, He JC, Claridge JA. Planned ventral hernia following damage control laparotomy in trauma: an added year of recovery but equal long-term outcome. Hernia. 2016;20:231–8.
50. Burlew CC, Moore EE, Cuschieri J, et al. Who should we feed? A western trauma association multi-institutional study of enteral nutrition in the open abdomen after injury. J Trauma Acute Care Surg. 2012;73:1380–8.
51. Divarci E, Karapinar B, Yalaz M, Ergun O, Celik A. Incidence and prognosis of intraabdominal hypertension and abdominal compartment syndrome in children. J Pediatr Surg. 2016;51:503–7.
52. Gutierrez IM, Gollin G. Negative pressure wound therapy for children with an open abdomen. Langenbecks Arch Surg. 2012;397:1353–7.

24 Soft-Tissue Reconstructive Considerations in the Damage Control Environment

Graham Lawton

Abstract

Trauma is a leading cause of mortality and morbidity accounting for 11% of the global burden of disease [1]. Worldwide 16,000 people succumb to injuries everyday [2] with a similar number of fatalities every year in England and Wales as described by the Office for National Statistics, London, in 2011. For every trauma death, there are two survivors with serious and debilitating injuries. In 2004, approximately 30 million Americans were treated for a nonfatal injury in emergency medicine departments, of these, 2 million required in-patient care [3]. In the landmark 1985 publication *Injury in America*, one in every eight hospital beds was occupied by an injured patient.

24.1 Introduction

Trauma is a leading cause of mortality and morbidity accounting for 11% of the global burden of disease [1]. Worldwide 16,000 people succumb to injuries everyday [2] with a similar number of fatalities every year in England and Wales as described by the Office for National Statistics, London, in 2011. For every trauma death, there are two survivors with serious and debilitating injuries. In 2004, approximately 30 million Americans were treated for a nonfatal injury in emergency medicine departments, of these, 2 million required in-patient care [3]. In the landmark 1985 publication *Injury in America*, one in every eight hospital beds was occupied by an injured patient.

Trauma can affect all ages but is principally a disease of the young. In the United States, unintentional injury is the commonest cause of death between the ages of 1 and 24 [3], and globally it is the leading cause of death for all ages up to 60 years old [1]. In the United Kingdom, 36 life years are lost per trauma death.

By affecting the young, the economic impact is huge. If you combine healthcare costs with future loss of economic productivity for all American injuries that occurred in the year 2000, the total is in excess of US $406 billion [4]. Increased survival from traumatic injury in the Western world has been multifactorial in nature. Integrated trauma systems [5], high-volume centres [6] and a more sophisticated understanding and approach to the clinical management of the critically injured patient as manifested in the damage control philosophy [7] have all contributed to decreased mortality. It is less clear from

G. Lawton, B.Sc., M.D., D.M.C.C., F.R.C.S.
Academic Department Military Surgery and Trauma, Honorary Clinical Senior Lecturer Imperial College, Imperial College Healthcare NHS Trust, St Mary's Hospital, Praed Street, London, UK
e-mail: grahamlawton@nhs.net

J. Duchesne et al. (eds.), *Damage Control in Trauma Care*,
https://doi.org/10.1007/978-3-319-72607-6_24

the literature if the approaches previously outlined decrease morbidity; what is certain is the major trauma survivor has increasingly complex reconstructive needs. "The quality of life must be worth the pain of survival" [8] is a mantra from the burn care community, and it's incumbent on us to provide the very highest functional outcomes for our trauma survivors.

Reconstructive surgeons have historically been consulted in the aftermath where they have been presented with a defect to correct often after initial efforts to solve the problem have been unsuccessful. The vogue in the military for smaller trauma teams is a logistical and tactical necessity with primary surgical efforts delivered "down range" by a "resuscitative surgeon"; it is essential in those circumstances that consideration is taken for future reconstructive efforts. In modern civilian systems, integration of the reconstructive surgeon into the provision of acute care provides the most elegant solution but is the most resource-intensive option.

Reconstructive surgery was born out of conflict, but reconstructive surgeons are not generally involved in the acute management and immediate decision-making concerning the poly-trauma patient. There is no body of work labelled "damage control soft-tissue reconstruction" despite the explosion in the trauma literature of damage control philosophies applied to a whole host of differing specialities and the deployment of reconstructive surgeons to recent conflict zones [9, 10].

The aim of this chapter is to highlight areas related to decision-making and technique that preserve potential reconstructive options and minimise the future burden on the trauma patient undergoing a damage control sequence of operations in order to maximise their final functional outcome. It will also comment on the timing of definitive care when one has decided to embark on a damage control philosophy of treatment and highlight the success of soft-tissue reconstruction, even if delayed, after the initial resuscitative efforts.

The father of UK plastic surgery, Sir Harold Gillies, published a number of commandments based upon his experience treating a large volume of military personnel wounded in the First World War. From his initial list, I've selected, and amended, a number of principles that every surgeon involved in damage control should have in the back of their mind at the outset:

- Make a reconstructive plan even if you know you will not be responsible for its delivery.
- Try and provide yourself and your patient with a lifeboat but plan B must not be the same as plan A.
- Do not throw away a living thing.
- Do not do today that which can be *honourably* put off until tomorrow.
- Do not have a routine.

24.2 Debridement and Dressings

Complete removal of all necrotic material and contamination from a traumatic wound is the foundation upon which all future reconstructive efforts rest. "The best antibiotic is good surgery" [11]. It is a key skill for all trauma resuscitative surgeons and should not be overlooked in the damage control setting. Although certain anatomical areas (the buttocks) are difficult to access in the standard cruciform position, every effort should be made to address wound contamination surgically as early as is practicably possible.

Delay in converting a contaminated uncontrolled wound into a surgically controlled wound predisposes the patient to the development of wound sepsis and makes future surgical efforts to regain control more difficult and physiologically more burdensome to the patient [12]. Whilst the early administration of antibiotics has been shown to reduce infective complications [13], sharp debridement and lavage are still essential especially in the damage control environment where high degrees of environmental contamination, necessary massive transfusion [14] and a high injury severity scores coexist causing immunosuppression and host susceptibility to sepsis.

Multidisciplinary team working allows concurrent debridement of wounds to the extremities/face at the same time as thoraco-abdominal control of bleeding and contamination. Potentially under tourniquet control, these adjunctive debridements can be performed in such a manner as to provide benefit to the patient without adding greatly to the physiological burden. A systematic "clock face" approach to wound debridement working superficial to deep with extensile exposures "creating a tunnel not a funnel" shortens the operative time and allows for a thorough wound assessment and formulation of the future reconstructive plan without unnecessary operative delays. This is the methodology taught to UK military surgeons prior to deployment.

Digital clinical photography is a useful adjunct for planning and discussion but essential when limb ablation becomes part of the resuscitative efforts [15]. Traditionally there was an intent to debride all open fractures within 6 hours of injury based on predicted bacterial growth [16]; however, there has been a move to delay the debridement of isolated open fractures of the lower limb provided it is accomplished within 24 hours of injury [17]. This has been shown to result in no increase in local infective complications [18]. In the damage control setting, any opportunity to debride wounds at the index procedure should be grasped in order to mitigate the deleterious effects outlined previously, and this advice forms part of the standards of care for open fractures in the United Kingdom [19].

Irrigation should be with copious quantities of warm saline with care taken not to cool the patient. The "solution for pollution is dilution", and whilst a whole of host of differing liquids have been proposed, normal saline delivered by a low-pressure system has been deemed to be effective minimising the rebound bacterial growth seen with high-pressure pulsatile devices [20] and the deleterious effects of some cytotoxic solutions to healthy tissue [21] despite their perceived attraction.

In the damage control environment, return to the operating theatre and the opportunity to examine traumatic wounds will be driven by the physiological condition of the patient and the desire for the resuscitative surgeon to examine the body cavities. Careful coordination of surgical logistics should be undertaken in order to maximise the benefit to the patient of each return to the operating theatre. The role of microbiological sampling of the wound at subsequent debridements is controversial in the absence of clinical infection except in military wounds when there is a suspicion or concern regarding invasive fungal infection [22]. Potentially contaminated traumatic wounds should never be directly closed in the damage control setting, and care should be taken in the choice and application of the most appropriate dressing that should be applied in a sterile manner to prevent introduction of microorganisms from the environment and clinical staff.

Topical negative pressure wound therapy (TNPWT) has become the mainstay in treatment of moderate to large traumatic wounds in the damage control setting. Prior to the introduction of TNPWT, wounds were dressed in a standard fashion involving a non-adherent barrier then dressing gauze followed by some form of bandage in order to fix this dressing to the patient. The high volume of exudate frequently overwhelmed this construct, with strike through onto the external aspect of the dressings and bedding. Malodour and skin complications due to moisture were common. The application of TNPWT sees either an open cell/pore foam or gauze placed in direct contact with the wound bed; a semi-occlusive dressing creates a seal (iodine impregnated may reduce wound colonisation [23]); negative pressure is applied via a pump to the wound/dressing interface and fluid from the wound collected in a canister.

TNPWT exerts beneficial effects in the damage control setting by preventing tissue from contracting (macro-deformation) creating a hypoxic stimulus at the centre of the wound that creates a gradient of vascular endothelial growth factor (VEGF) that drives angiogenesis and the formation of granulation tissue. The manner in which tissue within the wound bed is altered by mechanical forces acting across it is known as micro-deformation. Exudate is removed from the wound and collected allowing more accurate fluid balance calculations, whilst the semi-occlusive dressing helps create a moist environment that is beneficial for wound healing and helps to reduce oedema. They are also quick, simple to apply and require minimal training.

The efficacy of TNPWT in the management of the open chest and abdomen following damage control strategies will be dealt with in other chapters, but in the limbs, it has been shown to allow the earlier closure of fasciotomy wounds [24] and reduced the incidence of infection when used in the treatment of open fractures of the lower limb [25]. Care should be taken in interpretation of the Stannard study as the numbers were low, 59 patients with 63 open fractures; the study was funded by the makers of the TNPWT device (KCI San Antonio, TX), and perhaps unsurprisingly the investigators were not blinded to the dressings utilised.

In the military damage control environment and inclusive trauma systems, it also facilitates movement of the patient between differing medical treatment facilities with the wound sympathetically packaged.

24.3 Degloving and Delamination

Composite tissues subjected to stresses fail by delamination as layers of material are driven apart losing their strength. When stresses are applied to soft tissues, they also fail in a not dissimilar manner. Degloving is defined as the separation of the skin and subcutaneous tissues from the underlying fascia and muscle in such a way as to isolate it from its blood supply. These random pattern flaps are also themselves injured and contaminated.

Arnez has classified degloving into four different categories increasing in severity from limited degloving with abrasion/avulsion to circumferential multiplanar degloving [26]. This classification is useful in so much as it highlights the severe nature and extent of soft-tissue injury that can exist even in the absence of fracture. They proposed a limited treatment algorithm but utilised a very aggressive initial approach without recourse to TNPWT and observation that would be the author's preferred initial approach in the DCS environment.

In the context of traumatic injury, the resuscitative surgeon needs to be appreciative of that which has been caused by the injury and mindful not to add to it by further surgical exposure. Accurate documentation will aid future reconstructive surgical planning, as certain flaps will not be possible or reliable in the context of degloving; this is especially relevant in open tibia fractures where local fasciocutaneous flaps based on perforators from the posterior tibia artery have an important role.

Certain injury patterns are indicative of devolving, such as the Morel-Lavallee lesion associated with shear forces across the pelvis seen with some with pelvic ring and acetabular fractures. These are classically closed injuries and often underappreciated in the early post injury phase where recognition alone combined with removal of pelvic binder, drainage of the harmful hematoma [27] and meticulous pressure area care in the ICU can prevent devastating complications.

Clinical assessment of skin viability following degloving is often inaccurate, and there is no sensitive or specific investigation available. Whole body fluorescence has been described [28], and the more modern iteration of intraoperative laser angiography utilising indocyanine green is equipment/labour intensive, runs the small risk of anaphylaxis and is not appropriate in the damage control setting. Vessel thrombosis, fixed dermal staining and circumferentially degloved skin are indicative of the skin that will go on to become necrotic (Fig. 24.1).

Degloved skin should be handled gently and left where it wants to sit with no additional tension applied to the subdermal plexus of blood vessels causing compromise to the circulation and further necrosis. In privileged skin, such as glabrous skin of the palms/soles of the feet, less is more at the initial debridement, and we frequently advocate a policy of "observe to conserve" in the absence of an open fracture that requires coverage.

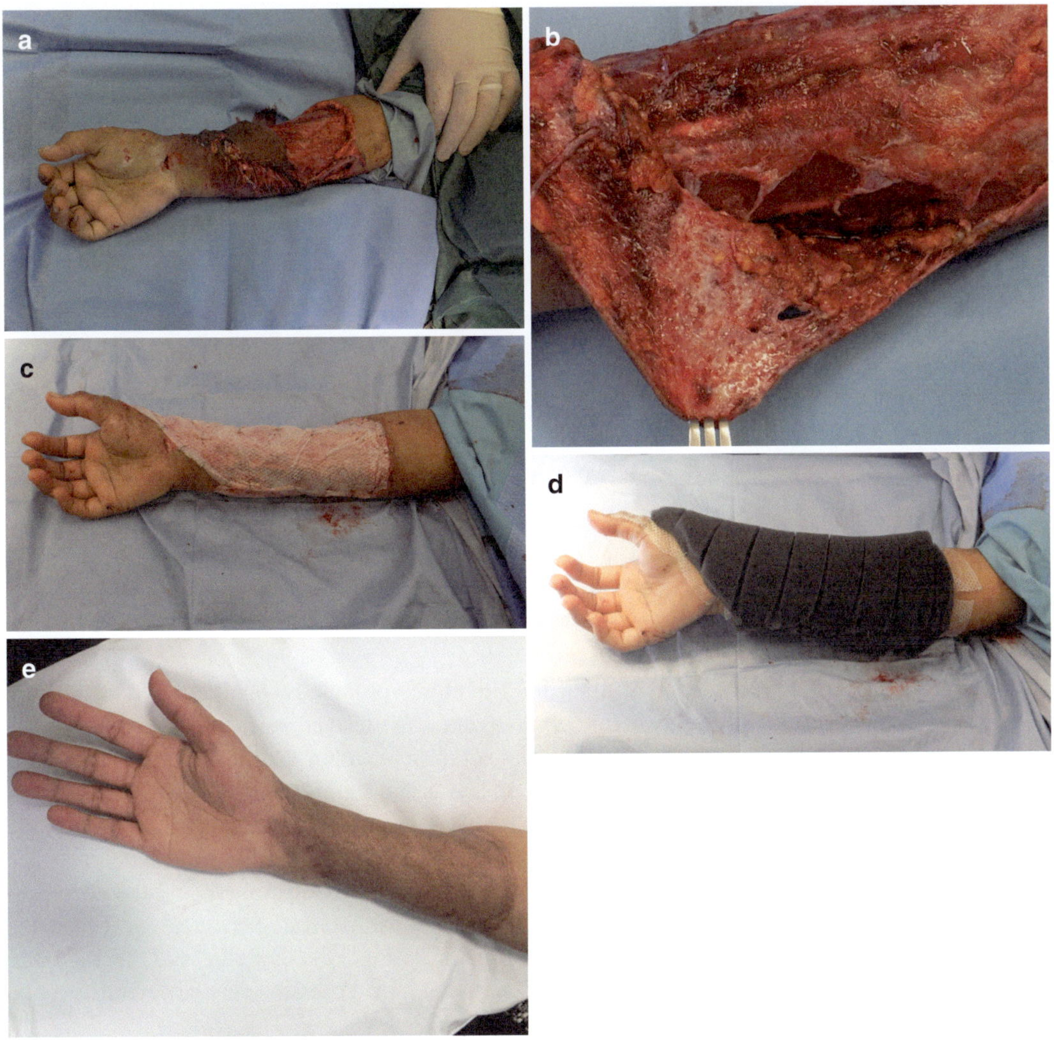

Fig. 24.1 (**a**) Demonstrating degloved skin. (**b**) Demonstrating damage to the subdermal plexus. (**c**) Dermal regeneration template in situ. (**d**) Topical negative pressure wound therapy. (**e**) Final result after skin graft

24.4 Extremity Injury

In recent conflicts, extremity trauma has accounted for 54% of all wounds suffered by those surviving to reach a medical treatment facility [29]; in European civilian trauma, 58.6% of 24 885 critically injured patients had a significant extremity injury [30].

Stabilisation of long bone fractures as part of a damage control orthopaedic procedure has physiological benefits to the patient [31] as does addressing the soft-tissue injury by decompression to avoid compartment syndrome and minimise reperfusion injury and debridement to avoid subsequent sepsis [32].

Better functional outcomes following blunt trauma are best achieved by an integrated trauma system [33], but the ideal approach to improving functional outcomes following open extremity

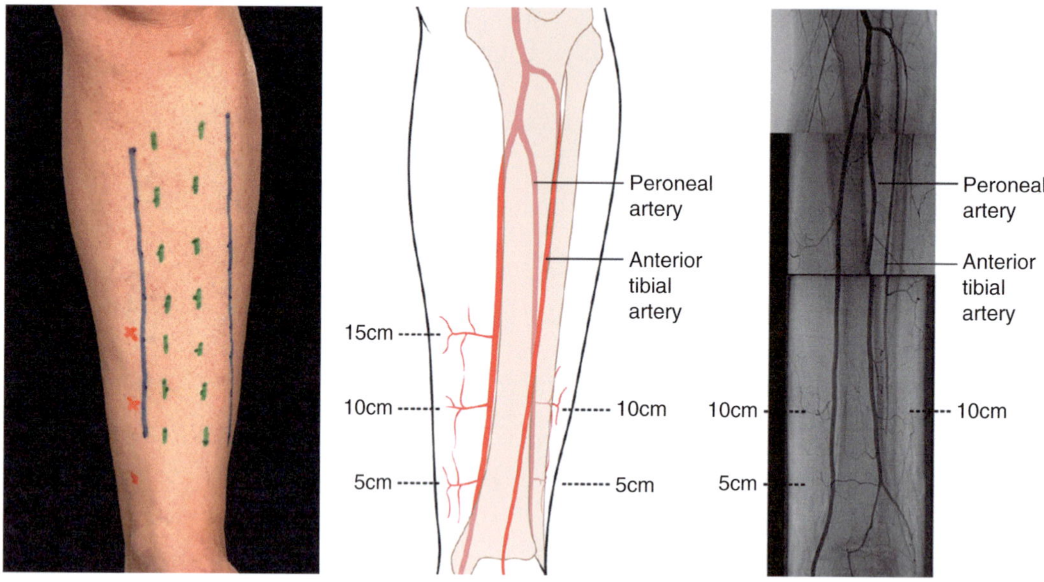

Fig. 24.2 Lower limb fasciotomy (British Association Plastic and Reconstructive Surgeons (BAPRAS))

fractures is less clear. If early infection is utilised as a marker of the quality of surgical care following open extremity fractures, then they are best managed by a combined orthoplastic approach [19] with further improvement if this is as part of an organised trauma system [34]. However, there is no good literature to support if this influences final functional outcome.

In extremity trauma, judgements regarding limb salvage are immensely challenging in the damage control environment. Decisions regarding amputation and limb ablation should be made by two surgeons preferably from differing specialities, supported by clinical photography and x-ray with appropriate note taking. Limb salvage scores should not be used in the military setting and nerve dysfunction distal to the injury should not be considered an indication for amputation [15].

24.5 Lower Extremity

Fasciotomy and limb decompression are essential to avoid the deleterious consequences of ischemia/reperfusion, myoglobinuria and the risk of renal failure. After 2–4 h of warm ischemia, there is histological evidence of tissue necrosis and reperfusion injury in muscle and nerve [35]. Therefore, prompt recognition and action are essential as delayed release risks exposing the dead muscle within the compartment to the risk of sepsis and significant morbidity [36].

In the leg, the four compartments are accessed via a two full-length incision technique. The superficial deep compartment and the deep posterior compartment are accessed via the medial incision, whilst the anterior and lateral compartments are accessed via the lateral incision (Fig. 24.2).

In the medial incision, care should be taken in the context of open tibial fractures to preserve perforating blood vessels from the posterior tibial artery in the skin flap distant to the tibia. By maintaining that flap as a composite fasciocutaneous tissue block with a recognised perforating vessel supplying it, local flap options are preserved. In the United Kingdom, an incision 15 mm behind the subcutaneous border of the tibia is taught in order to maximise the potential of capturing these vessels within the flap (Fig. 24.3).

The lateral incision is more controversial between differing surgical communities. UK orthopaedic and plastic surgeons advocate marking the incision 20 mm from the lateral subcutaneous border of the tibia, accessing the

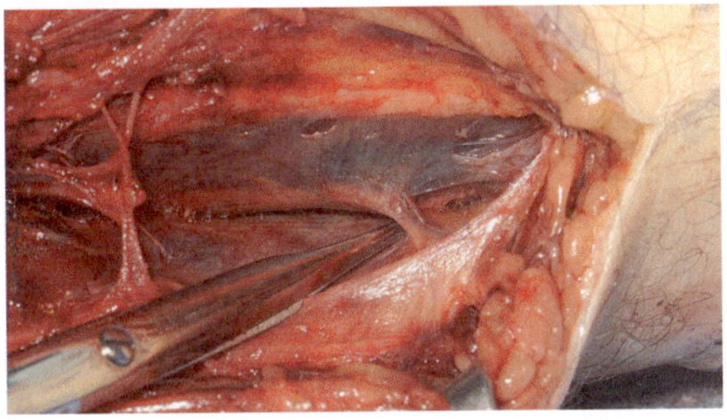

Fig. 24.3 Perforating vessels from the posterior tibial artery

anterior compartment and then decompressing the lateral compartment via the anterior in a subfascial manner. An alternative approach is making your initial incision more lateral, finding the septum and using this as the landmark to decompress both compartments. The challenge with this approach is with the initial incision; if it is not over the septum, then the skin has to be degloved in the subcutaneous plane in order to identify it. In fasciotomy for proximal vascular injury, this in itself is not particularly burdensome, but in the context of blunt lower limb trauma or open fractures, the further insult of degloving may cause skin necrosis.

Regardless of technique, the surgeon must perform a prompt, full and complete release of all compartments; application of TNPWT following fasciotomy has been shown to allow early closure of these wounds [24].

24.6 Upper Extremity

Ischemic fibrosis in the upper limb is a devastating complication with severe functional implications. Prompt recognition and decompression is imperative.

A multitude of different extensile exposures in the upper limb for fasciotomy have been described, and whilst a single dorsal incision to access the mobile wad and extensor compartments is uncontroversial, the Academic Department of Military Surgery and Trauma (ADMST) has advocated the following exposure to access the superficial and deep flexor compartments (Fig. 24.4).

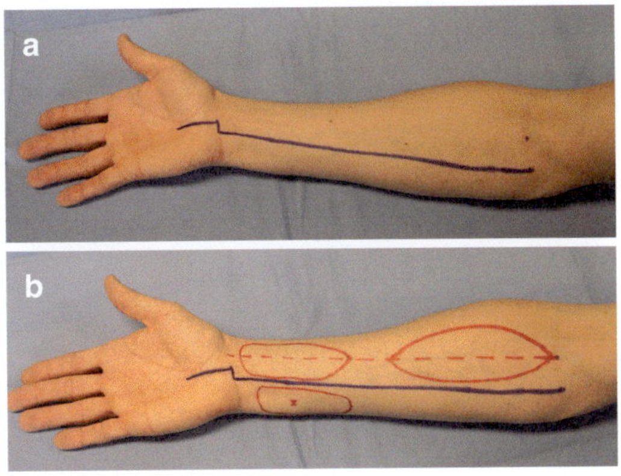

Fig. 24.4 (**a**) Markings for upper limb fasciotomy. (**b**) Markings to show common flap options preserved

Distally the carpal tunnel is accessed from Kaplan's cardinal line in an incision based on the radial aspect of the fourth ray terminating at the distal wrist crease. The wrist is crossed in a stepwise fashion by extending the incision ulnarly to a line drawn down from the ulna border of the fourth ray. This is then continued as a straight incision to a point midway within the medial half of the antecubital fossa.

This preserves a number of local and potential free flap donor sites for future soft-tissue reconstruction and provides excellent access to the volar aspect of the limb. The offset at the level of the wrist is a common modification not attributable to ADMST that allows for the median nerve to be remained covered by a skin flap in the event of marked swelling within the forearm.

External fixation in the upper limb is less commonly performed than in the lower limb, and great care must be taken in order to minimise the risk of upper limb iatrogenic nerve injury. At particular risk is the radial nerve in the distal humerus (Fig. 24.5). The author would advocate decompression, wound debridement and application of a gauze-based TNPWT system with plaster of Paris to immobilise and support fractures. The use of a gauze-based TNPWT system also allows for the hand to splint in the most sympathetic fashion to avoid contractures around the interphalangeal joints [37]. As once established, these contractures are very difficult to treat (Fig. 24.6).

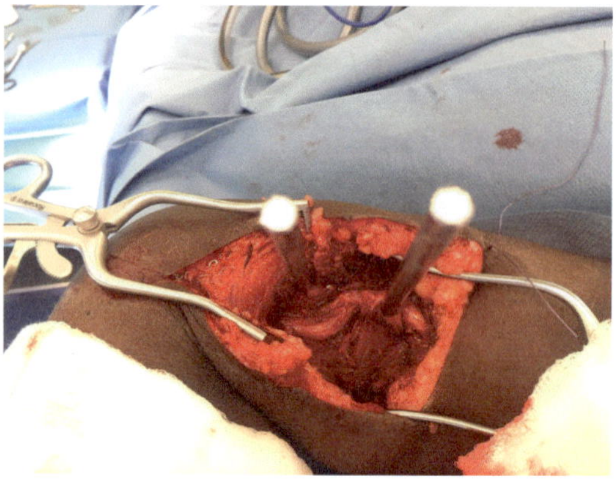

Fig. 24.5 Iatrogenic radial nerve injury

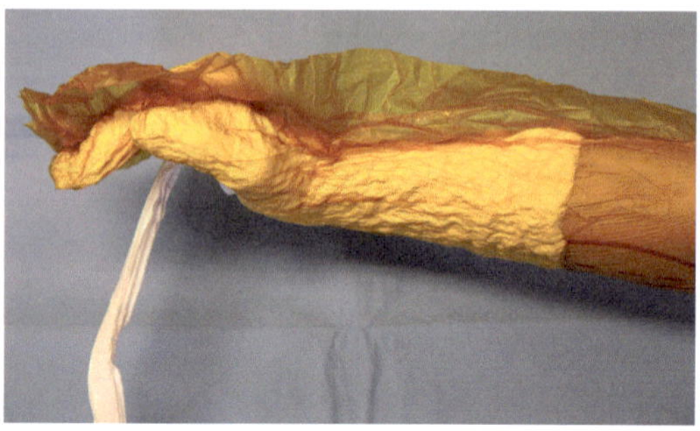

Fig. 24.6 Topical negative pressure wound therapy to splint hand

24.7 Timing of Reconstruction

When to perform flap reconstruction of the injured extremity has been driven by the pioneering work of Marko Godina who critically examined the results of free tissue transfer in three distinct groups based on time to coverage in 532 patients. The groups were divided into coverage in less than 72 h, coverage between 72 h and 3 months and coverage after 3 months. He found that those patients provided with suitable soft-tissue cover within 72 h had fewer operations, lower infection rates and lower rates of flap failure, saw their fractures unite more quickly and spent the least time in hospital [38].

This classic paper has influenced reconstructive surgeons thinking on the subject of timing ever since and has become incorporated into UK standards of care for open fractures [19]. Whilst there are undoubtedly attractions to combined early definitive skeletal and soft-tissue coverage, there is also the additional physiological burden on the patient to be taken into consideration.

In the DCO setting, consideration needs to be given as to when to perform any secondary procedures. Some centres consider surgery 2–4 days following a DCO procedure to be unwise due to the marked pro-inflammatory processes [39] they cite experience in their unit of 4314 patients who had protracted (>3 h) procedures before 4 days having a much higher chance of developing multi-organ dysfunction when compared to those who had definitive procedures delayed between 6 and 8 days [40]. The desire to avoid microvascular surgery during the period of systemic inflammatory response driven by danger associated molecular patterns from severe soft-tissue injury [31] makes physiological sense.

Godina was operating when microsurgical techniques, equipment and experience was still developing. How much does delay beyond 72 h adversely affect outcome in modern units? In the same North West German centre as Pape, 42 patients had limb reconstruction delayed due to delays in transfer and concomitant life-threatening injuries in 67%. Mean time to wound closure was 28 days, and wounds were temporised with TNPWT. They experienced three pedicled flap failures and only one free flap failure but did not comment on any other outcome measures [41].

A UK urban trauma centre examining 66 severe open tibia fractures in 65 patients reported very low rates of infection (1.6%) despite the median time to soft-tissue coverage being 5 days [34]. Fifteen of the cases waited 7 days, and two waited 28 and 30 days, respectively. The authors considered adequate debridement within 24 h key to the low incidence of infection as well as microbiological sampling at the time of definitive closure; again all of these wounds associated with open fractures were temporised with TNPWT. Perhaps the key message from this paper and earlier work from the same institution is that definitive orthopaedic fixation and soft-tissue cover need to happen at the same operation. Delayed coverage of indwelling metalwork at a second operation benefits no one.

The improvement in outcomes associated with high-ratio blood and blood product resuscitation [42] and anti-fibrinolytic therapy [43] has revolutionised resuscitation strategies, but would they predispose to thrombotic complications in future soft-tissue reconstruction? It would appear that use of tranexamic acid (TXA) did not increase the rate of complications, including venous thromboembolism, in those undergoing flap reconstruction, but only 11% of the 173 flap procedures reviewed had received TXA, and further work is needed TXA [44], or if its use predisposed to the development of wound infections [45].

Although less used in current practice, recombinant activated VII (rFVIIa) was well utilised before the CONTROL trial was unable to demonstrate a survival advantage. Potential adverse effects with regard to soft-tissue reconstruction are not discussed in the literature. However, the adjunctive use of rFVIIa in the setting of vascular repair combined with a damage control resuscitation philosophy has been examined by Fox et al. They postulated that vascular graft failure was not thought to be due to rFVIIa but caused by poor soft-tissue coverage and infection although the long-term outcomes with regard to limb salvage were not known [46].

24.8 UK Military Model

Previously I have commented that it may be challenging to involve reconstructive surgeons at the index operation. However, the UK military has recent experience of integrating a plastic surgeon into the deployed surgical team in recent conflicts. A single plastic surgeon was deployed to Camp Bastion Southern Afghanistan from 2008 until the conclusion of the British military mission in 2014. This coincided with the heaviest periods of coalition combat activity and casualties working alongside general surgical and orthopaedic colleagues to provide a balanced team and to help manage the "increase in the incidence of multiple, complex extremity injuries being sustained" [9].

Plastic surgeons were involved in 40% of all surgical cases, two-thirds of these were alongside another surgeon, most commonly orthopaedics. Approximately 70% of cases were debridement and surgical control of military wounds in the extremities and head and neck. No reconstructive procedures were performed on coalition troops due to the efficiency of the evacuation chain and the operational pressures of immediate work in the combat hospital.

No objective evidence of improved outcomes is available to demonstrate functional benefit in the survivors treated in this manner, but subjective discussions with deployed colleagues and those receiving injured UK service persons from this facility commented on the added benefit of the multidisciplinary team being involved from the outset.

Conclusion

Damage control philosophies of care have improved survival for severely injured trauma patients. It is every team member's responsibility to ensure that decisions taken in the pressurised initial moments do not prejudice future functional recovery.

Systems should be put in place to support the resuscitative surgeon either by early direct involvement of reconstructive surgeons or by easy access to remote decision support. This is the responsibility of the reconstructive surgical team within the trauma system to provide, test and continue to improve.

As mortality gives way to quantification of morbidity as a marker of trauma care effectiveness, then we all need to have the patient's ultimate functional requirements at the front of our minds.

References

1. Murray CJ, Vos T, Lozano R, Naghavi M, Flaxman AD, Michaud C, et al. Disability-adjusted life years (DALYs) for 291 diseases and injuries in 21 regions, 1990–2010: a systematic analysis for the global burden of disease study 2010. Lancet. 2012;380(9859):2197–223.

2. Krug EG, Sharma GK, Lozano R. The global burden of injuries. Am J Public Health. 2000;90(4):523–6.
3. Thacker SB, Stroup DF, Carande-Kulis V, Marks JS, Roy K, Gerberding JL. Measuring the public's health. Public Health Rep. 2006;121(1):14–22.
4. Corso P, Finkelstein E, Miller T, Fiebelkorn I, Zaloshnja E. Incidence and lifetime costs of injuries in the United States. Inj Prev. 2006;12(4):212–8.
5. Celso B, Tepas J, Langland-Orban B, Pracht E, Papa L, Lottenberg L, Flint L. A systematic review and meta-analysis comparing outcome of severely injured patients treated in trauma centers following the establishment of trauma systems. J Trauma. 2006;60(2):371–8. discussion 378
6. Minei JP, Fabian TC, Guffey DM, Newgard CD, Bulger EM, Brasel KJ, et al. Increased trauma center volume is associated with improved survival after severe injury: results of a resuscitation outcomes consortium study. Ann Surg. 2014;260(3):456–64. discussion 464-5
7. Duchesne JC, Kimonis K, Marr AB, Rennie KV, Wahl G, Wells JE, et al. Damage control resuscitation in combination with damage control laparotomy: a survival advantage. J Trauma. 2010;69(1):46–52.
8. Wood FM. Quality assurance in burn patient care: the James Laing memorial essay, 1994. Burns. 1995;21(8):563–8.
9. Maitland L, Lawton G, Baden J, Cubison T, Rickard R, Kay A, Hettiaratchy S. The role of military plastic surgeons in the management of modern combat trauma: an analysis of 645 cases. Plast Reconstr Surg. 2016;137(4):717e–24e.
10. Klem C, Sniezek JC, Moore B, Davis MR, Coppit G, Schmalbach C. Microvascular reconstructive surgery in operations Iraqi and enduring freedom: the US military experience performing free flaps in a combat zone. J Trauma Acute Care Surg. 2013;75(2 Suppl 2):S228–32.
11. Coupland RM. Technical aspects of war wound excision. Br J Surg. 1989;76(7):663–7.
12. Coupland RM. The role of reconstructive surgery in the management of war wounds. Ann R Coll Surg Engl. 1991;73(1):21–5.
13. Jackson DS. Sepsis in soft tissue limbs wounds in soldiers injured during the falklands campaign 1982. J R Army Med Corps. 1984;130(2):97–9.
14. Stephens CT, Gumbert S, Holcomb JB. Trauma-associated bleeding: management of massive transfusion. Curr Opin Anaesthesiol. 2016;29(2):250–5.
15. Clasper J, Lower Limb Trauma Working Group. Amputations of the lower limb: a multidisciplinary consensus. J R Army Med Corps. 2007;153(3):172–4.
16. Crowley DJ, Kanakaris NK, Giannoudis PV. Debridement and wound closure of open fractures: the impact of the time factor on infection rates. Injury. 2007;38(8):879–89.
17. Schenker ML, Yannascoli S, Baldwin KD, Ahn J, Mehta S. Does timing to operative debridement affect infectious complications in open long-bone fractures? A systematic review. J Bone Joint Surg Am. 2012;94(12):1057–64.
18. Srour M, Inaba K, Okoye O, Chan C, Skiada D, Schnüriger B, et al. Prospective evaluation of treatment of open fractures: effect of time to irrigation and debridement. JAMA Surg. 2015;150(4):332–6.
19. Naique SB, Pearse M, Nanchahal J. Management of severe open tibial fractures: the need for combined orthopaedic and plastic surgical treatment in specialist centres. J Bone Joint Surg Br. 2006;88(3):351–7.
20. Hassinger SM, Harding G, Wongworawat MD. High-pressure pulsatile lavage propagates bacteria into soft tissue. Clin Orthop Relat Res. 2005;439:27–31.
21. Owens BD, White DW, Wenke JC. Comparison of irrigation solutions and devices in a contaminated musculoskeletal wound survival model. J Bone Joint Surg Am. 2009;91(1):92–8.
22. Evriviades D, Jeffery S, Cubison T, Lawton G, Gill M, Mortiboy D. Shaping the military wound: issues surrounding the reconstruction of injured servicemen at the royal centre for defence medicine. Philos Trans R Soc Lond B Biol Sci. 2011;366(1562):219–30.
23. Jacobson C, Osmon DR, Hanssen A, Trousdale RT, Pagnano MW, Pyrek J, et al. Prevention of wound contamination using duraprep solution plus ioban 2 drapes. Clin Orthop Relat Res. 2005;439:32–7.
24. Yang CC, Chang DS, Webb LX. Vacuum-assisted closure for fasciotomy wounds following compartment syndrome of the leg. J Surg Orthop Adv. 2006;15(1):19–23.
25. Stannard JP, Volgas DA, Stewart R, McGwin G, Alonso JE. Negative pressure wound therapy after severe open fractures: a prospective randomized study. J Orthop Trauma. 2009;23(8):552–7.
26. Arnez ZM, Khan U, Tyler MP. Classification of soft-tissue degloving in limb trauma. J Plast Reconstr Aesthet Surg. 2010;63(11):1865–9.
27. Glass GE, Nanchahal J. Why haematomas cause flap failure: an evidence-based paradigm. J Plast Reconstr Aesthet Surg. 2012;65(7):903–10.
28. McGrouther DA, Sully L. Degloving injuries of the limbs: long-term review and management based on whole-body fluorescence. Br J Plast Surg. 1980;33(1):9–24.
29. Owens BD, Kragh JF, Wenke JC, Macaitis J, Wade CE, Holcomb JB. Combat wounds in operation iraqi freedom and operation enduring freedom. J Trauma. 2008;64(2):295–9.
30. Banerjee M, Bouillon B, Shafizadeh S, Paffrath T, Lefering R, Wafaisade A, German Trauma Registry Group. Epidemiology of extremity injuries in multiple trauma patients. Injury. 2013;44(8):1015–21.
31. Balogh ZJ, Reumann MK, Gruen RL, Mayer-Kuckuk P, Schuetz MA, Harris IA, et al. Advances and future directions for management of trauma patients with musculoskeletal injuries. Lancet. 2012;380(9847):1109–19.
32. Keel M, Trentz O. Pathophysiology of polytrauma. Injury. 2005;36(6):691–709.

33. Gabbe BJ, Simpson PM, Sutherland AM, Wolfe R, Lyons RA, Cameron PA. Evaluating time points for measuring recovery after major trauma in adults. Ann Surg. 2013;257(1):166–72.
34. Wordsworth M, Lawton G, Nathwani D, Pearse M, Naique S, Dodds A, et al. Improving the care of patients with severe open fractures of the tibia: the effect of the introduction of major trauma networks and national guidelines. Bone Joint J. 2016;98-B(3):420–4.
35. Labbe R, Lindsay T, Walker PM. The extent and distribution of skeletal muscle necrosis after graded periods of complete ischemia. J Vasc Surg. 1987;6(2):152–7.
36. Glass GE, Staruch RM, Simmons J, Lawton G, Nanchahal J, Jain A, Hettiaratchy SP. Managing missed lower extremity compartment syndrome in the physiologically stable patient: a systematic review and lessons from a level I trauma center. J Trauma Acute Care Surg. 2016;81(2):380–7.
37. Taylor CJ, Hettiaratchy S, Jeffery SL, Evriviades D, Kay AR. Contemporary approaches to definitive extremity reconstruction of military wounds. J R Army Med Corps. 2009;155(4):302–7.
38. Godina M. Early microsurgical reconstruction of complex trauma of the extremities. Plast Reconstr Surg. 1986;78(3):285–92.
39. Hildebrand F, Giannoudis P, Kretteck C, Pape HC. Damage control: extremities. Injury. 2004;35(7):678–89.
40. Pape H, Stalp M, Weinberg A, Dahlweit M, Tscherne H. Optimal timing for secondary surgery in polytrauma patients: an evaluation of 4,314 serious-injury cases. Der Chirurg; Zeitschrift Fur Alle Gebiete Der Operativen Medizen. 1999;70(11):1287–93.
41. Steiert AE, Gohritz A, Schreiber TC, Krettek C, Vogt PM. Delayed flap coverage of open extremity fractures after previous vacuum-assisted closure (VAC) therapy: worse or worth? J Plast Reconstr Aesthet Surg. 2009;62(5):675–83.
42. Pidcoke HF, Aden JK, Mora AG, Borgman MA, Spinella PC, Dubick MA, et al. Ten-year analysis of transfusion in operation Iraqi freedom and operation enduring freedom: increased plasma and platelet use correlates with improved survival. J Trauma Acute Care Surg. 2012;73(6 Suppl 5):S445–52.
43. Roberts I, Shakur H, Coats T, Hunt B, Balogun E, Barnetson L, et al. The CRASH-2 trial: a randomised controlled trial and economic evaluation of the effects of tranexamic acid on death, vascular occlusive events and transfusion requirement in bleeding trauma patients. Health Technol Assess. 2013;17(10):1–79.
44. Valerio IL, Campbell P, Sabino J, Lucas DJ, Jessie E, Rodriguez C, Fleming M. TXA in combat casualty care: does it adversely affect extremity reconstruction and flap thrombosis rates? Mil Med. 2015;180(3 Suppl):24–8.
45. Lewis CJ, Li P, Stewart L, Weintrob AC, Carson ML, Murray CK, et al. Tranexamic acid in life-threatening military injury and the associated risk of infective complications. Br J Surg. 2016;103(4):366–73.
46. Fox CJ, Mehta SG, Cox ED, Kragh JF, Salinas J, Holcomb JB. Effect of recombinant factor viia as an adjunctive therapy in damage control for wartime vascular injuries: a case control study. J Trauma. 2009;66(4 Suppl):S112–9.

MIX
Papier aus verantwortungsvollen Quellen
Paper from responsible sources
FSC® C105338

If you have any concerns about our products,
you can contact us on
ProductSafety@springernature.com

In case Publisher is established outside the EU,
the EU authorized representative is:
Springer Nature Customer Service Center GmbH
Europaplatz 3, 69115 Heidelberg, Germany

Printed by Libri Plureos GmbH
in Hamburg, Germany